# Diagnosis and
# of
# DIABETES
# MELLITUS

# Diagnosis and Management of DIABETES MELLITUS

*A Clinical Manual for Medical Students, Residents, and Primary Care Physicians*

---

O. CHARLES OLSON, M.D.
*Director, Diabetes Education Center*
*Deaconess Hospital*
*Spokane, Washington*

LEA & FEBIGER *1981* *Philadelphia*

Lea & Febiger
600 Washington Square
Philadelphia, PA 19106
USA

**Library of Congress Cataloging in Publication Data**

Olson, O Charles, 1913–
Diagnosis and management of diabetes mellitus.

Includes index.
1. Diabetes. I. Title. [DNLM: 1. Diabetes mellitus
—Diagnosis. 2. Diabetes mellitus—Therapy. WK 810
052d]
RC660.04 1981 616.4′62 80-27025
ISBN 0-8121-0790-X



PRINTED IN THE UNITED STATES OF AMERICA

Print Number: 3 2 1

*TO ALL THE DEDICATED RESEARCH AND CLINICAL<br>SCIENTISTS WHO BY VIRTUE OF THEIR LABORS,<br>OBSERVATIONS, AND CONCLUSIONS<br>HAVE MADE VALUABLE CONTRIBUTIONS<br>TO OUR KNOWLEDGE OF DIABETES MELLITUS.*

# Foreword

It is a delightful task to write a brief foreword for this excellent book on the management of diabetes mellitus.

What makes this an outstanding contribution is that it is both practical and scientifically well documented. It will prove helpful to both the physician and all the allied health personnel who treat diabetics. Beyond that, many of the sections in this book could be read by patients as well, with real benefit. That would be good, since it is true that only those diabetics survive a complete lifetime who thoroughly understand the disease and its management.

In the introduction, the point is made clear that the control of blood sugar levels is the single most important aspect of successful management. The modern diagnosis of diabetes is well described in terms of the latest classification for both major types of diabetics, those who require insulin and those who do not. There is a good chapter on dietary management that is both practical and accurate. The discussion on insulin is divided into a theoretic part and a practical one, with excellent details on the methodology of insulin administration. There follows a chapter on oral antidiabetic drugs, which covers a once controversial subject with recent and reasonable conclusions showing that there is a definite place for this medication when indicated.

The importance of urine testing is given a whole chapter with much useful detail.

The management of diabetes is well described in separate chapters for insulin-requiring and non-insulin-requiring diabetics and brings one right up to date.

The special chapter on exercise in diabetes is refreshing.

Hypoglycemia is covered in detail, and this discussion is good because hypoglycemia is, in fact, the hallmark of excellent control of blood sugar.

Obesity, so prevalent in older diabetics, has a special chapter. So do the management of the diabetic with surgical procedures and infections, the diabetic foot, and infections of the extremities, with many useful hints for treatment.

A discussion of pregnancy is most important because at present everyone agrees that only the most careful control of blood sugar levels will assure a normal baby.

Communications between the doctor and the patient are discussed in a novel fashion that should prove both lifesaving to the patient and reassuring to the doctor following the patient.

Information on urine testing and recording of results, office visits, and suggestions for asking for consultations are all well put.

The theoretic background and the management of complications are discussed. We learn about the etiology, the good and bad hormones in diabetes, some of the metabolic pathways in the breakdown of glucose, and details of the now-established relationship between diabetic control and the development of degenerative complications; various chapters discuss all the complications from the acute ones, such as lactic acidosis, to the more chronic ones, such as accelerated atherosclerosis and the unfortunate sexual dysfunctions in long-continued diabetes.

The book is completed by citing the latest advances in home glucose monitoring, insulin delivery systems, and above all, the glycohemoglobin determinations to evaluate the degree of hyperglycemia existent over a two-month period. Finally, the rare kinds of diabetes that come with other types of endocrine diseases, such as Cushing's syndrome, acromegaly, and hyperthyroidism, are covered.

As an insulin-requiring diabetic of some 56 years' standing and as a specialist in the field, I am happy to see this excellent book appear in press. It carries the hallmark of a vast experience acquired by Dr. Olson in managing diabetics for over 30 years, together with his expressing many admirable humanitarian feelings and a great sense of humor that make this volume readable indeed.

Peter H. Forsham, M.D.
Professor of Medicine;
Director, Metabolic Research Unit,
School of Medicine,
University of California,
San Francisco

# Preface

You will find this book unique and unorthodox compared with the usual medical text. Written primarily for medical students, house-officers, and primary care physicians, it is a manual that gives step-by-step procedures for treating the patient with diabetes and the acute and chronic complications of diabetes. It is not cluttered with a lot of "gingerbread," and I have purposely omitted numbered references which the practicing physician may not bother to look into, anyway. Although most of the advice follows accepted methods of treatment, some of the information may be controversial.

The manual is written to give the practicing physician a quick and easy desk reference to the general management of diabetes and its problems. The book is organized so that the busy doctor can quickly look up a procedure. The book is not intended to be a complete reference on diabetes and its complications, but does discuss related subjects in detail sufficient to allow the physician to manage the average diabetic patient satisfactorily. I hope it will fill in some of the gaps that were left in medical school, where in general the teaching of diabetes is far from adequate.

These are exciting times in diabetes because so much progress is being made in research into the serious and life-threatening complications of the disorder. It is time for the practicing physician to assume a more optimistic attitude about the future for all diabetics, since it is going to be better.

Statistics relating to serious complications and limited life expectancy for diabetics can be alarming and depressing, particularly to newly diagnosed diabetic teenagers. Emphasizing statistics to the new patient is neither advocated nor helpful. In many cases, it has "turned off" the desires and intentions of the patient to follow the principles of maintaining good control of his diabetes at all times, and thus has encouraged a feeling of futility.

The physician must realize that interpretation of statistics can take many pathways. First of all, some of the present statistics regarding morbidity and mortality are based on antiquated retrospective findings and on hospital diagnosis and/or death certificates, many of which have been shown to be deficient in detail and even erroneous in specific diagnosis. Additionally, one must remember that a portion of our diabetic population does not receive adequate medical care because of socioeconomic factors beyond their control. They probably never attain what we consider "good" diabetic control. Last, another segment of our diabetic population becomes so depressed with the facts and figures about their own prognosis that they prefer to "throw in the sponge" at an early stage and make no further attempt to attain and maintain good diabetic control. Both these segments of the diabetic population are included in the reported statistics.

On the optimistic side, we can show that many diabetics have a minimal decrease in life expectancy and that a substantial number are alive and well after having taken insulin for over 50 years. Such persons have usually followed the diabetic rules of living well.

The physician caring for diabetics should emanate optimism and counsel his patients, especially the younger Type I patients, with an attitude of encouragement and promise of improved health and extended life expectancy in view of many recent developments, which are discussed in detail in this book. We must boost the morale of our young diabetics who are already depressed and frightened of what the future may bring.

I suppose that the complacency of many attending physicians regarding the state of control obtained in the average diabetic, Types I and II both, is mainly because established hyperglycemia rarely produces symptoms in an otherwise healthy diabetic. As doctors we are attuned to providing relief to patients who have complaints. The average diabetic, especially the juvenile, may show constant blood sugar levels of 300 to 400 mg/dl and have neither symptoms nor complaints, unfortunately, until acute or chronic complications develop. It is too bad that any blood sugar level over 200 mg/dl does not produce a severe headache, for example, relieved only by reduction of the blood sugar.

Another factor may be that many doctors are not attuned to the recently reported studies showing without question that excellent control of hyperglycemia is an important factor in the prevention of life-threatening vascular complications. In most diabetics, it is possible to obtain good or excellent control with patience and perseverance.

I feel confident that the primary physician can do a satisfactory job of caring for most diabetic patients if he is knowledgeable, interested, motivated, and empathetic. Most of all, he must be willing to spend the extra time necessary in caring for persons with diabetes. He must also realize when to ask for consultation for the person with deteriorating vision, crippling neuropathy, vascular occlusions, or renal failure. Something can be done for almost everyone.

The basics involved in caring for diabetics now are no different from 25 years ago, but the methods have changed. We feel the diabetic patient should be knowledgeable regarding meal-planning, insulin or tablets, exercise programs, and complications. I am a strong advocate of in-depth education for the diabetic person and thereby direct a diabetes education center at Deaconess Hospital in Spokane, Washington. One-to-one education is often impossible for the busy doctor, so group education replaces it. One should take advantage of opportunities to send patients for diabetic education—it will make them easier to care for. It has been proved that the educated diabetic person is hospitalized far less often for problems associated with the disorder than the noneducated diabetic. Education probably extends the life of the student.

It is past time for physicians to take more interest in caring for diabetes. Ten per cent of office patients have diabetes, but they require more than 10% of the physician's time, without the added remuneration, except the satisfaction of a job well done. I have taken care of many diabetics for 35 years and still enjoy every challenge. I hope this manual will help the reader to become a better diabetologist and that he, too, will enjoy this challenge.

*Spokane, Washington* O. Charles Olson

# Contents


| | | |
|---|---|---|
| *Chapter 1* | Introduction | 1 |
| *Chapter 2* | Diagnosis of Diabetes | 9 |
| *Chapter 3* | Dietary Management | 18 |
| *Chapter 4* | Selection and Use of Insulin | 28 |
| *Chapter 5* | Injection Procedures for Insulin | 43 |
| *Chapter 6* | Oral Antidiabetes Tablets (Sulfonylurea Drugs) | 49 |
| *Chapter 7* | Urine Testing | 59 |
| *Chapter 8* | Care of the Juvenile Diabetic (Type I) | 68 |
| *Chapter 9* | Management of the Older Diabetic Patient | 76 |
| *Chapter 10* | Exercise | 86 |
| *Chapter 11* | Hypoglycemia | 93 |
| *Chapter 12* | Diabetic Ketoacidosis | 101 |
| *Chapter 13* | Immunologic Reactions to Insulin | 114 |
| *Chapter 14* | Obesity | 120 |
| *Chapter 15* | Surgery | 125 |
| *Chapter 16* | Infections and Skin Disorders | 131 |
| *Chapter 17* | Impaired Diabetic Limbs | 137 |
| *Chapter 18* | Pregnancy | 146 |

*Chapter 19* Relation of Diabetic Control to Degenerative Complications ..... 165

*Chapter 20* Diabetic Retinopathy and Other Eye Disorders .. 172

*Chapter 21* Diabetic Neuropathy ..... 179

*Chapter 22* Sexual Dysfunction ..... 188

*Chapter 23* Diabetic Nephropathy ..... 192

*Chapter 24* Risk Factors in Cardiovascular Disease: Hyperlipidemia and Hypertension ..... 197

*Chapter 25* Substitute Insulin Delivery Systems ..... 207

*Chapter 26* Home Blood Glucose Monitoring ..... 212

*Chapter 27* Substitute Sweeteners ..... 217

*Chapter 28* Glycohemoglobin ..... 226

*Chapter 29* Diabetes Secondary to Other Disease States and Rare Types of Diabetes ..... 230

*Chapter 30* Lactic Acidosis ..... 235

*Chapter 31* Hyperosmolar-Hyperglycemic Coma ..... 241

*Chapter 32* Etiology and Genetics of Diabetes Mellitus ..... 245

*Chapter 33* Multiple Hormones Involved in Diabetes ..... 251

*Chapter 34* Pathways of Glucose Metabolism and Glucose Homeostasis ..... 263

*Chapter 35* University Group Diabetes Program (UGDP) Study ..... 267

*Appendix* ..... 277

*Index* ..... 283

# 1

# Introduction

Diabetes mellitus (DM) is a fascinating disorder of metabolism that involves many physiologic systems other than glucose metabolism. Every author attempts to define diabetes, but a complete and satisfactory definition remains to be found. The important point, however, is that the physician treating diabetes understands what disorderly metabolic defects he is trying to correct or readjust in order to allow the person with diabetes to function physiologically as normally as possible. The physician must then be prepared to carry out these adjustments and corrections according to presently accepted practices.

Almost all diabetologists who write about diabetes start out by telling us what a heterogenous disorder diabetes is and then go on to describe the rare types that most of us never see in a lifetime. Some authors describe a complex picture. I prefer to refer to diabetes as a metabolic disorder rather than a disease. The types of diabetes that the primary care physician treats are not complex, and generally they are not difficult to understand. I am always astounded that the average physician does not show more interest and enthusiasm in diabetes, but maybe it is because much of the literature is conflicting. My reward for writing this book will be in clarifying the confusion facing practicing physicians and in simplifying the orderly and acceptable treatment of diabetes.

For many years there was much confusion about classifying the various stages of carbohydrate intolerance, and we have had to struggle with such terms as potential diabetes, prediabetes, chemical diabetes, juvenile-onset diabetes (JOD), maturity-onset diabetes (MOD), maturity-onset diabetes of the young (MODY), insulin-dependent diabetes (IDDM), non-insulin-dependent diabetes (NIDDM), and impaired glucose tolerance (IGT). It was obvious that the profession needed a simplified and understandable classification of diabetes that could be used worldwide and that would put us on common ground when talking or writing about the disorder.

## CLASSIFICATION OF DIABETES

In April of 1978, an international work group convened under the sponsorship of the National Diabetes Data Group of the National Institutes of Health and presented the following classification of diabetes, which has been considered by the American Diabetes Association.

The terminology and classification system had to fulfill the following requirements, quoted from the recommendations of the workgroup:

> "1. The classes should be defined so as to be mutually exclusive, that is, an individual at any time in his life can be placed in only one class, although with prospective follow-up he may change characteristics and need to be reclassified subsequently.
> 2. The classification should require only simple clinical measurements or descriptive observations which are readily obtainable and have biologic significance.
> 3. The classes should be as precise and well-defined as our current knowledge of the etiopathology of diabetes allows, so that each class contains a population as homogeneous as possible.
> 4. The terminology should be precise and well-defined and should, as much as possible, describe the phenotypic expression of the abnormality.
> 5. The classification should be adaptable and able to incorporate new research findings on the etiopathology of diabetes."

### Classes of Diabetes Mellitus

Type I, insulin-dependent type (IDDM), patients are characterized by the following:

1. They are dependent on injected insulin to prevent ketosis and to preserve life, hence these patients have insulinopenia.
2. In 90% of these patients, the onset of the disorder is in youth or young adulthood (to age 40).
3. They may have certain HLA types.
4. They may have islet-cell antibodies.

Persons who are not prone to ketosis and who use insulin only to correct hyperglycemia are not considered to be Type I patients.

Type II, non-insulin-dependent types (NIDDM), patients are not insulin-dependent or ketosis prone, although they may use insulin for correction of symptomatic or persistent hyperglycemia; this subclass is not autoimmune-related or HLA-associated. In most of these patients, onset of the disorder is after 40 years of age.

Subtypes are as follows:

A. Nonobese NIDDM (less than 120% ideal body weight (IBW), or body mass index (BMI) of less than 25 for women and 27 for men) patients may be either (i) insulin-treated for hyperglycemia or (ii) not insulin-treated.

B. Obese NIDDM (IBW or BMI greater than criteria for Type II-A) patients may be either (i) insulin-treated for hyperglycemia or (ii) not insulin-treated.

These 2 types comprise the majority of diabetics treated by the primary care physician. However, for the sake of completeness, the remaining classifications are listed.

### Gestational Diabetes (GDM)

The onset or recognition of this disorder occurs during pregnancy (see Chap. 18).

### Impaired Glucose Tolerance Test (IGT)

See section on diagnosis for details.

### Previous Abnormality of Glucose Tolerance (Prev. AGT)

This class includes those persons who have normal glucose tolerance but who previously had impaired glucose tolerance or, in some cases, diabetic hyperglycemia. Examples are patients with gestational diabetes or with hyperglycemia as the result of the stress of an accident, an operation, or an infection.

### Potential Abnormality of Glucose Tolerance (Pot. AGT)

This category includes persons with increased risk of developing DM because:

1. They have an identical twin with DM.
2. Both their parents have DM.
3. They have 1 parent and 1 sibling with DM.
4. Other first-degree relatives have DM.
5. They have given birth to a baby of 10 lbs or more.

### Glucose Intolerance Associated with Certain Conditions and Syndromes

These conditions and syndromes are hormonal or drug-induced disorders, pancreatic disease, insulin receptor abnormalities, and other genetic and chromosomal syndromes.

## AGE DISTRIBUTION

The primary care physician cares for diabetics in all age groups, and the statistics in Table 1–1 should be of interest.

Most of those patients with onset of the disorder before age 25 are Type I, insulin-dependent. Approximately 30 to 40% of those with onset of diabetes between 25 and 44 years are also Type I. Thus, about 20% of the diabetic patients of the primary care physician (excluding pediatricians) are Type I, whereas the remaining 80% are Type II. The pediatrician has mainly Type I patients.

About 5% of diabetes beginning in childhood is not Type I and can be controlled by diet alone or by diet and tablets. Dr. Fajans and colleagues, who first described these patients, have studied a group for more than 20 years. The researchers chose to call them maturity-onset diabetes of the young (MODY). Whether these patients are Type II diabetics is not clear.

Approximately 10 to 15% of diabetic adults develop Type I diabetes over age 45. The physician should look for it in the lean adult, particularly if there is a history of weight loss and muscle-wasting.

## PREVALENCE AND INCIDENCE

Figures given for the total number of diabetics in the United States are not exact, since diabetes is not a reportable disease. The most recent reliable information is published in the pamphlet entitled "Diabetes Data," compiled in 1977 under the direction of the National Diabetes Data Group established in the National Institute of Arthritis, Metabolism, and Digestive Diseases.

National Health Interview Surveys conducted by the National Center for Health Statistics of the United States Department of Health, Education, and Welfare of 120,000 persons in 1973 gave the prevalence of diabetes at 2%. Thus, in 1973, the total number of persons with diabetes was 4.2 million. A similar survey in 1975 reported 4.8 million. The rate increased with age, from 1.3/1000 (1 in

Table 1–1. Age of Distribution of Diabetes Mellitus.

| Age of Onset | % of All Diabetics | Type of Diabetics |
|---|---|---|
| Birth to 25 years | 8 | 95% Type I |
| 25 to 44 years | 22 | 30–40% Type I |
| 44 years and older | 70 | 85–90% Type II |

770 persons) for those under 17 years to 78.5/1000 (1 in 12) among persons aged 65 and older.

Based on the 1973 National Health Interview Survey, the incidence is approximately 0.3% of the total United States population per year, or 612,000 persons (3/1000).

A statistical study showed that between 1965 and 1973 there occurred a 50% increase in the total number of cases, meaning a 6% incidence increase per year. The increase was 26% for males, but 50% for females, and females under age 45 had a 79% increase.

The marked increase may only represent an increase in the recognition of diabetes, because the rapidly expanding automated chemistry reveals previously undiagnosed diabetic blood sugar levels. One doubts that the incidence could double every 15 years in the future.

## OCCURRENCE IN CHILDREN

Diabetes mellitus, fortunately, is an uncommon disorder in children. However, unfortunately, few physicians are familiar with all aspects of Type I diabetes in school-aged children simply because there are so few of them. A 1975 National Health Interview Survey report gave a total of 65,000 children under 17 years of age in the United States with DM, of which 37,000 were male and 28,000 female. The generally accepted figure is a prevalence of 1.3/1000 children, or 1 in 770. Recent surveys in Michigan and Minnesota gave comparable figures. The incidence of the disorder is 1 in 2,500 children 17 years or under.

## UNDIAGNOSED DIABETES

The figures given vary tremendously, and most are based on the glucose tolerance tests in a probability sample of the United States population in 1960 to 1962 in persons age 18 to 79 years taken during the National Health Examination Survey (HEW). Their figures showed a probability of twice as many persons with undiagnosed diabetes as with known diabetes, based on the results of a 50-g OGTT. Now there is reason to doubt the veracity of these findings. No doubt a number of Type II, mostly mild, diabetics go undiagnosed each year, but again, in view of automated chemistry determinations done on so many more persons now than in 1960, it is probable that a large percentage of those so-called "undiagnosed diabetics" have been added to the total of known diabetics. Diabetes detection drives carried on as community projects over the last 15 years have not found new diabetics in twice the number of known diabetics, and many such detection drives are generally regarded as being fraught with too many errors to be worthwhile. So, one can probably say there is one undiagnosed diabetic for every 2 known diabetics and be close to accurate, even though the figure itself is not important to the clinician.

## IMPORTANCE OF BLOOD SUGAR CONTROL AND COMPLICATIONS

All physicians who treat diabetes must intensify their counseling of diabetic patients in view of some recent findings regarding control and chronic complications. This counseling is particularly important to the insulin-dependent or Type I diabetic, who may be living with diabetes for 50 years or more.

Studies conducted since 1970 show conclusively that chemical control, i.e., maintaining blood sugar levels as close to normal as possible at all times, is a key to minimizing and/or preventing retinal and renal failure, as well as having a beneficial effect in avoiding neuropathy.

The present evidence indicates that the relationship of macroangiopathy (coronary-cerebral-peripheral arteries) is not so closely allied to chronic hyperglycemia as are complications involving the kidney and/or the retina. Neuropathy manifests itself in both Type I and Type II diabetes, but perhaps more severely in the long-standing Type I patient. A detailed discussion of the complications is found in other chapters of this book, as well as brief resumes of studies substantiating these premises.

Therefore, the new philosophy seems to be meticulous control of blood sugar levels at all times, and this, of course, requires more effort on the part of the physician and more cooperation on the part of the patient. The patient must be thoroughly educated in the importance and manner of attaining constant blood sugar control. There is no way for the physician to educate the patient adequately in a 15- to 20-minute office visit once a month or every 3 months. He must insist that his patient attend classes in diabetic education that are detailed and thorough in teaching all the important aspects of diabetes and how to control it.

## WHAT CONSTITUTES METICULOUS DIABETIC CONTROL?

Ideally, meticulous control means that there is no more than ¼% or a trace of sugar in the premeal urine test for Type I diabetics and in any pre- or postmeal urine specimen for Type II patients, assuming a normal renal threshold.

For Type I, insulin-dependent diabetics, excellent control of diabetes approximates as closely as possible the nondiabetic normals. Blood sugar levels in nondiabetics vary between a low of 80 to

85 mg/dl and a high of 120 to 130 mg/dl, thus with an excursion rarely above 50 mg/dl. Many diabetologists who have followed large populations of diabetics over the years have noted that if blood sugar levels never exceed 175 mg/dl, fasting, and 200 mg/dl, postprandial, severe microangiopathy rarely develops. The primary physician should use these figures as a guide. Diabetics who have worn infusion pumps with continuous 24-hour insulin delivery usually have almost normal (nondiabetic) blood sugar levels.

Every experienced diabetologist realizes that excellent diabetic control is frequently unobtainable in some Type I patients, in most cases owing to noncompliance of the patient. However, factors that increase stress hormone concentrations may affect control of the disorder. Most of the time, these patients are teenagers or persons in their twenties. The attitude of the patient toward his disorder is mainly responsible for the attainment of diabetic control when the program of insulin, diet, and exercise has been properly prescribed by the physician and dietitian. Many young diabetics are difficult to manage, and consultations with members of the family as well as with diabetologists are helpful. Group therapy may also be helpful, as may be a thorough understanding of diabetes gained by attending diabetes education classes.

For Type II diabetics, excellent control of diabetes means that blood sugar levels must be close to normal, nondiabetic levels, both fasting and postprandial. This control is obtained only when the obese diabetic loses weight, and if needed, takes oral antidiabetes tablets. The Type II patient of normal weight who controls his diabetes by diet and tablets or by diet alone should have blood sugar levels within or close to the nondiabetic range.

This is a strict edict and not always easy to attain or maintain, particularly in younger patients, especially if the insulin requirements are large. You must be sure that the patient does not experience severe hypoglycemic episodes as a result of a strict regimen. However, if we eliminate the 2 to 3% of Type I patients who are "brittle," a well-balanced program frequently attains this goal.

However, from recent studies using the "artificial pancreas," by which a "nondiabetic" state in a research metabolic unit can be attained for short intervals, it is obvious that even the most meticulous daily program of insulin, diet, and exercise often fails to achieve the normal physiology of blood sugar control present in the nondiabetic person.

We are all grateful to the 1974 Congress, which passed Public Law 93–354, the National Diabetes Mellitus Research and Education Act. As a result, research funds are now being provided to enable our scientists to perfect the "artificial pancreas" for all insulin-dependent diabetics, so that they may attain or approach that state of "nondiabetes." Further discussion of such devices is found in Chapter 25. Research funds are allocated for many projects other than these, of course.

In summary, then, we are dealing with a known prevalence of diabetes in 2% of our population, around 5 to 6 million persons, with perhaps another 2 to 3 million with some alterations in their carbohydrate tolerance that may or may not properly be labeled diabetes.

The majority of all diabetics in the United States are over 50 years of age; many of them were asymptomatic at the onset of the disorder, and glucosuria was found on a routine urinalysis. The danger of overdiagnosis is an obvious pitfall; the other unanswered question is whether benefits can be derived from vigorous treatment of mild or borderline hyperglycemia in the older person. We must keep in mind that carbohydrate tolerance decreases with age in all of us, and we allow a 10 mg/dl increase for postprandial levels and a 3 to 4 mg/dl increase for fasting sugar levels per decade beginning at age 50 when interpreting blood glucose levels.

Approximately 10% of the average office practice of the primary care physician is with diabetic patients, as are 10% of all hospital admissions. Therefore, it behooves the physician to improve and sharpen his knowledge and skills in caring for this important segment of his practice.

## FURTHER READING

Gorwitz, K., et al.: Prevalence of diabetes in Michigan school-age children. Diabetes, *25*:122, 1976.

National Diabetes Data Group: Classification of diabetes mellitus and other categories of glucose intolerance. National Institutes of Health, 1978. (Available from NIAMDD, Westwood Bldg., Room 605-B, Bethesda, Maryland 20016.)

United States Public Health Service: Diabetes data. NIH, 1977. (Available from NIAMDD, Westwood Bldg., Room 605-B, Bethesda, Maryland 20016.)

# 2

# Diagnosis of Diabetes

In response to an obvious need to reassess diagnostic blood glucose levels proposed by the American Diabetic Association in 1969, the National Diabetes Data Group of the National Institutes of Health convened an international workgroup in April of 1978, and they presented to the Statistics Committee of the American Diabetes Association in June of 1978 the diagnostic criteria paraphrased in the following section.

## CRITERIA FOR DIAGNOSIS

1. First is the presence of obvious symptoms such as polyuria, polydipsia, polyphagia, with weight loss. The fasting plasma sugar (FBS) level is grossly elevated on 2 or more occasions (greater than 160 mg/dl).
2. No obvious symptoms may be present, but FBS is elevated to 140 mg/dl or more (plasma), repeated 2 or more times.
3. If neither of the foregoing prevails, then one should do an oral glucose tolerance test (OGTT) under the careful, standardized conditions detailed in this chapter. One should note that the accepted standard dose of glucose is 75 g for an adult and 1.75 g/kg body weight for children, up to a maximum of 75 g.
   Diagnosis is positive if: (1) 2-hour plasma glucose concentration is 200 mg/dl or greater, and (2) at least 1 value between zero time and 2 hours is 200 mg/dl or more.
4. If the results of the first OGTT are positive, it should be repeated in 6 to 8 days.
5. Instead of repeating the OGTT, some diabetologists feel that a satisfactory method is to do a 1- and 2-hour blood sugar test when the patient has eaten a meal slightly loaded with carbohydrate. One should be sure that the potential diabetic patient has eaten a normal diet for 3 days prior to doing the postprandial blood sugar tests. Then one should advise him to eat a meal loaded in carbohydrate prior to coming to the laboratory.

Examples of such meals are:

*Breakfast:* Orange juice, hotcakes with syrup, sugar in tea or coffee.

*Lunch:* Sandwich and apple pie à la mode or candy bar, and a sweet soft drink.

One should draw blood samples exactly 1 and 2 hours after the patient has finished the meal.

**Interpretation.** Both samples should be 200 mg/dl or above to prove the positive diagnosis of the previous OGTT. If the readings do not agree with the results of the OGTT and are both under 200 mg/dl, then one must give careful thought to how vigorously to treat such a person. The degree of impairment based on the laboratory readings should be evaluated, always remembering that the results of any given OGTT are difficult to reproduce; one may need to repeat tests at more frequent intervals. The generally accepted normal plasma glucose level for those age 50 or under is:

Fasting, less than 125 mg/dl;
1-hour postprandial, less than 175 mg/dl;
2-hour postprandial, less than 150 mg/dl.

**Allowance for Age.** All of us develop progressive glucose intolerance with age. Therefore, it is accepted procedure to allow 10 mg/dl more glucose per decade after 50 years for postprandial readings, and 3 to 4 mg/dl for fasting readings. In its criteria for diagnosis, the National Diabetes Data Group makes no allowances for age, probably because "over 200 mg/dl" is generous.

## Impaired Glucose Tolerance

Based on the standardized oral glucose tolerance test, the diagnosis of impaired glucose tolerance would be made if: (1) the 2-hour plasma glucose concentration is more than 140 mg/dl, but less than 200 mg/dl, AND (2) at least 1 value between zero time and 2 hours is greater than 200 mg/dl.

## Gestational Diabetes

In this type of diabetes, the onset of the disorder occurs during pregnancy. One should give 100 g glucose for the OGTT in the pregnant patient. Gestational diabetes is present when 2 or more of the following plasma glucose values are met or exceeded:

Fasting, 105 mg/dl
1-hour, 190 mg/dl
2-hour, 165 mg/dl
3-hour, 145 mg/dl

It was suggested that one might consider a diagnosis of "impaired gestational glucose tolerance" if the 2-hour plasma glucose level was between 120 mg/dl and 164 mg/dl.

### OGTT Criteria for Children

One cannot at present apply exact criteria to children, since not enough long-range studies have been done. Fasting blood sugar levels are known to be lower in children than in adults. However, 95% of children do not need a glucose tolerance test for diagnosis because they come to the physician with marked symptoms accompanied by a gross elevation of fasting plasma glucose. When the physician feels an OGTT is indicated, one could apply the adult diagnostic values until standards are developed.

### Criteria for Normal GTT

Both fasting and 2-hour plasma glucose levels are under 140 mg/dl.

### Screening Test

Some physicians prefer to screen all their new patients, and there are occasional community screening projects in an effort to find those with asymptomatic diabetes.

A 2-hour post-carbohydrate-load plasma glucose level is suspicious if over 150 mg/dl. In this case, an OGTT should be undertaken for patients under 50 years of age.

### Procedures for OGTT

Following is the summary of recommendations for standardizing the OGTT as presented by the American Diabetes Association:

**Preparatory Phase.** Several factors are important.

***Diet.*** For the 3 days preceding the scheduled test, if the patient was on a normal diet previously, his diet should include, among other things, the following foods in at least the quantities given. More of these foods may be taken if desired, but the quantities given are the *least amounts* that should be eaten *each* day (250 g carbohydrate).

1. Three slices of white, rye, or whole-wheat bread.
2. Two tablespoonsful of jam or jelly.
3. One dish of breakfast cereal.
4. One cup of cooked corn, peas, or lima beans.
5. Fresh or canned fruit with cake or cookies for dessert.
6. Sugar freely used in tea or coffee.

***Acute Illness.*** There should be a delay of at least 2 weeks after a period of acute illness before performing the test. The patient should be ambulatory, not in bed or hospitalized.

***Medication.*** The patient should discontinue drugs proven or believed to influence the OGTT for at least 3 days prior to the test. These include hormones, oral contraceptive drugs, diuretics, salicylates, and all nonessential medications. Oral antidiabetes agents should be discontinued for at least 2 weeks.

***Fasting Period.*** There should be no intake of any food value for at least 8 and not more than 16 hours preceding the test.

***Miscellaneous Restrictions.*** The patient should avoid coffee, smoking, and unusual physical exercise for at least 8 hours prior to the test.

***Postponement of Test.*** One should omit the test in the event of unexpected illness (e.g., fever, gastritis) or if food has been ingested within 8 hours.

**Testing Phase**

***Time.*** One should conduct the test beween 7 A.M. and noon; i.e., taking the fasting specimen between 7 and 9 A.M.

***Glucose Load.*** The commonly used and recommended dose is 75 g for adults and 1.75 g/kg (up to 75 g) for children. Available commercial preparations generally contain 75 g. This dose should be consumed within 5 minutes of taking the FBS specimen.

***Specimen Timing.*** The antecubital venous blood specimen should be drawn at fasting. One should note zero time when the patient starts drinking the glucose and draw additional blood specimens 60 and 120 minutes after zero time. A 3-hour specimen may be helpful only if *reactive hypoglycemia* is suspected. One should not draw specimens at half an hour, 4 hours, and 5 hours. They are an added expense and are of no diagnostic value.

***Patient's Behavior.*** The patient should avoid physical exertion, emotional stress, and stimulants (tobacco, alcohol, coffee, tea).

**Processing of Blood Sample**

***Type of Sample.*** Plasma or serum are preferable to whole blood. Separation by centrifugation should be done within 30 minutes of drawing blood. RESULTS FROM PLASMA AND SERUM ARE 15% HIGHER THAN WHOLE BLOOD. Capillary blood, accurate only in the fasting state, is best not used, but if used, it is 10% higher than venous blood.

***Preservation of Sample.*** Freezing, or the addition of sodium EDTA (1 mg/ml blood) and sodium fluoride (2 mg/ml blood), are required if chemical determination is not performed on the same day the specimen was drawn. Thymol must not be present during the color development phase of the test.

***Chemical Methods.*** Any of the following methods are comparable when performed with adequate quality control procedures: glucose oxidase, hexokinase, *o*-toluidine, Somogyi-Nelson, AutoAnalyzer ferricyanide, or AutoAnalyzer neocuproine. All ferricyanide, neocuproine, and Somogyi-Nelson methods measure reducing substances other than glucose and are generally being phased out.

### Nondiabetic Causes of Abnormal OGTT

Abnormal OGTT results can arise from nondiabetic causes, most of which are obvious to the astute clinician. The most common causes are:

1. Acute stresses (fever-trauma-major operations-myocardial infarction-cerebrovascular accident) when even *fasting* hyperglycemia may exist.
2. Chronic illnesses; prolonged physical inactivity; starvation and malnutrition; there is no fasting hyperglycemia in these persons.
3. Potassium depletion from any cause; fasting hyperglycemia may be present.
4. Chronic renal disease with uremia, which can indicate pseudohyperglycemia due to non-glucose-reducing substances.

### Tests Other Than OGTT

Other infrequently used tests for the diagnosis of abnormal glucose tolerance include the intravenous GTT, the cortisone GTT, and the tolbutamide tolerance test. The reader is referred to detailed textbooks on diabetes for further information and procedures.

### When *Not* To Do an OGTT

There is no indication for doing an OGTT on a patient who has an obvious diagnosis of diabetes, based on his fasting plasma glucose level. The glucose tolerance test is not a satisfactory criterion of severity, nor do the results offer any scientific guidance as to the amount of insulin necessary. One should do an OGTT only when there is a definite indication that one will gain more information.

### Disagreement Regarding OGTT

For many years, leading diabetologists have disagreed on the wisdom of making a diagnosis of diabetes based on the OGTT. Even after acceptance of these new diagnostic standards, disagreement will remain. However, it is logical to have some standard procedure for establishing the diagnosis, and until newer and more reproducible methods are devised, we shall continue to use the OGTT. For those patients in whom the diagnosis is "borderline," or who clearly fall into the classification of "impaired glucose tolerance," several studies have shown a link between even mild hyperglycemia and vascular disease, particularly of the coronary and peripheral arteries.

## OVERDIAGNOSIS

One must beware of labeling a patient with the diagnosis of diabetes unless one is certain that it exists. All diabetologists see the occasional patient who has been diagnosed and treated, including treatment with insulin, for the disorder when actually no diabetes exists. This inexcusable error is easy to avoid if one is familiar with the standards of diagnosis. To saddle a patient with a false diagnosis leads to personal frustrations, including insurance "riders," in some states driver's license limitations, and possible limitations in employment opportunities.

One must beware of making the original diagnosis of diabetes in an adult who is hospitalized for any reason. The stress of illness, bed rest, operations, fractures, fever, myocardial infarction, and stroke is frequently severe enough to cause marked hyperglycemia temporarily. Many of these patients show a normal carbohydrate tolerance a few days or weeks after recovery; at the same time, the stress itself may be the precipitating factor of a true diabetic state. In the case of a coronary occlusion, an interval of at least 6 weeks is recommended before further testing. However, one should remember that frank diabetes can be precipitated by an illness or an operation, and if the patient's routine glucose level on the SMA-12 test is unusually high, one must do further laboratory studies to make the differential diagnosis.

## POSSIBLE REMISSION

Undue embarrassment may be avoided by realizing that an adult coming to a physician's office for the first time, with diabetes having been diagnosed by another physician, may not have present evidence of diabetes after proper laboratory tests. This patient may well be in a complete remission, and one must be tactful so as not to cast any doubt on the prior diagnosis. It is prudent to ask for a copy of the previous physician's records to appraise the situation properly.

## DIAGNOSTIC CLUES IN TYPE II PATIENTS

A small percentage of Type II patients initially have symptoms of diabetes, with glucosuria and significantly elevated blood sugar levels, both fasting and postprandial, making the diagnosis obvious. The majority, however, are discovered during the course of routine examinations for other conditions or complaints. These clues may arise during the taking of the patient's history or the physical examination. One should keep these points in mind:

1. Random glucosuria, which indicates a high probability index; further investigation is always in order.
2. Abnormal obstetric history, including repeated abortions, stillbirths, congenital deformities, toxemia, birth weight over 10 lb, and "renal glycosuria" of pregnancy. (One must be sure the urine sugar is glucose—see Chap. 18.)
3. Postprandial hypoglycemia, 2 to 4 hours after eating, in addition to family history of diabetes mellitus. (See Chap. 11.)
4. Obesity and family history, especially after age 40.
5. Premature macroangiopathy (coronary, cerebral, etc.) before age 50.
6. Recurrent skin infections after adolescence.
7. Unusual eye problems—blurred vision, frequent changes of eyeglasses, cataract before age 50.
8. Peripheral neuropathy after age 50; one should be alert to paralysis of third or sixth cranial nerve—50% of the time the patient has diabetes.
9. True "renal glucosuria"—the question of how many such persons eventually become diabetic is controversial.

In these patients and any others in whom diabetes mellitus is suspected, one should proceed as follows:

1. The patient should be instructed to eat a normal diet for at least 3 days prior to blood sugar tests.
2. An FBS test should be done. If it is 140 mg/dl or more, the cause is *probably* diabetes. One should repeat the FBS test at least twice more, at 5-day intervals.
3. Before starting treatment on the person with moderate elevation of FBS (140 to 175 mg/dl), it is wise to do an additional 2-hour postprandial blood sugar test for the physician's records and satisfaction. This is best done after a loaded carbohydrate meal. One must be sure that the blood is drawn exactly 2 hours after completing the meal.
4. If the FBS test result is normal (less than 140 mg/dl), one may proceed to a 2-hour postprandial blood sugar test as mentioned, or a complete OGTT.

## CLASSIFICATION OF "IMPAIRED GLUCOSE TOLERANCE"

When a patient has blood glucose levels that are between normal and diabetic, what steps should be taken in counseling him? One must remember that persons in this category are not diabetic by the new criteria, but up to 5% per year may develop overt diabetes. Likewise, many will return to a normal glucose tolerance level spontaneously; some will remain that way for many years. There is evidence that these persons are at a higher risk than the general population of experiencing cardiovascular complications.

Physicians should discard from their vocabulary all those unscientific and confusing terms so often used in the past, such as chemical diabetes, latent diabetes, borderline diabetes, subclinical diabetes, asymptomatic diabetes, prediabetes, and potential diabetes. The term "impaired glucose tolerance" replaces all these terms.

At the present time, there is no known way to prevent progression to overt diabetes in persons with impaired glucose tolerance except by their attaining normal weight when obese. Patients in this category should receive instructions on weight loss when indicated, education as to what impaired glucose tolerance means, and follow-up monitoring at proper intervals. This monitoring includes requesting the patient to do urine tests for sugar at least weekly, 1 to 2 hours after the largest meal, and to report any evidence of glucosuria. The physician should schedule him for a 2-hour postprandial (loaded-carbohydrate meal) plasma glucose test every 6 months or so, based on his judgment of the situation and the patient's anxiety. The patient should be told that most persons in this category either remain so or revert to normal. If the physician feels the need for more assurance than given by a properly administered 2-hour postprandial blood sugar test, he should do a complete OGTT annually.

## QUICK SUMMARY OF DIAGNOSTIC PROCEDURES

1. Patients of any age, but more often those under 25, who have obvious symptoms and a fasting plasma glucose level of over 160 mg/dl (usually much higher), need no further testing to diagnose diabetes mellitus. One should start treatment at once. This patient is a Type I diabetic.
2. For a patient, usually over 25 years of age, with a suspicious history, possibly glucosuria, probably obese, with mild symptoms, if any, one should do the following:
   - A. Order a fasting plasma glucose test.
     1. Over 140 mg/dl means diabetes, but if barely over 140 mg/dl (145 to 155 mg/dl), proceed to step "B."
     2. Whatever the result, repeat in 7 days.
   - B. Order a plasma glucose test 1 and 2 hours after a carbohydrate-loaded meal or 75 g glucose.

1. If both are 200 mg/dl or more, diagnose diabetes (no allowance for age).
2. If glucose level at 1 hour is 200 mg/dl or more and at 2 hours is between 140 and 200 mg/dl, diagnose impaired glucose tolerance.
3. Repeat the test once, in 1 week.

C. If results of testing are borderline suspicious, (level at 1 hour over 175 mg/dl and at 2 hours over 150 mg/dl), then order an oral glucose tolerance test, following directions in text. It is a poor and irreproducible diagnostic test, but the best we have so far. Insurance companies and employers may request that it be done. Make allowances for age in the "borderline" patients.

D. OR skip the OGTT and explain to the patient the state of impaired glucose tolerance and what it means. Do follow-up studies as explained in text. Emphasize to the patient that any degree of impairment of glucose tolerance carries some cardiovascular risk.

### Announcing the Diagnosis

The word "diabetes" means the end of the world to some persons who know little or nothing about the disease. The physician should announce the diagnosis without expressing alarm and with assurance that everything will be fine once control of the disorder is established. He should use tact and thoughtfulness. Patients have read untruths and partial truths about diabetes, and the worst always is remembered, such as that blindness will overtake them in a few years, they will lose their limbs to gangrene, and in due time men will all be impotent. The physician must reassure them that this course is not necessarily inevitable and the future has never been more promising, especially for young Type I diabetics. Optimism works much better than pessimism, and there is now real cause to be more optimistic.

# 3

# Dietary Management

## IMPORTANCE OF DIETARY EDUCATION

All diabetics, regardless of their age or the severity of their diabetes, must be aware of the importance of dietary management and must be instructed in suitable meal planning. Caloric intake and the composition of the diet must be a relative constant, against which is computed the necessary medication and the individual's exercise habits.

It is indeed unfortunate that most of our medical schools almost entirely neglect dietary education. As director of medical education in a 300-bed hospital, I am appalled by the house staff's lack of knowledge of diet therapy. I would suggest that medical schools take a hard look at their dietary teaching curriculum and take more time for such education.

The worst approach to diet a practicing physician can take is to pick from a stack of American Diabetes Association (ADA) or similar diabetic diets one of appropriate or inappropriate caloric value, hand it to the newly diagnosed patient, and say, "Here's your diet—go home and read it and follow it." Another frequent admonition by the physician is, "Watch your diet." No other instruction is given. This happens frequently, according to the diabetic students who come to our education center. The physician either must become proficient at dietary teaching on a one-to-one basis or must refer his diabetic patients to a teaching dietitian, particularly one well educated in diabetic counseling. This second approach may mean sending the patient several hundred miles from home, but it is certainly worth the trip. All large cities have available dietitians capable of instructing patients in adequate meal planning, and the physician owes it to his patients to see that they avail themselves of this service.

With the advent of the oral antidiabetes tablets, there arose an erroneous belief among some physicians that their Type II patients could take the tablets and eat "almost anything." This is not true, and physicians have been criticized for not being more demanding of their patients in the field of diet therapy. One can speculate that perhaps over 80% of all Type II diabetics could be controlled by diet therapy alone, but we shall never know, since few obese Type II patients stay on a reducing diet long enough to attain their ideal weight. This problem is discussed in Chapter 14.

The patient's compliance with the diet involves considerable effort and cooperation and usually involves marked changes in eating habits. We do not use the term "diet" in instructing our patients, since this term connotes a weight-losing regime to the average person, and certainly this is not always the case with the diabetic. A much better term is "meal plan" or "meal planning."

## VARIABLES IN MEAL PLANNING

What does the dietitian want to know about the patient prior to prescribing the meal plan?

1. Is he Type I, insulin-dependent or Type II?
2. What is his age, occupation, economic status?
3. What is his present weight and his ideal weight for his age and body build?
4. How motivated is the patient regarding diet therapy?
5. Dietary history—what are his customary eating habits (how much? what kind of food? when?).

A simple rule for calculating ideal weights is shown in Table 3–1. It might be well to post it next to the scales so the nurse can compare these figures with the patient's weight.

Table 3–1. Calculation of Ideal Weights for Adults.

<table>
<tr><th></th><th>Medium Frame</th><th>Light Frame</th><th>Heavy Frame</th></tr>
<tr><td>Men</td><td>106 lb—first 5 ft, plus 6 lb each additional inch</td><td rowspan="2">Subtract 10% from ideal weight for medium frame</td><td rowspan="2">Add 10% to ideal weight for medium frame</td></tr>
<tr><td>Women</td><td>100 lb—first 5 ft, plus 5 lb each additional inch</td></tr>
</table>

NOTE: These figures apply to persons of average build. Heavily muscled persons may be 20–40% heavier.

## CALORIC REQUIREMENTS

The basal caloric requirement for adults is approximately 10 times the ideal weight in pounds or 22 cal/kg. To this basal requirement one should add 6 cal/kg of ideal weight for sedentary persons, 12 cal/kg for moderately active persons, and 24 cal/kg for physically active persons. Caloric requirements for children are usually calculated according to this formula: 1000 calories baseline plus 100 calories for girls and 125 for boys per year of age up to 12 years. This formula is for average physical activity, so the athletic youngster requires considerably more. The additional calories needed for physical activity vary from 10 to 100%. For instance, the moderately physically active adult under 60 years of age probably requires 15 to 25% more calories, whereas the young school athlete may require 50 to 100% more. Since energy expenditure is so variable, even in persons of the same body weight, it is necessary frequently to review and to readjust diabetic diets to maintain ideal body weight.

It is important to remember that we no longer "starve" the insulin-dependent Type I diabetic, but we do attempt to reach and to maintain ideal weight or a few pounds over it. Continual weight loss in the young diabetic means either that the caloric intake is not sufficient or that hyperglycemia is uncontrolled, with marked caloric loss through glucosuria. Neither situation should be allowed to continue.

## DIETARY GUIDELINES FOR THE TYPE I INSULIN-DEPENDENT GROUP

These guidelines are more easily understood when broken into age groups.

**Birth to 4 to 5 Years of Age.** It is difficult to maintain any type of constant caloric intake, although it is surprising how many children in a given age group do consume about the same amount each day. The main concern is the avoidance of concentrated sweets and the assurance that the total caloric intake is sufficient and the diet is nutritionally adequate. Parents need much counseling, since their frustration seems to be the main problem.

An excellent article by Benz and Kohler, "Baby food exchanges and feeding the diabetic infant," is published in Diabetes Care (3:554, 1980). All who instruct parents of diabetic infants and young children should refer to this article.

**Five to 10 Years of Age.** A gradual trend into measured food portions should take place in these years, with dietary discipline emphasized by the parents and learned by the child. Again, it is important to make at least semiannual adjustments in the total

Table 3–2. Effect of Diet on Diabetic Complications.

| Research Group | Number of Patients | Diet* | Age at Onset | Duration of DM years | Retinopathy % | Proteinuria % | Hypertension % |
|---|---|---|---|---|---|---|---|
| Knowles | 78 | NM | 17 | 10 | 64 | 33 | 28 |
| Constam | 12 | NM | 17 | 20 | 100 | 66 | 50 |
| Constam | 41 | M | 17 | 20 | 44 | 7 | 0 |

* NM = nonmeasured, M = measured

caloric intake to provide for growth and development as well as increased physical activity. The physician must weigh and measure all diabetic children at every office visit.

**Ten to 18 Years of Age.** Dietary discipline and education can be completed in these years. Girls generally have reached full physical growth by age 14, whereas boys continue to grow and develop through 18 years, and thus require continued caloric adjustments for a longer time.

Many pediatricians prescribe more liberal diets for their diabetic youngsters in order to minimize disturbance at mealtimes for all the family. Perhaps they feel that a measured, balanced diet is not really necessary. However, pediatricians do not have their patient for long enough to observe and to treat the microvascular complications. It is interesting to note the statistics in Table 3–2.

## New Type I Patients

Most new Type I patients are hospitalized for a few days to establish control and for preliminary education, which includes dietary instruction. This means that the hospital dietitian, following the physician's diet prescription, instructs the patient and his parents. It is well for the physician to discuss the diet with the dietitian to compare ideas prior to instructing the patient. If the physician does not know much about diets and really does not care about learning diet therapy, he should be frank with the dietitian and should give her free rein to take over the calculations and instruction. In most cases, the dietitian does a good job. One must remember that most patients and/or parents simply do not learn dietary management in one sitting. It is best to have at least 3 sessions of 60 minutes or more, and occasionally a fourth, before the patient or parents feel confident about the diet. A refresher session with the dietitian should be scheduled in 6 weeks.

Many physicians in smaller communities are not utilizing the services of their dietitians, probably because they are not fully aware of their capabilities. If one practices in such a community and has access to good dietitians, one should by all means use their services for diabetic diets as well as other special diets.

One must always remember that frequent dietary adjustments must be made in growing children. A diet adequate at age 9, for instance, is not going to be adequate at age 11. This means a visit to a dietitian at least yearly during the growth years. However, in many families, it seems that intuitive parents learn rapidly about the need for additional calories for growth and development and gradually increase the food portions sufficient to maintain normal growth and weight. Frequently, all that is needed is a short discussion between patient, parent, and physician to review growth, weight, and caloric intake.

### Between-Meal Snacks

Each snack generally furnishes about 150 to 250 calories. Children through grade school usually require midmorning, midafternoon, and bedtime snacks; older children usually do well with afternoon and bedtime snacks only. All diabetics who take insulin should have a bedtime snack because the time span between the evening meal and breakfast is too long to expect normoglycemia without additional intake of food.

Composition of the snacks can vary considerably, but generally the midmorning snack may be all carbohydrate in the form of fruit, while the afternoon and bedtime snacks should provide some protein with carbohydrate, such as a sandwich and 1 to 2% milk.

## DIETARY GUIDELINES FOR TYPE II PATIENTS

Approximately 80% of Type II adult-onset patients could control their disorder by diet alone if we knew the magic formula to keep them on such a diet. Since almost 75% are overweight at the time of the onset of diabetes, most of their diets are restricted in calories. Discussions of the obese diabetic and reducing diets are found in Chapter 14.

The Type II patient who is not obese should be instructed in a meal plan that furnishes sufficient calories to maintain normal weight, strength, and working capacity. A bedtime snack should always be included for the Type II patient who takes insulin.

The Type II patient with mild diabetes who never shows glucosuria can generally follow a well-balanced general diet, but should omit concentrated sweets, including raw sugar, jellies, jams, syrups, honey, and frosted baked goods. These patients should be instructed in the composition of a nutritious diet.

### Diet Composition and Meal Division

Recent changes in diabetic diets have allowed for more carbohydrates and less fat and cholesterol, a change that many diabetologists made over 20 years ago when first told that high-cholesterol and saturated-fat diets were possibly harmful. A further discussion of the fat and cholesterol content of the diabetic diet is found in Chapter 24.

The accepted composition of the ideal diabetic diet today is as follows:

carbohydrate: 40 to 55% of total calories
protein: 20 to 25% of total calories (for growing children, in pregnancy and lactation, give at least 1 g protein/lb ideal weight)
fat: not over 30% of total calories, of which one-third is saturated, one-third monounsaturated, one-third polyunsaturated
cholesterol: not over 300 mg daily, ideally.

The calculated total calories are divided to provide around 150 to 200 calories for each between-meal snack; the remainder is for the 3 main meals, with approximately one-fifth for breakfast and two-fifths each for lunch and dinner. However, variations from this formula are frequent when planning meals for special or unusual situations, including work and vacations. The insulin dosage can be easily adjusted to compensate for variable caloric intakes, especially if 2 daily doses are taken.

## WHETHER TO WEIGH OR TO MEASURE FOOD PORTIONS

Generally, the use of common household measurements is satisfactory, except in the case of meats, cheese, fish, and poultry, for which it is difficult to estimate the weight in ounces of a given serving. For Type I diabetics who are on a closely controlled program, it may be advisable to use an ounce scale (a postage scale is satisfactory) for this purpose for 6 months or so. Beyond that time, use of the scale becomes tiresome.

## EXCHANGE LISTS

The exchange system, almost universally used, has the advantage of providing daily consistency while allowing considerable choice and variety. It is relatively simple to teach and to learn. The system includes 6 fundamental groups of food, shown in Table 3–3. Most of these foods are listed in common household measurements. Exchange lists are available from the American Diabetes Association, many drug companies, and the American Dietetic Association.

Table 3–3. Exchange System.

| Exchanges | Basic Amounts | Carbohydrates g | Protein g | Fat g |
|---|---|---|---|---|
| 1. Milk (Skim) | 8 | 12 | 8 | 0 |
| 2. Vegetable | ½ c (cooked) | 5 | 2 | 0 |
| 3. Fruit | variable | 10 | 2 | 0 |
| 4. Bread | 1 slice | 15 | 2 | 0 |
| 5. Meat | 1 oz | | | |
| | lean | 0 | 7 | 3 |
| | medium fat | 0 | 7 | 5 |
| | high fat | 0 | 7 | 8 |
| 6. Fat | 5 g | 0 | 0 | 5 |

Dietary instruction books for patients have the detailed information that diabetics must understand in order to adhere to a prescribed diet (see Appendix). Diabetic patients need such a book, and it is best for the physician to make it available to them.

## SPECIAL DIET FOODS AND "HEALTH" FOODS

Fruits packed without sugar, sugarless soft drinks, and artificial sweeteners such as saccharin are acceptable and useful in making the diabetic diet more palatable.

So-called diabetic candy found in "health food" stores is not recommended, except as a special treat. Any claims by health food stores as to the benefit of certain foods for diabetics must be carefully investigated.

### Fructose

In recent years, there has been renewed interest in fructose as a sweetening agent, and several studies have proved its usefulness in this capacity. For a detailed discussion on fructose, see Chapter 27.

## DIETARY FIBER

Dr. James W. Anderson of the University of Kentucky pioneered in the study of the effect of high-fiber diets on glucose, cholesterol, and triglyceride levels. Dr. D. J. A. Jenkins and colleagues have carried on similar research in England. Some plant fibers, especially gums and pectins, are water-soluble, whereas others, such as lignin and cellulose, are water-insoluble. Apparently, water-soluble fibers are the most valuable in lowering glucose and cholesterol levels. Guar gum is the most effective in lowering glucose levels, and to this end Jenkins and his group have incorporated this substance into a crisp bread. It is necessary to consume about 25 g/day guar gum as crisp bread in order to show a significant lowering of glucose values. This bread is not generally available in the United States.

Anderson's approach has been to make use of foods that are commonly and easily available to add to the diabetic's diet in an effort to accomplish the same lowering of blood glucose and/or cholesterol levels. Anderson used an experimental diet containing high carbohydrates and high plant fiber (HCF) composed of: 70% of calories from carbohydrate, of which 75% was complex carbohydrate; 19% of calories from protein; and 11% from fat; 35 to 40 g plant fiber/1000 cal food. He reported that 20 insulin-treated men maintained on such a diet for 16 days showed a 58% reduction in insulin requirements. This reduction was thought to be due mainly to the change in diet composition and, to a small degree, to the content of plant fiber. These studies indicated that such a diet increased the number of insulin receptors.

Anderson's studies also showed an average decline of 30% in cholesterol levels in diabetic patients studied on the HCF diet. This decline was attributed to both the low-fat and low-cholesterol contents of the diet as well as to the specific effect of the plant fiber. He noted that oat bran was specific in its ability to lower low-density lipoprotein cholesterol levels and to raise high-density lipoprotein cholesterol levels. He also reported that fasting triglyceride levels are lower in patients following the HCF diet, particularly in patients who started the study with marked elevations of triglyceride levels. The exact mechanism by which plant fibers have a triglyceride-lowering effect is not clear.

Anderson's group devised an acceptable out-patient diet that uses commonly available high-fiber foods (see Appendix). The diet provides 55 to 60% of the calories as carbohydrate, 20% as protein, and 20 to 25% as fat, with 25 to 30 g plant fiber/1000 calories. The diet contains foods such as raw fruits, whole grain cereals and crackers, bran cereals, shredded wheat, grapenuts, and beans of all kinds. Most of the patients studied by Anderson had a preliminary period of intensive hospital treatment for 1 to 10 days prior to instituting the out-patient program. This hospitalization apparently is most advantageous in bringing about the initial drop in glucose and lipid levels.

Even though the primary care physician may feel that the cost of this initial hospitalization is not warranted, there is certainly good reason to believe that an out-patient, high-fiber diet would prove to be valuable to the average diabetic patient. Other benefits from high-fiber diets are appearing in the literature, especially as related to neoplastic disease of the colon. Future studies will be of value in substantiating existing reports. Meanwhile, one should consider the inclusion of commonly available high-fiber foods in the diabetic meal plan.

## COMPLIANCE OF THE PATIENT

No one knows how many patients are continuously conscientious about their meal plans, but the consensus is that about 60% neither understand nor follow their diets. There are many reasons for this, such as:

1. Lack of understanding and motivation by the patient.
2. Physicians' indifference to dietary compliance.
3. Physicians' lack of knowledge of basic nutrition.
4. Resentment by the patient of drastic change in living habits.
5. Juvenile diabetics' attachment to "junk foods."
6. Obese adults' emotional attachment to food as well as complete lack of motivation.
7. Lack of parental motivation and supervision.

Compliance can be drastically improved with adequate education of patient and parent, dietary counseling by a skilled dietitian, including frequent follow-up and review sessions, and encouragement by the physician who realizes the importance of long-term diabetic control.

## INSTRUCTION BOOKS

Every physician prescribing diabetic diets should also recommend a good book on diabetic meal planning for his patients. Many excellent books are on the market, and I enthusiastically suggest the one that I use, written by dietitians, in the Diabetes Education Center of Deaconess Hospital in Spokane, Washington. The reader is referred to the Appendix for information on this and other books on diabetic meal planning.

In summary, practicing physicians' opinions about diabetic meal plans vary. This ambiguity complicates their ability to organize an effective control program, since a constant daily caloric intake is basic. Except in the mildest Type II patients, the "free diet" approach should be condemned. However, some mild Type II diabetics can be instructed in a nutritionally adequate diet that avoids concentrated sugars, such as raw sugar, jellies and jams, honey and syrups, frostings and candy, and sugary desserts. Mastering an exchange diet for a 75-year-old patient with mild Type II diabetes may not be possible, so the instruction to avoid "raw sugars" simplifies his dietary management.

Dietary compliance by the patient probably occurs less than we like to believe. Perhaps fewer than 50% of all patients adhere strictly to a diabetic meal plan. Every diabetic is entitled to instructions in meal planning by a competent person, either a physician or a dietitian. Review and reinforcement is necessary at regular intervals to encourage compliance. The diet must be nutritionally adequate, fat should not furnish more than 30% of the calories, and the diet should not include more than 300 mg cholesterol. It should have calories sufficient to attain and to maintain normal weight and strength and, in the case of children, adequate growth and development. Meal planning for young diabetic children (under age 8) must frequently be modified from rigid exchange diets in order to assure a nutritionally adequate intake.

# 4

# Selection and Use of Insulin

## TYPES OF INSULIN

Table 4–1 outlines the fundamental characteristics of the available insulins. Protamine zinc (PZI) is long out-dated. Globin is used infrequently in the United States, but is popular in England and in some European countries. NPH, Lente (L), and regular (R) insulin comprise the 3 basic types; we could manage without the others. NPH and Lente insulin are almost identical in time-action curves, but NPH is modified by the addition of protamine. The Lente family has no added protein. Regular insulin is a standby for treating acute diabetic situations as well as for mixing with NPH or Lente. Most diabetes can be controlled by multiple doses of regular insulin. Indeed, many patients experienced good control until physicians started deviating from this discipline in 1936, when PZI came on the market.

When I was a medical student, the only available insulin was regular, and the diabetic ward was one of the busiest places in the hospital. Diabetes was controlled with multiple doses of regular insulin, usually 3 per day, but patients who had a tendency toward hyperglycemia overnight sometimes had an additional midnight dose. Patients stayed in the hospital for 6 weeks, and when they went home, their disorder was well controlled and they were well disciplined and educated in diabetic management. Some who were periodically examined in the diabetic out-patient clinic had been taking multiple doses of regular insulin since 1923. Almost none had evidence of severe microangiopathy.

Table 4–1. Physical and Chemical Characteristics of Various Insulins.*

| Type | Onset of Action hours | Peak of Action hours | Duration of Action hours | Mixable with Regular | pH | Comments |
|---|---|---|---|---|---|---|
| Rapid-Acting | | | | | | |
| Regular | ½–1 | 2–4 | 5–8 | — | 7.2 | used for supplemental injections, in emergencies, and for mixing with NPH or Lente |
| Semilente | 1–2 | 4–8 | 12–16 | no | 7.2 | can be mixed with Lente; occasionally satisfactory alone if 2 doses are given daily |
| Intermediate | | | | | | |
| Globin | 2–4 | 10–14 | 14–24 | yes | 3.5 | not popular in the United States |
| NPH | 1–2 | 8–14 | 24–28 | yes | 7.2 | important basic insulin |
| Lente | 1–2 | 8–14 | 24–28 | yes | 7.2 | important basic insulin |
| Prolonged-Action | | | | | | |
| Protamine-zinc | 4–8 | 14–24 | 24–36 | yes | 7.2 | obsolete and should be discontinued |
| Ultralente | 4–8 | 20–26 | 24–36 | no | 7.2 | long-acting; rare indications for use, except when mixed with Lente to provide sufficient overnight insulin |

* These time-action statistics were derived from studies on both volunteer nondiabetic subjects and stable, well-controlled diabetics generally taking low doses of insulin. In clinical practice, the physician may see marked variations from these time-action figures when treating patients with long-term insulin therapy. It is necessary to prescribe the insulin or combination of insulins that results in the best control of hyperglycemia for each patient, using this table only as a general guide.

Few patients now can afford to be hospitalized for 6 weeks, and fewer would tolerate the idea of 3 to 4 injections of insulin per day. Physicians try to release diabetics from hospitals as soon as possible because of the cost, and there is not really sufficient time to educate them properly. Thus, out-patient education is a must.

In order to duplicate partially the normal physiologic mechanism that takes place in the nondiabetic person (namely, a rise of insulin following meals that reaches its peak in about 30 to 60 minutes, and then a slow decline, with the accompanying rise in blood sugar to not more than 130 mg/dl average), it would be necessary to give multiple premeal injections of regular insulin plus a dose of NPH or Lente for overnight coverage. There are many diabetics living and well who have followed comparable programs for more than 50 years and have minimal evidence of retinal or renal disease and little neuropathy.

It really is too bad that we were not happy with multiple injections of regular insulin.

The following quotation is taken from a paper by Dr. Peter Forsham, an outstanding diabetologist who heads the Metabolic Department of the University of California Medical Center in San Francisco.

> "Only rapidly acting regular, soluble insulin given before meals will blunt the hyperglycemia and only food intake with six meals can buffer the hypoglycemia following injection. The importance of high plasma levels of insulin with meals is that insulin receptors on muscle, fat, and connective tissue have to be saturated in order for the cell to be enzymatically, fully activated."

It is obvious that few diabetics would be happy with 4 or more injections of insulin daily, even though it might establish more physiologic control of the diabetes.

Because the daily injection of multiple doses of regular insulin posed problems of time and convenience, diabetologists felt strongly about a need for a 24-hour insulin, one that could be injected once each morning and would gradually release an adequate amount of insulin from the injection site throughout the following 24-hour period. So,the search began for compounds to mix with insulin that would give it these characteristics. The ideal insulin has not yet been found.

Table 4–2 gives the availability of the currently used insulins. One should remember that U-80 strength was phased out early in 1980 and that U-40 will likewise be discontinued later.

## INSULIN PURIFICATION

In 1968 it was noted that commercial insulins contained proinsulin, and subsequently other proteins were noted as contaminants, including glucagon, pancreatic polypeptides, somatostatin, and vasoactive intestinal peptide. In the present methods of insulin purification, the content of proinsulin is used as the index of purity.

Two chromatographic methods are used separately or in combination to assure maximum purification. Gel filtration chromatography separates proteins according to molecular weight, and ion exchange chromatography separates proteins according to ionic exchange.

The older USP insulins contained 10,000 to 40,000 parts per million (ppm) of proinsulin; "single peak" contains 300 to 3000 ppm; "improved single peak" contains fewer than 50 ppm; and "purified" contains fewer than 10 ppm. The "purified" insulins are currently marketed in this country by Eli Lilly and Company in purified pork and pure beef, by Nordisk in purified pork only, and by Nova in purified pork and purified mixed beef-pork insulin.

## Use of Purified Pork Insulin

Are there any advantages to using the "purified" (fewer than 10 ppm) insulins as compared with those containing higher amounts of other proteins? Purified pork insulin is almost identical to human insulin and thus is the least antigenic. It becomes obvious that there are definite indications for the use of this insulin, i.e., (1) the presence of insulin allergy, either local or systemic (see Chapter 13), (2) immunoresistance when insulin requirements exceed 100 units daily, (3) lipodystrophy, either atrophy or hypertrophy, and (4) whenever insulin is to be used on an intermittent or interrupted basis, such as its temporary use in Type II diabetes when surgical procedures or major illnesses indicate the need, and in gestational diabetes. The purpose is to minimize future allergic reactions or immunoresistance.

It has been recently reported that in a group of patients using purified pork insulin, none of them showed lipodystrophy or allergic reactions to insulin. In addition, almost all patients with previous lipoatrophy showed improvement after using purified pork insulin.

The clinical importance of insulin antibodies has never been clearly defined. It has been shown that antibodies can interfere with the time of onset of action of regular insulin. However, a correlation between metabolic control and insulin antibodies has never been demonstrated. It is possible that insulin antibodies may interfere with endogenous insulin secretion by an unknown mechanism.

Several studies have reported a significant reduction in insulin dosage with an accompanying decrease in antibody titers after switching from conventional beef or beef-pork mixtures to purified pork insulin. More studies are needed before one can recommend the use of purified pork insulin for all diabetics. Perhaps the future

Table 4–2. Insulins Currently Available in the United States.

| Species Sources, Purity, Action | Manufacturer | | | |
|---|---|---|---|---|
| | Eli Lilly & Co.* | E. R. Squibb & Sons | Novo Industri A/S (Copenhagen) | Nordisk Insulinlaboratorium (Gentofte) |
| **Pork** (purified, <10 ppm) | | | All types in U-100 | All types in U-100 |
| Rapid-acting | Regular U-100 | | Actrapid (regular) | Quick (regular) |
| | U-500 | | Semitard (Semilente) | |
| | | | | Mixtard† |
| Intermediate-acting | NPH U-100 | | | NPH |
| | Lente U-100 | | Monotard (Lente) | |
| Long-acting | PZI U-100 | | | |
| **Beef** (purified, <10 ppm) | | | | |
| Rapid-acting | Regular U-100 | | | |
| Intermediate-acting | NPH U-100 | | | |
| | Lente U-100 | | | |
| Long-acting | PZI U-100 | | | |
| | | | Ultratard (Ultralente) | |

| | | | |
|---|---|---|---|
| **Beef Pork** (purified, <10 ppm) | | | |
| Intermediate-acting | | | Lentard (Lente) |
| **Beef-Pork** (USP, improved single peak, <50 ppm) | All types in U-40 & U-100 | | |
| Rapid-acting | Regular | | |
| | Semilente | | |
| Intermediate-acting | NPH | | |
| | Lente | | |
| Long-acting | PZI | | |
| | Ultralente | | |
| **Beef-Pork** (USP, conventional, >10,000 ppm) | | All types in U-40 & U-100 | |
| Rapid-acting | | Regular | |
| Intermediate-acting | | NPH | |
| | | Globin | |
| Long-acting | | PZI | |
| **Beef** (USP, conventional, >10,000 ppm) | | All types in U-40 & U-100 | |
| Rapid-acting | | Semilente | |
| Intermediate-acting | | Lente | |
| Long-acting | | Ultralente | |

* In 1980, Eli Lilly & Co. introduced "improved single peak" insulins in all their beef-pork mixtures. Prior to this they had introduced improved pure pork and pure beef insulins. For details see the discussion in this chapter.
† Mixture of 30% regular and 70% NPH.

availability of human insulin via the *E. coli* route will make future studies utilizing animal insulins unnecessary.

The insulin needs of the majority of diabetic patients can be well met by the use of mixed beef-pork insulins, either conventional (circa 10,000 ppm) or improved single peak (fewer than 50 ppm). The use of purified pork insulin should be reserved for those patients previously discussed.

Control of hyperglycemia is the most important factor in minimizing complications of diabetes and not the purity of the insulin nor the species source.

One word of caution is necessary for the patient who might wish to switch brands of insulin. Because of the difference in purity, there exists the possibility of a reduced (or increased) insulin requirement. Generally, it is advisable to stay with the same brand unless specific indications exist for changing to a more purified insulin. The highly purified insulins are much more expensive.

The following discussion is useful in enabling the physician to choose the proper dosage and type of insulin, as well as to make the necessary adjustments in the size of the dose, in order to attain optimal diabetic control.

## ADULTS REQUIRING FEWER THAN 25 UNITS DAILY

It is generally accepted that the average nondiabetic adult produces around 25 to 35 units of insulin per day and that the requirements would be even less if insulin were not beset with hormone antagonists and degradation by the kidneys. If an adult diabetic can be controlled with 15 to 20 units of insulin per day, the chances are good that there remains some secretion of endogenous insulin. Such an individual can usually control his diabetes with a single small morning dose of either NPH or Lente. Generally, his urine is sugar-free, and blood glucose fluctuations are minimal, with most determinations in the excellent category (not to exceed 50 mg/dl over nondiabetic, normal levels). This patient's diabetes is easy to control, and he will rarely have major problems.

## CHILDREN REQUIRING FEWER THAN 25 UNITS DAILY

It is probably best to start most children with a single morning dose of an NPH-regular insulin mixture, although the rare patient does well with NPH or Lente alone, if he absorbs insulin evenly throughout the 24 hours. There is no question, however, that most children eventually have better control with 2 doses per day. Discussion of 2 doses per day is best done after the first few months of insulin therapy, when the patient and parents are more apt to accept the physician's reasoning about the advantages of such a program. Most diabetologists feel that even though the total daily insulin requirement may be less than 20 to 25 units, 2 doses give better control. See Chapter 8 for further discussion.

## CHILDREN AND ADULTS REQUIRING MORE THAN 25 UNITS DAILY

Over the years that NPH and Lente insulins have been used, it has become obvious that only about 25% of patients attain good control of diabetes for the entire 24-hour period with a single morning dose of either NPH or Lente insulin. This conclusion is more evident as the required dose becomes larger. The other 75% of diabetic patients usually show a marked insulinopenia in the first 6 to 8 hours after injection; then they may have a plethora of insulin overnight, with a resulting hypoglycemic episode. This situation is a far cry from physiologic control, and modifications of the insulin program have to be made. An attending physician may not always be aware of this situation if he orders *fasting* blood sugar tests only, since test results are frequently in a satisfactory range. The physician must look at the urine record and must also order blood sugar tests 2 hours after breakfast and lunch to see the true picture. A determination of hemoglobin A-1c (HbA-1c) is also helpful in evaluating control of the disorder.

If the patient shows hyperglycemia and glucosuria in the first 6 to 10 hours of the day, he should add regular insulin to the Lente or NPH morning dose, the exact amount to be determined by the extent of the hyperglycemia. (Semilente may be added to Lente for accelerated action if preferred, but Semilente should not be added to NPH.) It is best to start moderately with regular insulin and increase as needed. Example: Patient presently takes 40 units of NPH, but shows control in the last half of the day only. One should start with NPH 30 and regular 10 and take an 11 A.M. blood glucose test in 7 days. At another time, the physician should obtain the blood glucose level 2 hours after lunch and should adjust the dose of regular insulin accordingly. If second-voided urine samples before breakfast are showing 1 to 2% glucose, the NPH should be increased. One should not make changes every few days, but rather every week or two for fine tuning, unless the disorder is severely out of control, in which case speed is of essence.

### Two Injections Daily

Some diabetes can be well controlled by the foregoing mixture given as a single morning dose, especially if the total needed is 40 units or less. However, there is no doubt that the majority of Type I patients, especially those whose insulin requirements exceed 30 to 40 units daily, do much better on split doses of mixed insulin. The formulas in the following sections may serve as a useful guide. Many pediatricians feel it is wise to begin 2 injections shortly after the onset of diabetes, even though the total daily requirement may be much less than 30 units.

Dr. Peter Forsham, at a symposium on diabetes, expressed his views on the need for 2 daily doses of insulin, stating that anyone who required over 20 units per day for adequate control should receive 2 injections daily. Each injection should contain a mixture of rapid-acting and intermediate-acting insulin in the proportions that give the best control of hyperglycemia, and about two-thirds of the total is given before breakfast and one-third before supper. Dr. Forsham further went on to say that the prevention of chronic hyperglycemia will certainly prevent many of the serious complications that may result in death at a relatively early age.

### *Morning Dose*

Judgment mainly determines the composition of the dose as well as total units required. Physically active young persons, especially school children who participate in daily sports, may need less regular insulin in the morning dose, whereas sedentary office workers may need considerably more. One should give the dose at least 30 minutes before breakfast.

**Composition.** All the experts have a different idea as to the composition, from 60% regular and 40% NPH or Lente insulin to the opposite—60% NPH or Lente and 40% regular. A good starting point is 60% NPH or Lente and 40% regular.

**Percentage of Total Daily Dose.** The morning dose should ordinarily consist of 60 to 70% of the total 24-hour insulin requirements, although occasionally 50 to 60% works better.

**Adjustment.** If a double-voided urine test shows a high sugar level before lunch, and midmorning blood sugar levels are also high, one should increase the regular insulin dose by about 20%, not more often than every 5 to 7 days. If the urine shows a sugar level of 1 to 2% before the evening meal, the Lente or NPH insulin is increased by about 10%, not more often than every 5 to 7 days. If hypoglycemia occurs before lunch, one should reduce the regular insulin dose, and if hypoglycemia occurs before supper, the Lente or NPH dose should be reduced.

### *Afternoon/Evening Dose*

Under most circumstances, this dose is best given 30 minutes before the evening meal. It is not advised to give it before bedtime, since then one misses the advantage of the regular insulin in controlling postprandial hyperglycemia.

**Composition.** Generally, about 60 to 70% NPH or Lente and 30 to 40% regular insulin should assure one of adequate nighttime coverage.

**Percentage of Total Daily Dose.** About 35 to 40% of the total daily dose should be given in the afternoon or evening. Again, this must be tailored to suit the individual.

**Adjustment.** The same sort of logic applies to adjustments in the afternoon/evening dose, realizing that the regular insulin's activity is manifested mainly in the first 4 hours after injection.

Note: When changing from a single morning dose of insulin to 2 doses per day, one may find that the total daily requirement is less, so some precaution is in order. Example: If the total single dose of insulin is 60 units, NPH 40, regular 20, mixed, and control is only fair, then one may start with 2 injections totaling 50 units and increase as indicated by urine and blood sugar levels. On the other hand, if control is poor with a single daily dose, more total insulin is required when changing to 2 doses per day.

Galloway recently reported studies in normal fasting subjects showing that the effects of regular insulin seemed better maintained when it was mixed with NPH rather than with Lente insulin (Diabetes Care, 3:615, 1980).

When regular insulin is used in combination with either NPH or Lente, the regular insulin's activity is usually maximal and total in the first 8 hours after injection. However, the occasional patient may show a longer duration of action of the regular component that might result in presupper hypoglycemia, the correction of which is accomplished by reducing the units of regular insulin rather than the NPH or Lente.

## SUPPLEMENTARY INSULIN INJECTIONS TO COVER DIETARY INDISCRETIONS

For many years, I have advised my patients to take small doses of regular insulin prior to an expected dietary indiscretion. Diabetics, like all of us, love holiday dinners, including dessert, and a night out on the town now and then, and thus are not always "dietary angels." I do not encourage this sort of indiscretion, but occasionally it happens. Taking insulin after hyperglycemia has occurred only shortens the length of the hyperglycemic episode. This procedure is better than nothing, but one had best take an injection of regular insulin before indulging and thus prevent marked hyperglycemia. The physician should instruct those patients who are apt to be indiscreet about diet to take a small injection of regular insulin not more than 15 minutes prior to starting their meal. Ten to 15% of their usual total daily dose should be about right. This usually means about 5 to 10 units. Ordinarily, one would not give more than 10 units.

## SENSITIVITY REACTIONS TO INSULIN INJECTIONS

For a complete discussion of problems associated with immunologic reactions to insulin, including localized and general allergic reactions, insulin resistance, and fat atrophy and hypertrophy, see Chapter 13.

## HELPFUL INFORMATION ABOUT INSULIN

One should refrigerate only the insulin not being used currently. Insulin for daily injection should be kept at room temperature because it is less painful when injected. Regular insulin is stable for 18 months at room temperature. NPH, all Lentes and PZI, are all stable for 24 months at room temperature. All insulins are stable for 36 months under refrigeration. L-Reg, NPH-Reg, L-SL, L-UL, and SL-UL may all be mixed in any proportion. Mixtures are stable for 3 months in glass containers, but not in individual plastic syringes. If insulin doses are premixed in plastic syringes, they are stable for up to 7 days. Twenty-milliliter premix sterile vials are available from pharmacies for premixing larger amounts. Recent studies suggest that mixtures of Lente and regular are stable for a relatively short time and should be injected within 5 minutes after mixing.

If during a perusal of the literature on diabetes one is confronted with the reporting of blood glucose results in mmol/L instead of in mg/dl, the conversion factor is 18; i.e., 8 mmol/L equals 144 mg/dl.

## TIMING INSULIN AND DIET FOR VARIABLE WORKING HOURS

A few diabetics work where there is a recurring change of working hours every week or several weeks. This pattern means that they change from so-called day shift to "swing shift" (3 to 11 P.M.) to "graveyard" (night) shift. Whenever possible, the attending physician should discourage such alterations and should help the patient to let his employer agree to keeping the diabetic on a straight day shift. Metabolic control is much simpler, and diurnal rhythms are not upset. However, if variable hour shifts are unavoidable, these patients need suggestions on how to arrange insulin and food intake to accommodate the hour changes. The following scheme has worked well for my patients over the years.

**Patients Taking 2 Daily Doses of Insulin.** This is the best system for revolving shift workers.

***Day Shift.*** No problem is posed because this is the usual and customary routine.

***Swing Shift.*** With most patients, this shift poses no problem, since they are in bed by midnight and sleep until 8 A.M. or so, at which time they can take their morning dose before breakfast. Since they start work around 3 P.M., they frequently have their largest meal at noon and carry a lunch for suppertime and evening snack. Therefore, in some cases it is wise to increase by a small fraction the morning insulin dose to cover the extra caloric intake at noon. However, the patient should have a few weeks of presupper urine tests before the physician makes a decision. The patient can prepare the suppertime dose of insulin in a disposable syringe and take it at work at the proper time preceding the evening meal. The evening snack had best be eaten before leaving work, to avoid any possible chance of hypoglycemia while driving home.

***Graveyard Shift.*** This is the most difficult shift for which to tailor the insulin and food intake for satisfactory diabetic control. The patient usually works from 11 P.M. to 7 A.M. or from midnight to 8 A.M., then goes home, eats breakfast, and goes to bed for 7 to 8 hours. I have found the following routine to work best:

The patient should take the usual morning dose of insulin before breakfast and sleep. The diurnal rhythm of the body apparently does not shift hormonal secretion in as short a time as a week, although little study has been done on this important problem in working diabetics. One assumes that the usual larger amount of insulin is required in the morning whether the patient is ambulatory or sleeping. In some cases, the patient feels better if he takes the smaller evening dose before breakfast during the time he is working night shifts, so one could try that if there is a problem.

On arising, usually at 4 P.M. or so, the patient takes the evening dose of insulin and eats his meal, which ordinarily is the biggest meal of the day.

The evening snack is to be eaten before going to work. If necessary, a small snack can be taken to work to eat at coffee-break time. Depending on the type of work, the before-supper insulin dose may have to be altered. It is necessary for the patient to carry urine-testing material with him to order to test himself at work.

**Patients Taking 1 Daily Dose of Insulin.** The rule of thumb here is to take the insulin before the meal that the patient considers to be his first meal for the ambulatory portion of the day. In other words, for normal day and swing shifts, this can be as always; i.e., before morning breakfast. With the graveyard shift, the insulin is given on awakening from sleep, which will be before the first meal after awakening, and is usually around the regular suppertime.

**Change from Working to Nonworking Days.** This change creates a problem with the graveyard shift worker who takes 1 dose of insulin daily. If he takes his insulin at 4 P.M. Friday, works on Friday night, but then is off on Saturday and Sunday, there is a change in his mealtimes. The physician can work out a schedule based on this information if the patient shows marked hyperglycemia during his days off. I again urge the physician to prescribe 2 doses of insulin per 24 hours in shift workers. Better yet, one should make sure that diabetics work continuously on day shifts.

## LONG-DISTANCE TRAVEL FOR PATIENTS TAKING INSULIN

The patient should take all the insulin and other supplies needed for the entire trip with him, since foreign insulin is unlike American insulin by name and strength. Insulin does not need to be refrigerated. If one uses only NPH or Lente, one should take a bottle of regular insulin along in case of emergency. Sufficient syringes and urine-testing equipment should also be packed, as well as a generous supply of hard candy and 2 packages of glucagon for treatment of hypoglycemia. The patient should take some easy-to-carry snack foods: raisins, nuts, crackers. A dog-tag or identification bracelet should be worn, and detailed information about the patient's diabetes should be carried in the wallet or purse. It is wise to carry at least half the needed supplies in carry-on baggage, to avoid being stranded if checked baggage is lost or delayed.

If crossing 6 or more time zones (hour changes) either east or west, some minor adjustments will have to be made in time of insulin injection for the first 24 to 30 hours after departure. The patient should keep his watch on "home time" for the first 24 hours after leaving home. If traveling east, one is "shortening" the day. It is safe to take about two-thirds of the usual morning insulin dose before breakfast either on the plane or at the destination, thus avoiding any overlap with possible hypoglycemia. The patient should test his urine for sugar before dinner that evening, and if he shows a 1 to 2% sugar level, he should take the remaining one-third of the usual morning dose. The next morning he can resume the usual before-breakfast dose.

If traveling west, one is "lengthening" the day. The patient should check his urine 18 hours after the previous morning injection, and if it shows a 2% sugar level, he should take one-third of the usual morning insulin dose, followed by a snack. He should take the rest of the morning dose before breakfast at his destination. If the urine test results are clear or show only minor amounts of sugar at 18 hours, the patient can well wait until the first morning at his destination to take his full morning dose before breakfast, even though it is more than 24 hours since the previous dose. If one is taking 2 doses per day, a similar schedule can be calculated. The patient should discuss his schedule with his physician before departing.

In case of emergency, it is important to try to find a university hospital emergency room or to call the United States embassy. The best thing to do is to call the patient's home physician if the situation is not an immediate emergency, since he can give the best advice. Frequently, the call is cheaper than a visit to a strange and foreign physician.

## POSSIBLE CAUSES FOR A PRECIPITOUS DECREASE IN INSULIN REQUIREMENTS

The physician is occasionally confronted with a Type I diabetic whose disorder was well controlled by a given dose of insulin for several years and who gradually, over a period of weeks or months, notes increasing episodes of hypoglycemia, not due to obvious causes, that require a marked reduction of insulin, sometimes as much as 50 to 60%. This situation is not the so-called honeymoon period that may occur early in the course of Type I diabetes (see Chap. 8).

The following list serves as a reminder of factors that may cause such a situation:

1. The patient reduces his caloric intake without reducing the insulin dosage and without informing the physician.
2. Without consulting the physician, the patient begins a vigorous exercise program and does not reduce the insulin dosage.
3. If the patient has had diabetes for 10 years or more, progressive renal decompensation may be occurring. The physician should look for persistent, marked proteinuria and an elevated serum creatinine level. Not all investigators agree that renal decompensation reduces insulin degradation and results in a decreased requirement, but clinically the situation certainly occurs frequently enough.
4. The association between diabetes and adrenocortical insufficiency or Addison's disease is rare; if it occurs and is not recognized clinically, the patient may lapse into acute adrenal failure and die suddenly. Coma accompanied by hypoglycemia that does not respond to intravenous (IV) glucose alone is always a clue, and large doses of IV cortisone can be lifesaving. One should be alert to early signs of adrenocortical failure such as weakness, lethargy, hypotension, weight loss, and possibly early pigmentation.

5. Other so-called autoimmune diseases occur rarely and cause marked decreases in insulin requirements. These disorders include primary hypothyroidism as well as panhypopituitarism.
6. The occurrence of an islet cell tumor (insulinoma) has been reported in diabetes, but this is an extremely rare combination.
7. Spontaneous recovery of beta cell function has been reported in a few patients who have taken insulin injections for relatively long periods of time. No satisfactory explanation has been reported.

# 5

# Injection Procedures for Insulin*

## STRENGTH AND MEASUREMENT OF INSULINS

At present, all types of insulin are prepared in solutions of 2 different strengths, designated as U-40 and U-100. The number after the U indicates the number of units in a milliliter. The most widely used insulin syringe holds 1 ml insulin when filled to the top line. It is helpful to remember that there are about 5 ml per teaspoonful.

The insulins of all strengths that are now marketed are the finest and purest ever available, thanks to the untiring efforts of the pharmaceutical companies who prepare insulin.

U-40 insulin bottles are marked with a red top; U-100 with orange. It is important for the patient to learn to read the labels properly, since it is easy to confuse these types of insulin. Insulin manufactured by Lilly carries a trademark, "ILETIN," which has caused misunderstanding. This word "ILETIN" does not indicate the kind of insulin, but only that it is Lilly's trademark. Both the cartons containing the bottles and the bottles themselves are clearly marked with a large initial, above which appears the strength of that insulin (e.g., U-100). R means regular; N means NPH; L means Lente; U means Ultralente; and S means Semilente. The patient must make certain that his order is correct, both in type and in strength.

---

*This chapter is modified from the Diabetes Education Center textbook (Deaconess Hospital, Spokane, Washington) for patients, "Diabetes Instruction Book" (see Appendix), and is included here to provide an opportunity for the physician and/or nurse to review the contents with the patient who requires insulin.

## INSULIN SYRINGES

Both permanent glass syringes and disposable plastic syringes are available for use with U-40 and U-100 insulin. These 1-ml syringes, when filled to the top mark, hold either 40 or 100 units of insulin. In addition, there is now available a ½-ml disposable syringe for use with U-100 insulin, which when filled holds 50 units of U-100 insulin. This half-sized syringe is for measuring small doses of U-100 insulin. There is also on the market a 35-unit glass syringe for use with U-100 insulin only. The patient must never use an insulin syringe that does not match the strength of the insulin he is taking. If he has some old syringes around that do not match the strength of insulin he is using, he should throw them away.

It is more economical to use the permanent type of glass syringe with disposable needles for the daily administration of insulin. The disposable syringes are fine for traveling and other special occasions. Glass syringes cost more originally ($8.00 to $10.00 each), but unless dropped or broken, they last indefinitely, providing good care is taken of them. A disposable needle attached to the glass syringe can be used several times, until it is too dull to be comfortable.

## PREPARATION FOR INJECTION

If the patient is using glass syringes, he should have the following equipment:

1. Two glass syringes, one as a spare.
2. Disposable needles, available in both 25 gauge, ⅝″ long, and 26 and 27 gauge, ½″ long. The patient should have at least 6 such needles on hand.
3. A cylindrical glass tube with cork stopper.
4. A block of wood with holes in it, to hold the glass tube and the insulin bottle.
5. Alcohol, 90% isopropyl. (One should never use rubbing alcohol.)
6. Cotton.
7. Insulin.
8. Traveling case for syringe, needles, etc. (optional).

If the patient prefers to use the disposable unit (syringe with needle permanently affixed), these are now available in 27-gauge needles, both ½″ and ⅝″ long, and the newest one is a 27.5-gauge, ½″ needle.

The following directions apply to glass syringes and to disposable needles.

When the patient prepares his injection kit for the first time, he must boil the test tube and syringe (with plunger out of barrel) for 5 minutes. He should allow them to cool. Then he should place about an inch of packed cotton in the bottom of the tube and fill the tube to about an inch from the top with isopropyl alcohol. The plunger should be placed in the syringe and the needle on the syringe when ready to use. The patient should tie an 8″ length of linen thread, light-weight string, or dental floss around the neck of the syringe and then place it in the alcohol-filled tube. The string should come out over the top. The tube should be corked, and the syringe is now ready to use at any time.

When preparing to take insulin, the patient should wash his hands thoroughly, and then empty the syringe and needle of all alcohol by pulling the plunger back and forth several times. If protamine zinc, NPH, Lente, or Semilente insulin is used, he should gently invert the bottle several times until the sediment in the bottom is in solution. Another technique is to roll the bottle between his hands. (One should not shake, since shaking causes the insulin to foam.) The patient should wipe the top of the insulin bottle with a piece of cotton wet with alcohol. Then, having looked at the unit marks on the syringe, he should fill the syringe with an amount of air equal to the amount of insulin to be withdrawn. He should then push the needle through the rubber cap of the bottle, force the air contained in the syringe into the bottle, and invert the bottle on top of the needle. He must be sure that the insulin in the bottle covers the point of the needle. Then he should withdraw the required amount of insulin into the syringe, taking care to expel air bubbles, by pressing the plunger in and out, if they appear in the syringe. The plunger should then be readjusted for the proper dose of insulin. The patient should place the needle of filled syringe on a cotton ball, alcohol swab, or suitable cradle. If a disposable syringe is used, the protective cap should be replaced.

### Mixing of Insulins

If a mixture of 2 kinds of insulin is used, the following instructions apply. Certain precautions are necessary to prevent the transfer of insulin from one bottle into the other.

The patient should wipe off the top of each bottle with alcohol as previously instructed. Then he should pull back the plunger of the syringe to the number on the scale corresponding to the units of the quick-acting insulin (regular or Semilente). He should insert the needle into the bottle and inject this amount of air and then withdraw the needle without taking out any insulin. Next, he should pull back the plunger to the number on the scale corresponding to the number of units of NPH or Lente insulin to be taken and inject this amount of air into the bottle; then he should invert the bottle and withdraw the proper amount of insulin. The next step is to insert the needle into the first bottle, invert, and withdraw the proper number of units of this insulin. The patient must be sure not to inject any of the insulin already in the syringe into this bottle. Then he should withdraw the needle. A small bubble of air should be drawn in and the syringe should be inverted several times to allow the air bubble to go up and down. This procedure mixes the 2 insulins in the syringe. If a disposable syringe is used, the patient must take in an air bubble considerably larger, and then he must snap the side of the syringe with his finger in order to mix the insulins properly. Insulin may stick to the wall of the plastic syringes.

If the patient is using a glass syringe, he should rinse the syringe and needle in the alcohol in the test tube and replace it in the tube when he has injected the insulin. He is then ready for tomorrow's injection. Glass syringes should be cleaned about once a month by replacing the cotton and alcohol and by boiling the tube and syringe. Do not boil disposable needles, since the plastic will become deformed. If at any time the syringe or needle is dropped, or left out of the storage tube for a period of time, it can become contaminated and the syringe must be sterilized again, and one must use a new needle. Touching the needle with one's hand, or on any other surface, also renders it unsterile, and it should be soaked in alcohol for 10 minutes to resterilize it.

## INSULIN INJECTION TECHNIQUE

Proper insulin injection technique is essential in order to assure uniform and constant absorption of insulin from the injection site into the blood stream, which then carries the insulin throughout the body.

Insulin injections are to be made subcutaneously. In order to do this properly, 2 hands must be used, one to pinch a fold of skin and the other to inject the insulin. Thus, the sites for insulin injection must be on parts of the body that can be reached easily and comfortably with both hands, if the patient is injecting his own insulin.

When an injection site has been selected (see following section), the patient should pinch up the skin with his thumb and forefinger, feeling for a soft spot. He should wipe the skin with an alcohol swab, and should pick up the syringe, holding it horizontally with 3 fingers underneath and his thumb on top.

Then the patient should slip the needle swiftly into the skin pocket, holding the syringe at a 45 to 90° angle. He should slowly press the plunger in with his forefinger or thumb and should release the pinch of skin slowly as the insulin is injected. Then he should place a cotton ball or alcohol swab over the needle site and withdraw the needle quickly. Gentle pressure may be applied if needed to prevent oozing of insulin or to stop capillary bleeding. The patient must not massage the injection site.

## Choice of Injection Area

There is reliable evidence that the rate of absorption of subcutaneously injected insulin can vary, depending on the anatomic site used. A recently reported study from Yale showed that absorption is most rapid from injection sites in the anterior abdominal wall, whereas absorption from injection sites in the arm is intermediate and from the thighs is slowest. During a 135-minute observation period, it was shown that absorption from the abdominal site was 86% greater than from the thigh. However, if the patient is a runner or a jogger, and he injects himself in the thigh, the absorption rate is increased considerably on the days that he runs. In view of these facts, I recommend that all diabetics follow this practice:

1. The patient should use one anatomic site at all times if possible, the abdomen being the preferred area. He should inject himself in a new spot each day, approximately 1 to 1½″ from the previous injection site, starting just above the pubic hairline and approximately 1″ out from the midline and proceeding upward to just below the rib margin. Then he should start a new line approximately 1 to 1½″ outward from the previous line and advance downward to just above the pubic hairline. Another line of injections should be repeated, starting outward 1 to 1½″ further and advancing upward again. This same procedure should be repeated on the opposite side of the abdominal wall. Following this technique, it is easy to fit 12 and occasionally 15 injections on each side, thus obviating the need to change to a different anatomic site.
2. If the patient prefers to use his thighs, the technique is similar. He should start with the first injection about 3″ above the kneecap. On the outside line of the thigh, he can go upward for about 10″, in the canter line about 8″, and in the inside line only about 6″ in order to avoid the groin area.
3. If parents are injecting a child, they must make every attempt to use the same anatomic area continuously, always avoiding daily injection into the same spot.
4. If for some reason it is absolutely necessary to switch from one anatomic area to another, adjustments in the insulin dose may be necessary to maintain good control. The patient should check with his doctor.
5. Again, the patient must avoid daily rotations to different anatomic areas of the body. This procedure could result in marked variation in his diabetic control.

6. Under no circumstances should he inject insulin into the same spot each day, since fibrosis (scar tissue), which occurs under the skin in time, alters the rate of insulin absorption.
7. When taking 2 insulin injections per day, it is preferable to choose one anatomic site for every morning injection and another anatomic site for every afternoon/evening injection. Example: morning injections will always be given in abdominal wall and afternoon/evening injections in thighs, unless the patient jogs or bicycles after the evening meal, in which case the sites can be reversed.
8. I discourage injection of insulin into the buttocks, as is sometimes done in infants and young children, since absorption rates of insulin may vary because of pressures applied from sitting. The back of the thighs may be a better choice. However, the upper-outer arms seem to be the best areas for insulin injection in an infant or young child. As the child grows older, the abdominal wall or thighs may be utilized, as in an adult.

In conclusion, it is important to remember to rotate the sites of injection, to use a pattern of rotation for each area, and to follow a definite plan for injection, so that the same site is not used too frequently.

# 6

# Oral Antidiabetes Tablets (Sulfonylurea Drugs)

This chapter deals with the clinical usefulness of the oral sulfonylurea agents. A discussion of the controversial University Group Diabetes Program (UGDP) study is found in Chapter 35.

In the early 1940s, Dr. Auguste Loubatières and co-workers in France first noted by chance the hypoglycemic effect of a sulfonylurea compound when studying its antibiotic effects. It was not until after World War II that the Germans synthesized carbutamide (B-Z 55), the first of many similar sulfonylurea drugs.

Four such compounds, the so-called first-generation drugs, are now commercially available in the United States. Three second-generation compounds have been studied extensively, but are not available for general clinical use. Their potency is much greater than their first-generation cousins. These second-generation drugs are glibenclamide, glipizide, and glibornuride. Many other antidiabetic compounds are being investigated, most of which are not sulfonylureas. The reader is referred to Table 6–1 for pertinent characteristics of the 4 available compounds. This information is of value when prescribing these drugs.

There have now been over 25 years of clinical experience with the oral antidiabetes drugs, during which time clinical results by and large have been satisfactory. The incidence of side effects has been low. Acceptance of these drugs by the patient has been enthusiastic, and most patients whose diabetes is controlled by tablets would not choose to change to insulin. Injecting insulin can be physically

Table 6–1. Oral Sulfonylureas and Their Actions.

| Name of Drug | Metabolism | Duration of Action hrs | Serum Half-life hrs | Effectiveness hrs after ingestion | How Supplied mg | Dosage Range and Max. Dose g | Mean Effective Dose | Doses per Day |
|---|---|---|---|---|---|---|---|---|
| Tolbutamide (Orinase) | oxidized in liver; metabolite excreted in urine | 6–12 | 4–5 | 3–5 | 500 | 0.5–3.0 | 1 g | 2–3 |
| Chlorpropamide (Diabinese) | minimal breakdown; primarily excreted in urine | 60 | 35 | 2–4 | 100<br>250 | 0.1–0.5 | 250 mg | 1 |
| Acetohexamide (Dymelor) | metabolized in liver; 75% excreted in urine and 25% in stools | 12–24 | 4–6 | 1½–5 | 250<br>500 | 0.25–1.5 | 500 mg | 1–2 |
| Tolazamide (Tolinase) | metabolized in liver and excreted in urine | 10–15 | 6–8 | 4–6 | 100<br>250<br>500 | 0.1–1.0 | 500 mg | 1–2 |

difficult for older patients and may be a constant source of worry. Control with the tablets seems easier, hypoglycemia is uncommon, and the patient is happy. Physicians with the greatest experience and knowledge in treating diabetes have mostly continued to use the oral antidiabetes agents in properly selected patients despite the UGDP controversy.

## MODE OF ACTION

All the antidiabetes drugs are readily absorbed from the gastrointestinal tract; then about 5% of the drug remains free in the blood, while 95% binds to serum albumin. The initial action of sulfonylurea drugs is to stimulate the beta cells to secrete insulin. For this process to take place, there must be functioning beta cells.

Long-term administration does not result in continuing beta cell stimulation, but there is evidence that endogenous insulin becomes more effective. Exactly how this occurs is unclear. It has been postulated that the following changes may take place: (1) there may be a positive effect on insulin receptors, with an increase in number or affinity, similar to what probably happens in the obese diabetic following weight loss; this benefit may take place in muscle, adipose, and hepatic cells, and perhaps even in the basement membrane of the beta cell; and (2) changes may take place in cyclic adenosine monophosphate (AMP) metabolism and in prostaglandin metabolism; one effect would be suppression of hepatic glucose production.

## INDICATIONS FOR USE

1. Adult, stable diabetics with the onset of diabetes at more than 40 years of age, generally. Over 60% are obese at the time of onset of the disease.
2. Patients who cannot adequately control the diabetes on diet alone, after a fair trial of 6 to 8 weeks. Adequate control by diet alone means a fasting plasma sugar level close to normal and a 2-hour postprandial level not over 150 mg/dl.
3. The Type II patient taking small-to-moderate doses of insulin (usually fewer than 40 units) may respond to sulfonylureas.
4. When evaluating the new adult-onset patient, one must be aware that the person with a history of weight loss (when not on a caloric-deficient diet) who looks lean, with even some evidence of muscle-wasting, may be a Type I patient and needs exogenous insulin from the start; 10 to 15% of adult-onset patients are Type I.

## CONTRAINDICATIONS

1. Acidosis or preacidotic states.
2. Severe infections accompanying the onset of diabetes.

3. Before, during, and immediately after major operations. During this time, it is best to change to insulin temporarily for adequate control.
4. Pregnancy. Several large series of pregnant diabetics treated successfully with tolbutamide have been reported, but the general consensus at present is that not enough is known about possible deleterious effects.
5. Patients with impaired hepatic or renal function, since the metabolism and excretion of the drugs may be impaired.
6. Patients with chronic debilitating disease of any type.
7. Type I diabetes, obviously.

## WHICH SULFONYLUREA IS BEST?

No one drug is "best," and they all have a similar mode of action, as described previously. Tolbutamide has the longest history, chlorpropamide the next. Tolazamide and acetohexamide are newer. Chlorpropamide and tolazamide are the most potent per mg. For reasons unknown, a patient who fails to respond to a certain sulfonylurea may respond to another, but probably not in more than 15 to 20% of cases. Starting doses can be as shown in Table 6–1, under the column headed "Mean Effective Dose." In some patients, however, the dose must be increased or decreased, depending on response. It is best to wait at least 1 week before increasing the dosage, and maximum response probably occurs within 2 weeks of beginning therapy in most patients. One must not exceed the maximum dosage shown in Table 6–1 because there is no added benefit. One must not use an initial loading dose, nor should one ever give 2 sulfonylurea drugs simultaneously. Formerly, a combination of a sulfonylurea and phenformin was frequently effective, but this is no longer possible because phenformin was taken off the market by the United States Department of Health, Education, and Welfare, in 1977. Many diabetologists objected strongly to this decision.

If the physician is not thoroughly familiar with the use of the sulfonylureas, he should study the detailed information published by the manufacturers and/or refer to the information published in the *Physicians' Desk Reference*. It is best to become thoroughly familiar with 1 or 2 available compounds and then to continue to use only these.

Approximately 80% of patients properly selected for treatment with these agents respond favorably to one or another. Over a period of 2 to 6 years, about 65% continue to control their disorder satisfactorily. Of the total failures, about 15 to 20% are primary failures, and a similar number are secondary failures. DeLawter and Moss reported a study of 200 patients who started taking tolbutamide in 1956. Twelve years later, in 1968, only 9 patients (4.5%) were still controlled with tolbutamide. The researchers reported 44 primary failures and 92 secondary failures. Fifty-five patients were lost to the study for various reasons. This study generally substantiates the predicted secondary failure rate of about 10% per year. This rate might indicate that by the end of 10 years of therapy, all patients would be secondary failures.

## CHANGING FROM INSULIN TO SULFONYLUREAS

In the carefully selected Type II adult patient who is taking fewer than 40 units of insulin to control hyperglycemia only, and who is thus not ketosis-prone, one can expect that many can control their diabetes by oral agents. Frequently, the patient expresses a desire to "get off the needle" and questions the physician about that possibility. In other cases, it is clear that injecting insulin is difficult, worrisome, and objectionable to the patient, and that a change to oral agents would be welcome.

The following procedure uses a stepwise decrease in insulin dosage. If followed carefully, it is a safe procedure. There is no need to hospitalize a patient for this procedure.

1. Assuming that the patient is taking 40 units or less of insulin, one should decrease this dosage by 50% on the morning the tablets are initiated.
2. One should instruct the patient to test his urine for glucose q.i.d.
3. If the patient's urine remains negative for sugar for 48 hours, he should decrease the insulin dose by another 50% and continue to take the prescribed dose of tablets.
4. Again, if the urine is sugar-free for the next 48 hours, insulin can be discontinued when a plasma glucose reading is in satisfactory range. (Some older diabetics have a high renal threshold.)
5. If in 1 to 2 days the urine tests again become positive, one should resume the last insulin dose for several more days and repeat step 4. It may be necessary to increase the dosage of the oral agent.
6. One must continue to check blood sugar levels about every 4 to 5 days for a few weeks until diabetic control is well established. If the patient cannot control his diabetes with a maximal dose of the chosen oral agent, he must return to the insulin regimen.
7. If the patient objects strenuously to insulin administration, and if the physician feels that he might respond favorably to another sulfonylurea compound, the patient should control his diabetes carefully for several weeks with insulin, and then repeat the procedure with another oral agent. It is claimed by the manufacturer that tolazamide is frequently effective in patients who have failed to maintain control with tolbutamide or chlorpropamide. If one desires to change to tolazamide, the following are dose equivalents:
   tolbutamide: 1g = tolazamide 100 mg
   chlorpropamide: 250 mg = tolazamide 250 mg
   acetohexamide: 250 mg = tolazamide 100 mg

### New Patient with Marked Hyperglycemia

It may be prudent to start the new Type II patient who has an initial blood glucose level of over 350 mg/dl with a small dose of NPH or Lente insulin until the blood glucose level is reduced to 200 mg/dl or less. Such an approach may better prepare the patient for the action of a sulfonylurea drug by permitting regranulation of the beta cells. The patient may then start the oral agent of choice while reducing the insulin dose by small increments until the diabetes is controlled by the tablets.

## ADVERSE SIDE EFFECTS

Fortunately, side effects are rare, with about a 3 to 5% incidence:

1. Skin rash, usually sensitivity-type, but occasionally becoming serious.
2. Gastrointestinal, consisting of nausea, vomiting, diarrhea, and flatulence.
3. Hematopoietic. Rare cases of leukopenia, thrombocytopenia, agranulocytosis, and anemia have been reported.
4. Hepatic toxicity, manifested by alterations in liver function tests. Rare cases of cholestatic jaundice have been reported, mainly associated with chlorpropamide. It may be dose-related, so one must never exceed 500 mg.
5. Alcohol sensitivity occurs in a few patients, manifested by a disulfiram-like reaction.
6. Chlorpropamide-induced water retention and hyponatremia with natriuresis has been described in the occasional diabetic patient. It develops as a result of an antidiuretic hormone (ADH)-like action of chlorpropamide. This apparently occurs most often in patients who have impaired water excretion due to renal or cardiovascular disease. In such persons, the drug must be discontinued. The physician should be alert to this possibility when faced with unusual water retention in a patient taking chlorpropamide.

Most side effects are relieved when the drug is discontinued, although some clinicians have reported continuing the drug and noting disappearance of the milder side effects. Discontinuing the drugs seems more logical.

## HYPOGLYCEMIA

Severe hypoglycemia to the extent of convulsions and unconsciousness is rare, although it has been reported. Most hypoglycemic episodes are a result of:

1. Too large a dose.
2. Patients who repeat the daily dose when there is uncertainty as to whether the morning dose was taken.
3. Patients who continue to take oral drugs even though food intake is reduced or sometimes discontinued.
4. Patients who develop liver or kidney impairment.
5. Drug interactions (see next section).

Hypoglycemia in the older diabetic patient poses a special threat of cerebrovascular accidents, and thus should be avoided. One occasionally sees a typical "stroke pattern" during a hypoglycemic episode, which may last several hours, with spontaneous recovery of full function after a period of normoglycemia. This rare type of reaction is most often seen in the older patient taking exogenous insulin.

The physician must carefully instruct the patient as follows:

1. Never to skip entire meals or omit prescribed snacks unless he is able to reduce or to omit his dose of medicine on the advice of his physician.
2. To increase his food intake if unusual exercise is undertaken.
3. To have a positive system of recording the daily medication taken, so that there is no chance of repeating a dose.
4. Always to contact his physician if he becomes ill from any cause.

## DRUG INTERACTIONS

Certain medications can sometimes contribute to hypoglycemia by their ability to bind protein and thus to displace the sulfonylurea to become free in the blood. The list of drugs includes anticoagulants, phenytoin (Dilantin), monoamine oxidase (MAO) inhibitors, sulfonamides, phenylbutazone (Butazolidin), and sometimes high doses of salicylates.

## CONTROL DURING ILLNESS OR SURGICAL PROCEDURES

It is frequently necessary to discontinue the oral agent and to prescribe small doses of insulin when a patient enters the hospital because of illness or for a surgical procedure. For short-term therapy (24 to 48 hours), the use of multiple doses of regular insulin is indicated. For longer periods, one should start with small morning doses of NPH or Lente. Under these circumstances, it is best to use purified pork insulin, since there is less chance of sensitizing the patient than if one uses mixed beef-pork insulin. In other words, any time a patient uses insulin on an intermittent basis, pork insulin is preferred. For details of insulin sensitivity reactions, see Chapter 13.

One must not overtreat the patient with insulin; many older patients are controlled well with small doses—5 to 8 U b.i.d. or as indicated. The physician should remember that these patients have endogenous insulin secretion to help them. Blood sugar levels should be checked daily if in doubt, since renal thresholds are often high in some older Type II diabetics.

For relatively minor surgical procedures, such as a cataract extraction or a prostate operation (T.U.R.), for which food is discontinued for a short period only, insulin by injection is not always needed. When oral agents are resumed on the first postoperative day, one should make certain that the patient has an appetite and is eating the necessary calories. Otherwise, he may become hypoglycemic.

## CONTINUING CARE

When good diabetic control has been established, one expects the blood sugar levels to be close to nondiabetic levels. The patient should be free of sugar in the urine both before and after meals. This goal is not always attainable, however. One should maintain excellent control with the smallest possible dose of sulfonylurea. The physician should try to decrease the dosage at 3- to 6-month intervals, always doing blood sugar tests approximately 1 week after reducing the dose. Many patients have maintained good control after discontinuing the oral agents, following 1 to 2 years of administration, particularly if they have brought their weight down to normal or at least have lost some weight. Others, who were not obese at the start, usually must be continued on an established dose to maintain excellent control. When one cannot establish excellent or even good diabetic control after a trial of oral agents and adherence to a diabetic diet, one should not hesitate to start the patient who is of normal weight or who is slightly overweight on insulin. The physician should not attempt to control any patient's diabetes with *both* insulin and an oral agent. If oral drugs alone are not effective, then insulin alone will certainly attain control, and the addition of oral agents is an unnecessary expense without contributing to diabetic control. The use of insulin in the obese Type II diabetic is discussed in Chapter 14.

The patient who has been well controlled with oral agents for a variable period and who then becomes a secondary failure also needs to be started on insulin promptly. This patient is reluctant to start injections, since he has been comfortable for so long while taking oral medication. The physician must be firm and must explain to him the consequences of continued high blood sugar levels. His endogenous insulin supply is becoming exhausted and needs help.

Older patients may cancel appointments if they feel well and have no complaints, partially to save money and also because they do not feel compelled to see the physician. Many would come for a "check-up" once every few years, if they had their way. Therefore, in order to avoid losing control of the patient, it is well to prescribe just enough oral medication to last until the next office visit. The interval at which the physician wishes to see his patients varies, but it is probably adequate to see the well-controlled Type II patient about every 4 months, and the patients with the mildest cases every 6 to 12 months.

## PHENFORMIN

Phenformin is no longer generally available, having been removed from the market as an "imminent hazard" on October 23, 1977 by the Department of Health, Education, and Welfare. The Food and Drug Administration (FDA) said that this action was taken because of the "unacceptably high risk of lactic acidosis associated with the use of this drug." This decision left about 350,000 patients in the United States without support. Phenformin and comparable drugs are widely used to control diabetes in Europe. Many clinicians felt that the drug was valuable, particularly when combined with a sulfonylurea, to establish excellent control, especially in obese Type II patients. As with any other drug, indications and contraindications had to be understood before prescribing.

Any physician whose patients' diabetes was well controlled with phenformin and who wishes to continue such medication can request the drug from the Food and Drug Administration, Rockville, Maryland 20857. He will then be furnished with forms to complete. When and if approval is given, the medication will be furnished by Geigy Pharmaceutical Company directly to the prescribing physician. As of this writing, this procedure is still in effect, but I do not vouch for continuation of any FDA policy.

In view of the many years of controversy surrounding the UGDP study, most physicians ask patients taking the oral antidiabetes agents to sign an informed consent form. This procedure is recommended.

## THINGS TO COME

The so-called second-generation agents that have been studied for many years (and may or may not ever be on the market) are far more potent than the original agents. However, they are all sulfonylurea drugs, and their action is the same as the agents in current use.

Another group of compounds of variable chemical composition is being studied in research centers here, in Europe, and in England. It is too early to know exactly the mechanism of their hypoglycemic effect or to be sure they are without adverse side effects.

# 7

# Urine Testing

## IMPORTANCE OF URINE TESTING

Home urine testing for the presence of glucose was found to be neglected in approximately 35% of diabetic students questioned while attending diabetes education classes. Another 15 to 20% of those students asked stated that they tested their urine rarely, mainly when they were not feeling well. Of the remaining 50% questioned, some were conscientious, whereas others tested their urine "off and on." Part of this indifference is the physician's fault, since it is apparent that many physicians do not realize the importance of urine testing for glucose. Others may feel that because the amount of glucose found at any given time does not correlate well with the blood sugar levels, one need not bother with urine testing. I hope that the material in this chapter convinces physicians that urine testing is worthwhile. Indeed, many diabetologists feel that, if they were given a choice of managing the patients' blood sugar levels on the basis of properly done and honestly recorded q.i.d. urine tests, or plasma glucose determinations done every 3 months or so, the urine glucose records would provide better guidance. I prefer both, as will be discussed later.

Detailed instructions for patients on urine testing procedures may be found, for example, in my Instruction Book for Diabetic Patients and in the Joslin Diabetes Manual (see Appendix).

Which method of urine testing should physicians recommend to their patients? Three satisfactory tests are available, each with some shortcomings: Clinitest, Diastix, and Tes-Tape. Table 7–1 compares the 3 methods. There is little doubt that Clinitest is the most accurate for glucose content, and it always indicates glucose when it is present. However, the time and preparation required to do the test

Table 7–1. Comparison of Methods of Urine Testing.

| | Comparative accuracy | Cost (1980) | False-positive reactions | False-negative reactions | Convenience for travel | Reaction with sugars other than glucose | Do ketones in urine change reading? |
|---|---|---|---|---|---|---|---|
| Clinitest (copper-reduction) 5-drop and 2-drop | The most accurate of all for actual glucose content; color changes easy to read, except when glucose exceeds 2%[1] | 3.7¢ each | YES [2] | NO; never misses glucose when present | poor; must have bottle, test tube, dropper, urine receptacle | YES; will give positive reaction with galactose, lactose, fructose, maltose, pentose | NO effect |
| Tes-Tape (glucose oxidase) | The least accurate, and underreads at 2%; best to read 1% as 2%; color changes difficult to read | 3.7¢ each | NO | YES; with some drugs, which cause a "partial" false-negative reaction[3] | most convenient | NO | YES, can inhibit color tones with large amounts[4] |
| Diastix (glucose oxidase) | good; accuracy between that of Clinitest and Tes-Tape; color changes easy to read up to 1%; change to 2% may be difficult to read | 5¢ each | NO | YES; complete false-negative reactions caused by a few drugs[3] | convenient; would be better if bottle were flat instead of round | NO | YES, as above[4] |

[1] If the urine contains over 2% glucose, the color phase will "pass through" the orange and become brick red or muddy brown. Then, the 2-drop method should be used.

[2] High-dose antibiotics, to include penicillin, cephalosporins, streptomycin, and nalidixic acid (NegGram); barbiturates; chloral hydrate; L-dopa; probenecid (Benemid); salicylates, in large doses (35 grains or more of aspirin daily), and para-aminosalicylic acid (PAS). False-positive reactions also occur if peroxide detergents remain in the vessel used to catch the urine.

[3] A "partial" false-negative reaction occurs with Tes-Tape when the ascending "wet" rim of green color leaves a yellow or negative color below. One should read the strip as "positive" without trying to ascertain the percentage. With Diastix, there will be a complete false-negative reaction. Drugs causing this phenomenon would include high-dosage salicylates (aminosalicylic acid (ASA) over 35 grains daily) and possibly large doses (over 1 g) of ascorbic acid (vitamin C). Other substances that may cause false-negative reactions include serotonin, 5-hydroxy-tryptophan, 5-hydroxy-indole acetic acid, and L-dopa.

[4] Ketone must be present in relatively large amounts (50 to 100 mg/dl), and will cause 1 color change less, or an underreading. When ketones are present in the urine, one should advise patients to check their urine with Clinitest tablets.

are a distinct disadvantage in this age of always "rushing," which means that many diabetics will skip doing regular tests. All insulin-dependent diabetics who frequently show large amounts of glucosuria should be instructed to do the "2-drop Clinitest," since this has the added advantage of registering up to 5% glucosuria, whereas the usual 5-drop method will register accurately only up to 2%. The procedure for both tests is the same, except 2 instead of 5 drops of urine are added, and a different color chart is used for interpretation. This same 2-drop testing is done when quantitative measurements are requested, which will be discussed later in this chapter.

Diastix is the test of choice for the average, well-controlled diabetic who rarely has a urine sugar level of more than 2%. This test is convenient and more accurate than Tes-Tape. It is also cheaper than Tes-Tape, if one instructs patients to slit the plastic stick lengthwise with sharp scissors, thus obtaining 2 for the price of 1.

Tes-Tape is the third choice because of its inaccuracy at high glucose content, as well as its false-negative reactions with certain medications.

## TIME SCHEDULE FOR URINE TESTING

How often urine tests should be done depends on the severity of the patient's diabetes and his control of it.

**Type I.** Insulin-dependent diabetics under good control should always test b.i.d., before breakfast and before supper, preferably. During times of insulin adjustment, stress from any cause, or fluctuations in control, tests should be done q.i.d., before each meal and bedtime.

**Type II.** Persons whose diabetic control is borderline should test b.i.d., and those whose control is good to excellent can test once daily, if they vary the time of testing each day, e.g., prior to breakfast one day, after supper the next day. Good to excellent control infers that they will not show glucose in the urine either before or after meals.

Persons controlled by minor dietary restrictions, who rarely show glucosuria, can check weekly as a matter of personal assurance. Urinary glucose frequently appears long before any other evidence of rising blood sugar levels.

## FIRST-VOIDED OR DOUBLE-VOIDED SPECIMENS

There is not complete agreement among physicians as to whether the first-voided urine specimen or a second specimen secured 15 to 30 minutes after drinking a glass of water is preferable for urine testing. If the object of urine testing is to correlate the glucosuria with the blood glucose level in a given time bracket, then it seems obvious that urine that has been in the bladder from 11 P.M. until 7 A.M. probably does not accurately reflect the patient's blood sugar level between 6 and 7 A.M. However, the first-voided specimen does tell you something about what happened overnight. On the other hand, studies were done several years ago that showed that the second-voided specimen is almost always dilute, and dilute specimens registered higher on all 3 testing methods in some, but not all, of the urine specimens tested. Studies by Diana Guthrie indicate that in 61% of urine specimen pairs, the same amount of glucose was found in both, whereas in 33%, more was found in the first specimen, and only in 6% was more found in the second.

Another real problem is in obtaining a second-voided urine specimen from children and even from some teenagers. They simply cannot produce a second specimen before it is time to eat, so in those patients the first-voided specimen is the one to test.

**Advice to the Physician.** The patient should test his first-voided morning urine specimen, since it gives valuable information concerning overnight spill. If it usually shows a 1 to 2% sugar level, one should try to obtain second-voided morning specimens 2 to 3 times a week. These specimens are an indication of the fasting blood glucose level. For other tests, the first-voided specimen is satisfactory and gives information about the patient's overall control. According to Guthrie's studies, the specimen would only have been potentially misleading less than 6% of the time. In patients who have continuous, severe glucosuria, the physician should do frequent quantitative tests, discussed in the following section of this chapter.

In the case of young children who are not toilet-trained, parents must test any specimen they can "catch." Diaper urine can be tested with Diastix or Tes-Tape.

## QUANTITATIVE URINE GLUCOSE MEASUREMENT

This is one of the most important measurements available to the patient and the physician, particularly in the Type I juvenile diabetic who has marked fluctuations in urinary glucose output. This procedure is so often neglected and is so rarely discussed with patients that it is obvious many physicians do not realize its value and advantages. Quantitative tests can be done in any of 3 ways: (1) total 24-hour collection of urine; (2) 2 12-hour urine specimens, usually divided thus: 7 A.M. to 7 P.M. and 7 P.M. to 7 A.M.; and (3) 4 6-hour urine specimens, usually divided starting at 6 A.M.

The following instructions are given to the patient:

1. On the day of collection, empty the bladder upon arising and discard this specimen. Note the time.

2. Have containers available for collection of all the urine passed in the following 24 hours. Two 2-quart containers are adequate for either a 12- or 24-hour collection and 1-quart containers are adequate if 6-hour collections are requested. Keep containers in refrigerator or add 1 teaspoon of boric acid crystals to each container.
   a. If only a total 24-hour collection is requested, collect all the urine passed for the 24-hour period in a single 2-quart container.
   b. If 2 12-hour specimens are requested, put all urine passed in the first 12 hours in one container and the second 12-hour urine specimens in a second container. Make sure they are labeled properly as to time of collection.
   c. If 4 6-hour collections are requested, put each 6-hour collection in separate bottles. Timing of these collections is from 6 A.M. to noon; noon to 6 P.M.; 6 P.M. to midnight; midnight to 6 A.M. Again, accurate labeling is necessary.
3. When the total collection has been made, measure the amount in ounces, using an ordinary household measuring cup, and record this for each bottle.
4. Clinitest tablets are the preferred method for testing the urine since the 2-drop color chart (available from the druggist) will be used. If Clinitest tablets are not used for daily urine testing, small amounts can be purchased in foil-wrapped, 24-tablet packages from the druggist. Test the urine from each collection bottle separately and write down the percentage found—remember to use the 2-drop method and read out on the 2-drop color chart.
5. Now, multiply the number of ounces by 30 to give the total in milliliters and multiply this number by the percentage shown on the test to give the total grams of sugar. Report this number to the physician.

Example:

30 ounces of urine passed in 12 hours
Testing shows 2% sugar level
30 × 30 equals 900 ml urine
900 × 2% equals 18 g sugar total in 12 hours

Ordinarily, a request for total urine collection does not bring forth strong objection from young patients if the procedure is not done more than once a month. During the school year, it has to be done on Saturday or Sunday, and that limits activities away from home for that 24-hour period.

The advantages of quantitative urine glucose measurement are obvious, since it not only checks the accuracy of premeal urine tests, but also tells the physician the amount of the total urinary loss of glucose. Total glucose in grams should not exceed 5% of the dietary carbohydrate intake, so ordinarily the patient's glucose level is under 15 g if diabetic control is fairly good. It is best to split the urine collection into at least 12-hour divisions, and then for even more information concerning the time of most severe glucosuria, 6-hour samples can be collected separately.

One must make certain that the urine for quantitative testing is not unusually dilute by checking its specific gravity if it appears light in color. Dilute urines overread with Clinitest; in some cases, there can be a 100% overreading.

Many diabetologists feel that quantitative urine measurements are far superior to blood sugar tests in furnishing information regarding diabetic control, and they ask their patients to do such testing at least weekly if control is poor. Blood glucose determinations tell only what the level was at a given time; 2 hours later, it may be 100% changed. Because blood is drawn under stress, as a rule, and timing is not always accurate as regards fasting or postprandial specimens, home monitoring of blood glucose levels obviates many objections.

## RECORDING URINE TESTS AND KEEPING A DIABETIC DIARY

Since the advent of testing the urine for sugar, patients have been taught to record the results in plus marks, from 1 to 4. This method was acceptable in the days when the only test available used Benedict's solution; unless a physician is over 50 years of age, he probably does not even know about Benedict's test. As illustrated in Table 7–2, the continued use of plus marks is confusing because of the variation in the correlation of plus marks with the actual percentage of glucose in each of the 3 testing methods. It is obvious from studying Table 7-2 that all 3 testing methods agree only when the urine tests 4+. The 2+ reading can mean ¾% with Clinitest, ¼ % with Tes-Tape, and ½% with Diastix. Recording test results in percentages solves the problem. The 2-drop Clinitest records only percentage, and the color chart shows ½%, 1%, 2%, 3%, and 5%

Table 7–2. Comparative Results of Urine Testing Methods (% Versus Plus Marks).

| | Trace | 1+ | 2+ | 3+ | 4+ |
|---|---|---|---|---|---|
| Clinitest 5-Drop | ¼% | ½% | ¾% | 1% | 2% |
| Tes-Tape | — | 1/10% | ¼% | ½% | 2 |
| Diastix | 1/10% | ¼% | ½% | 1% | 2% |

glucose. Most clinics now teach patients to record urine test results in percentages, and I hope that physicians will follow suit.

When instructing patients regarding urine testing, it is also important for the physician to emphasize the need for honesty and accuracy in recording test results. Human nature is such that, when one omits a test for any reason, it seems easier to enter a zero on the chart than to leave it blank. In addition, each test result must be recorded right away; unless the patient has all negative readings, it is difficult to remember from day to day how much sugar was present. To this end, I suggest that patients keep a diabetic diary. Physicians can have small books printed to give to their patients, or the patients can make them out of an ordinary notebook. A sample diary sheet is shown in Figure 7–1.

Other notations in the diary besides urine test results are of value to the physician. Patients should record the occurrence of hypoglycemic episodes, with some estimation of severity. Minor illnesses, menstrual periods, emotional upsets, and unusual exercise should also be recorded, since it may help to explain fluctuations in the degree of glucosuria.

Urinary metabolites of many drugs can affect the accuracy of results with all 3 methods of urine testing. Table 7–1 summarizes the effects of the drugs most commonly used. The list may not be complete, since new drugs have not all been evaluated from this standpoint. Because the physician is usually aware of the medications his patients are taking, he can easily understand sudden changes in the results of urine tests.

At each office visit, the physician must take the time to review carefully the patient's diabetic diary, noting not only the results of urine testing but also other significant notations that have a bearing on the patient's overall control. It may give one a clue as to when to check a plasma glucose level. If, for instance, there is 2% urine sugar level at noon each day, the physician should ask for a plasma glucose reading at 11 A.M. If mild hypoglycemic episodes occur frequently during the night, the evening dose of insulin may have to be adjusted, or the patient's bedtime snack may have to be increased. Other clues become obvious as the physician studies the diary.

## Urine Testing and Recording—General Guidelines

1. The physician should be specific and definite about the home testing of urine, including the number of times one expects the patient to test, the methods of recording tests, and the reminder to bring the record book when the patient comes for an office visit.
2. One must always take the time needed to review the record with the patient, answering any questions that arise and verbalizing one's

DIABETES RECORD BOOK

TAKE THIS BOOK WHEN YOU

VISIT YOUR DOCTOR

Diabetes Education Center
Deaconess Hospital
West 800 Fifth Avenue
Spokane, Washington 99210

| Date | Medication | | URINE TESTS | | | | Notes* |
|---|---|---|---|---|---|---|---|
| | AM | PM | BRKFST | LUNCH | SUPPER | Bedtime | |
| 1/1 | N50 R25 | | 1/2 | 1 | 2 | 1 | |
| 1/2 | N50 R25 | | 1 | 2 | 1 | 1 | Doctor called Advised 2 doses |
| 1/3 | N30 R15 | N12 R6 | 1/4 | 0 | 0 | 0 | |
| 1/4 | N30 R15 | N12 R6 | 1/2 | 1/2 | 1 | 2 | Getting a cold Temp 100° |
| 1/5 | N30 R18 | N12 R10 | 1 / 0 | 3/4 / 0 | 1 / | 1/4 / | Called doctor |
| 1/6 | N30 R18 | N12 R8 | 1/4 | 0 | 0 | 0 | Improved |
| 1/7 | N30 R15 | N12 R6 | 0 | 1/4 | 0 | 0 | |
| | | | | | | | |
| | | | | | | | |

**Fig. 7–1.** Diabetes diary and sample page.

impression of the urine tests. Not only does this give the physician important information, but it impresses upon the patient that one really utilizes the urine record in management of the diabetes.

3. For the patient whose urine records and control vary greatly, one should arrange for a review of the record every week or so, either by telephone report or by the patient's mailing a copy of the record. This reinforces the patient's confidence.

## RENAL THRESHOLD

Sugar appears in the urine in amounts detectable by the usual testing methods when the blood sugar level exceeds 200 mg/dl on the average. However, test results of many diabetics vary considerably from this figure, particularly the older Type II patients whose renal threshold might be as high as 300 to 350 mg/dl. Some younger diabetics, as well as pregnant diabetics, may show lower thresholds, showing glucosuria at levels as low as 130 mg/dl. Such special situations must first of all be recognized by the physician by correlating the record of urinary glucose with blood sugar levels drawn at different times of the day. The patient's insulin dose must be carefully regulated, based mainly on periodic plasma glucose determinations. The most reliable program is home blood sugar testing, and indeed, in some instances this is being done with an astounding improvement in control of blood glucose levels.

Home glucose monitoring has revealed that a high percentage of postpubertal females have poor correlation between urine sugar content and blood sugar content, particularly when the urine shows only a ½ to ¼% sugar level. For this reason, many physicians are instructing such patients in home glucose monitoring.

For details on home glucose monitoring, see Chapter 26.

# 8

# Care of the Juvenile Diabetic (Type I)

This category mainly includes children and young persons up to 25 years of age, the age group that presents the greatest challenge to physician, parents, and patient. Fortunately, unless one is a pediatrician, the minority of diabetic patients are in this age group, since the prevalence is 1 in 770 children up to age 18. The incidence is 1 in 2,500 children under the age of 17 years.

The primary goals of a therapeutic program for juvenile diabetics are as follows:

1. To minimize hyperglycemia and glucosuria while avoiding serious hypoglycemia.
2. To avoid preacidosis and frank ketoacidosis at all times.
3. To maintain normal growth and development with an adequate control program.
4. To encourage full physical and social activity appropriate for patient's age and stage of development.
5. To counsel patient and parents regarding emotional problems related to diabetes.
6. Most important, to make certain that patient and parents are educated in depth about the pathophysiologic and psychologic aspects of diabetes mellitus. If the physician does not have the time or facilities for such education, he should send them to a reputable diabetes education center.

## NEW JUVENILE PATIENTS

The onset of juvenile diabetes is most often explosive, with rapid weight loss, polyuria, polydipsia, fatigue, pruritus, and blurring of vision. Random blood sugar levels are frequently over 300 mg/dl. The patient may even have symptoms of preacidosis or frank ketoacidosis.

New juvenile patients should always be hospitalized, even though they may have only hyperglycemia without acidosis. In the hospital, the physician can promptly start and continue adequate treatment. The hospitalized patient also has the added advantage of trained personnel. The other advantages of hospitalization of juvenile diabetics are to the parents, who are usually alarmed and anxious and are thus unable to cope with the situation immediately.

The physician should immediately order a blood sugar test, unless he has just done one in his office. An evaluation for preacidosis or frank acidosis, if clinically suspected, should include tests for urine ketones, plasma bicarbonate, and pH (optional). If ketoacidosis is present, one should proceed as directed in Chapter 12.

### Insulin Requirements in Hospital

The physician should order a first dose of insulin for the nonketotic patient to be given immediately. For the first 24 hours, regular insulin should be given at 6-hour intervals until the hyperglycemia is reduced and the patient can be evaluated.

How much insulin should be given? The amount required may vary, and an educated guess by an experienced diabetologist is usually satisfactory. However, since most physicians are not diabetologists, they need some guidance. Approximately 1.0 to 1.5 U/kg body weight are beginning daily requirements, but in the first few days the dosage may be greater, depending on the blood sugar readings.

**First Hospital Day.** On admission, the patient should receive one-fourth to half the suggested dose in units of regular insulin every 6 hours, based on urinary glucose and blood sugar levels. One should reduce or increase subsequent doses as indicated. The last dose should be around midnight. Food should be given approximately 30 minutes after each insulin injection, so that it can be timed with breakfast, lunch, supper, and midnight snack. (The midafternoon snack should be given without preceding insulin injection.) In the first 24 hours of hospitalization, it is helpful to ascertain the patient's blood glucose level 5 hours after each insulin injection.

**Second Hospital Day.** The physician should order a fasting blood sugar test. Assuming the sugar level has dropped, he should give the patient a morning dose of Lente or NPH insulin, the total number of units to be based on 70 to 80% of the first day's requirements. Additional injections of regular insulin should be given before each meal, based on urinary glucose levels. Additional regular insulin should be administered only when the patient's urine glucose level is 1% or more. The dose should be about 0.2 U/kg, depending on blood sugar test results.

**Third Hospital Day.** The physician should give a base dose of NPH or Lente insulin, calculated from the patient's requirements of the day before. A 2-hour postprandial breakfast blood sugar test should be ordered. One should continue to give extra regular insulin as indicated by urine sugar levels, but only at noon and suppertime, thus minimizing the chances of hypoglycemia.

**Fourth Hospital Day.** If the patient's midmorning blood sugar level from the day before was high, and it easily could be, then one should begin mixing regular with NPH or Lente insulin for the basic morning dose. A good initial dose is two-thirds NPH or Lente and one-third regular insulin. The physician should continue to administer extra regular insulin at noon and suppertime, if there is 1 to 2% glucosuria. He should also order blood sugar tests 2 hours after the patient's evening meal.

**Fifth Hospital Day.** The physician should continue to increase or decrease the insulin dose depending on the patient's total daily requirements and the urinary glucose output as well as blood sugar levels. Blood sugar tests should be ordered 2 hours after lunch.

## Other Orders Pertinent to Diabetic Management

**Urine tests.** Tests for glucose in the urine should be taken q.i.d., before each meal and bedtime, if the patient is old enough to cooperate. Some physicians prefer to collect all urine; this procedure may be easier in younger patients. Urine collection can be divided either into 2 12-hour periods or into 4 periods, ending at 6 A.M., noon, 6 P.M., and midnight. The patient's urine should be tested with the 2-drop Clinitest method. Ketone levels can be checked with Acetest or Ketostix.

**Control of Hypoglycemia.** The physician should instruct nurses to watch carefully for signs of hypoglycemia and to treat it promptly themselves. If desired, he can leave standing orders for a blood sugar test if hypoglycemia is suspected, but not at the expense of a long delay in administering sugar. I have never found that knowing whether a patient's blood sugar level was 35 or 24 mg/dl was valuable. The important move is to raise that blood sugar level. I always teach nurses this rule of thumb, "If in doubt, give sugar." One never harms a diabetic with 15 g sugar, but a physician could harm his reputation if convulsions occur as a result of neglected or delayed treatment of hypoglycemia, especially in the first few days of treatment.

**Diabetic Diary.** It is important to keep an accurate diabetic diary, and most hospitals have such printed sheets, listing urine tests, blood chemistry, insulin administration, and hypoglycemia episodes, for example. The physician should discuss record-keeping with the charge nurse if the routine is not satisfactory.

**Diet.** It is best to discuss the dietary requirements with the hospital dietitian who will do the teaching. It is customary to divide the diet into 6 feedings, which include a midmorning, midafternoon, and bedtime snack. Caloric requirements of the diabetic child are no different from those of the nondiabetic child; roughly they are 1000 basic kcal plus 125 kcal per year of age for boys and 100 for girls (see Chap. 3).

**Exercise.** One must not make an invalid out of the diabetic child—he should be up and around from the first hospital day. Exercise is important.

**Education.** The physician should start education at once for both child and parents. This includes:

1. Insulin mixing and injection techniques. Any child over 9 years should learn to inject his own insulin.
2. Urine testing for sugar and ketones as well as record-keeping.
3. Dietary instruction, intensive and thorough.
4. Recognition and treatment of hypoglycemia.
5. Instruction on ketoacidosis, recognition of preacidosis and steps to take.

## Release From Hospital

Ideally, a patient should be hospitalized for 3 to 6 weeks, but in most places without research funds, long hospitalization is an unbearable financial burden. As a compromise, I generally plan to discharge the patient as soon as I feel that child and parents feel confident about their ability to cope on their own, with assurance that the physician will be available at all times to help to solve any problems that may arise. This discharge usually comes after 6 to 8 days of hospitalization. Before discharge, the physician should sit down with the patient and his parents and explain that the insulin dose the child is taking will need to be changed every few days, for "fine-tuning." The parents should report urine tests to the physician by telephone at regular intervals for this purpose. One must remember that the child is going home with blood sugar levels higher than they will be after he resumes normal physical activity. *One should never do the "fine-tuning" in the hospital.*

The physician must also make it clear that the parents are to report any sudden changes in urine sugar levels, either up or down, as well as any hypoglycemic episodes or intercurrent illness. He must make certain that they understand the meaning of both hypoglycemia and ketoacidosis.

The physician should also make arrangements to send the patient's parents to an intensive and thorough diabetic school. For children under 9 years, diabetic school is not that impressive, so the parents should be encouraged to attend without the child. Similar education for the child should be undertaken at the age of 9 to 10 years.

Both child and parents should visit the physician's office within 4 to 7 days of discharge from the hospital.

### First Office Visit on Release from Hospital

At this time, the physician should discuss the "honeymoon period." He should point out that many children experience this, but certainly not all of them, and that this phenomenon is definitely not cured diabetes. This period occurs after several weeks or even months of diabetes, when the patient's beta cells again function adequately and insulin requirements drop, sometimes precipitously. Repeated hypoglycemic reactions with glucose-negative urine tests usually herald the approach of this wonderful period, and of course, insulin dosage must be reduced as indicated, usually 10% to 15% every 3 to 4 days. During this time, the physician has 2 choices, both satisfactory: (1) He may discontinue the patient's insulin entirely if possible and advise that b.i.d. urine tests should be continued. Additionally, he should test blood sugar levels once a month as indicated and resume insulin when hyperglycemia occurs. (2) By continuing small daily insulin injections, some physicians feel that one avoids the possibility of sensitizing the patient to insulin, as has been reported to take place occasionally when insulin is given intermittently. Intermittent injection can result in the formation of large amounts of insulin antibodies that would then necessitate administration of large doses of insulin. In addition, daily small insulin doses may reduce the stress on the beta cells and prolong the "honeymoon period." Some clinics have reported maintaining young diabetics for several years with tiny doses of insulin. I have never experienced such good fortune in my practice, since most "honeymoons" end in 1 to 4 months.

The physician should also explain that soon, maybe after the honeymoon period (if it occurs), he may advise that the child will attain more physiologic control with 2 doses of insulin per day. This advance warning allows the patient and his parents to discuss the suggestion. Strong objections are rare if the physician explains the advantages of this regimen. Some clinicians start their juvenile diabetic patients with 2 doses a day in the hospital, but I believe that trauma can be minimized by adding the second dose a few months later. The patient who maintains partial endogenous insulin production may do well with a single small injection of mixed insulin per day. Some physicians feel that most of their patients do well with a single daily dose. The physician must make his own decision. The average daily stable insulin requirement in children is 0.75 U/kg/day.

### Follow-Up Office Visits

The physician had best see his new juvenile diabetic patient at 2- to 4-week intervals for the first 6 months and more often if problems arise.

At each visit, he must carefully review the patient's diabetic diary. If it is accurate and honest, it provides valuable information. A 12- or 24-hour quantitative measurement of urine glucose should be done weekly.

The physician should check blood sugar levels at each office visit, and after 2 to 3 months of excellent diabetic control, he should order a glycohemoglobin test (HbA-1c) (see Chap. 28).

At this time, the physician should briefly test one phase of the patient's knowledge by asking questions on diet, reactions, and urine testing technique.

One must always remember that it takes more time and patience to treat diabetics, and it is so important to gain the patient's full confidence. If a physician does not have the time for these patients, he should refer them to someone who does.

## INSULIN REQUIREMENTS THROUGH PUBERTY

Insulin requirements continue to increase during the period of physical growth and development. Indeed, it has been shown that chronic hyperglycemia serves as a growth retardant, whereas well-controlled diabetic children enjoy normal growth patterns.

In girls, insulin requirements increase rapidly after 10 or 11 years in association with their prepubertal growth spurt; then they decrease with cessation of rapid growth and the menarche. Boys do not have rapid increases in insulin requirements until around age 12. Similarly, requirements decrease after full growth is attained.

## BRITTLE DIABETICS

Much has been written about the so-called brittle diabetic, but no one has really defined the term. The young diabetic who undergoes rapid swings in blood sugar levels from hyperglycemia to hypoglycemia and whose diabetes seems almost impossible to control fits the definition of "brittle." It has been suggested that these persons have no remaining endogenous insulin secretion, but if this were the case, there would be far more brittle cases than appear to be presently under treatment. My observations over a period of 30 years lead me to believe that many such situations occur in young persons who are indifferent about their diabetic control. Some are suffering the Somogyi effect, but many are hyperactive individuals who partake in too many activities; some older adults are over their heads in business activities. Excessive stresses stimulate secretion of stress hormones, which make adequate control difficult. I do not wish to suggest that there could not be other unknown hormonal factors that make control difficult, but until our knowledge of such factors is more complete, the physician should try to regulate all aspects of the life of a hyperreactive patient.

## SOMOGYI PHENOMENON

Excessive insulin is responsible for the wide fluctuations in blood sugar levels seen in some young diabetics. Hypoglycemic episodes provoke surges in secretion of the insulin-antagonists and cause hyperglycemia. Glucosuria and ketonuria are then commonly seen. The patient may gain weight too rapidly. Hypoglycemic episodes may be brief, nocturnal, and almost asymptomatic, and thus are not easily recognized. The physician usually sees the patient in the hyperglycemic stage and promptly advises an increase in the insulin dosage. This increase worsens the problem. Most such patients take large daily doses of insulin, exceeding 1.5 U/kg/day. The treatment is to lower the insulin dose in small steps until optimum control is obtained.

## PSYCHOSOCIAL PROBLEMS OF JUVENILE DIABETICS

Although there is no intent to discuss in depth the various aspects of this subject, some of them that receive most attention are as follows:

The diabetic child may exhibit overt hostility. He may demand unusual attention by manipulating his diabetes or his parents. This child may actually deny the presence of diabetes to himself and friends, and he is frequently insecure and depressed.

Tension between parents frequently exerts a deleterious effect on the diabetic child. He may become indifferent about diabetic control, even to the point of ketoacidosis, a result of his deliberate discontinuance of his insulin injections.

Adolescents, often rebellious, turn not only against parental guidance, but also against the state of their health. Diabetic control can deteriorate rapidly in such a situation.

Parents may be affected more than the diabetic child by guilt, if there is a positive family history of diabetes. They may also act almost with hostility in pressuring the child into rigid control of the diabetes. They may have a constant fear of diabetic complications. Parents frequently become overprotective, especially if the child's diabetes starts between 3 and 6 years of age.

The family physician should discuss these issues with the parents if it is obvious that things are not going well at home.

In 1975 the Upjohn Company printed a helpful brochure entitled "The child with diabetes mellitus," written by 2 prominent experts in juvenile diabetes, Drs. Robert Jackson and Richard Guthrie. This pamphlet is available gratis from Upjohn representatives.

# 9

# Management of the Older Diabetic Patient

## NEW ADULT DIABETICS

In Chapter 8, I discuss hospital management of the Type I diabetic whose condition and/or age dictates hospital management. All other new diabetics who are not threatened with ketoacidosis and who do not have an accompanying illness can be managed better as office patients than as in-patients. In the average primary care physician's practice, about 10% of patients have diabetes. A few are children, but most are adults over 40 years of age. It is much easier to establish good diabetic control on an out-patient basis because patients are generally able to carry on their normal activities. In addition, there are definite psychologic advantages. A new meal plan is still "home cooking," and acceptance of it is generally better. Fewer stress hormones are secreted, since most patients are more comfortable at home than in the hospital.

### Nonobese Adults

With these patients, the physician must first determine whether they are Type I diabetics and are thus insulin-dependent and prone to ketosis or whether they are Type II diabetics who may need insulin only to control hyperglycemia. As a general rule, when the onset of diabetes occurs after middle age (circa age 50), only about 10 to 15% of such persons will have Type I diabetes—the others will have Type II. Patients' medical histories and laboratory findings are generally indicative.

### Diagnosis of Type I Adult-Onset Diabetics

A history of weight loss with frequent evidence of muscle wasting should arouse the physician's suspicions. These patients are usually symptomatic, as are children with Type I diabetes, but the symptoms generally are not as pronounced and appear more slowly. This does not mean, however, that these patients cannot experience an explosive onset of the disorder. The fasting plasma glucose levels of these patients are elevated, as are postprandial plasma glucose levels. One never needs a glucose-tolerance test to make the diagnosis. (For further diagnostic information, see Chapter 2.)

## MANAGEMENT OF TYPE I ADULT-ONSET DIABETICS

The physician should prescribe insulin for these patients immediately, with an average starting dose of around 20 to 30 units of NPH or Lente insulin, given once each morning. The occasional patient whose glucose levels exceed 300 mg/dl may need extra regular insulin before meals for the first few days. However, the physician must be cautious about treatment until he has had a chance to evaluate the patient's response to insulin. Ordinarily, a premeal injection of 5 to 8 units of regular insulin when the urine tests show a 1 to 2% glucose level is sufficient. The physician should be careful about the amount of insulin ordered prior to lunch if he has already instructed his patient to take an extra injection before breakfast. Midafternoon hypoglycemia can occur easily under those circumstances. In some instances, it is better to give the extra regular insulin only before breakfast and supper until a suitable total dose has been established.

Patients should be instructed to test urines for sugar q.i.d. (before each meal and bedtime) and to keep a diabetic diary.

The physician should prescribe a diet and should make sure that these patients have several consultations with a dietitian. All diabetics taking insulin should have bedtime snacks. (See Chapter 3 for information on diet.) The patient's original blood glucose level is not a true indication of the severity of the diabetes nor of the amount of insulin that will eventually be needed for good diabetic control. It is prudent to repeat a blood glucose test (preferably postprandial morning and evening) daily or every other day during the first few weeks of treatment for guidance.

The physician should see these patients daily in the office for the first 4 to 5 days until he is assured that they are out of danger and that they understand the fundamentals. (They, too, are prone to ketosis.)

Starting with the first day, the physician's nurse should begin instruction in insulin-injection technique. During the few days required to learn the technique, it is best to have patients eat breakfast at home at the usual time and then come in for the instruction and injection of insulin. This procedure is more convenient for both nurse and patients. However, it must be made clear that ordinarily they will take their insulin injection 30 minutes before mealtime.

The physician must make certain that his nurse is knowledgeable about diabetes and insulin injection technique, since wrong advice is worse than none. He may send his nurse to a diabetes education center for proper education or furnish him with suitable books on the subject. If the physician does not have a nurse, he must instruct the patient himself.

It is important to send patients to a diabetes education center as soon as possible and meanwhile to make certain that they are instructed in the recognition and avoidance of ketoacidosis and hypoglycemia.

The physician should make sure that these patients do not have their eyeglasses changed until their diabetes is under control.

## Follow-up

For the first 6 to 8 weeks, the physician should see these Type I patients weekly for a plasma glucose test, evaluation of urine tests, weight check, and general health examination. At the first weekly visit, the physician should obtain a 2-hour postprandial morning blood sugar level reading and make the necessary insulin adjustment based on those findings. Ordinarily, it is best to raise the Lente or NPH insulin only if urinary sugar levels are equal around the clock. However, if the patient's urine before breakfast contains no sugar, but there is 2% glucosuria at noon and perhaps at suppertime, then he needs more insulin activity in the first 6 to 10 hours after breakfast. He should then be instructed to mix regular insulin with the NPH or Lente. A good starting proportion is one-quarter regular to three-quarter NPH or Lente. Further adjustments depend on midmorning and midafternoon plasma glucose findings.

The physician should make no dietary changes in the first 2 to 3 weeks unless there is a continued weight loss that is not the result of glucosuria. On a second weekly visit, one should follow the same procedure, with whatever change is indicated in insulin dosage.

If, after 6 to 8 weeks, 24-hour control of plasma glucose and urinary sugar levels is not completely satisfactory, then one should consider switching to 2 injections per day of mixed insulins, with approximately five-eighths to two-thirds before breakfast and three-eighths to one-third before supper. Ordinarily, the morning dose is from one-half to two-thirds NPH or Lente and the rest is regular insulin, while the evening dose should be two-thirds to three-quarters NPH or Lente, with the remaining regular insulin.

## OFFICE MANAGEMENT OF TYPE II DIABETICS

It takes time to care for diabetics adequately, and a physician must be willing to give that time. These patients, who are bewildered in the first 6 months of their "new disease," need reassurance and help at every office visit. I give them 30 minutes for a routine office visit, and sometimes that is not enough. If one is a 60-patient-a-day physician, there is no way that one can do a good job with diabetic patients unless evenings or certain days are set aside for them, to give them each 30 minutes. First one must listen to them, then one has to review their urine records, then one will need to check any physical complaint, and finally, one has to alter the program as needed. Last but not least, the physician should have a social chat with them—how are the kids, the crop, the business, or the duck hunting or whatever—they are the physician's cares and they expect to be his friends. The art of practicing medicine is the fun of practicing medicine, and patients come to love one as a friend and physician.

As mentioned earlier, the majority of diabetic patients are in the Type II category, and of those, about 65% are obese Type II diabetics. Most are over 40 years old, but there are a few young adults with Type II diabetes. It should be emphasized that in older-onset, Type II diabetics, the absolute level of the blood glucose at the time of diagnosis is not crucial and does not say much about treatment needed to restore blood sugar levels to normal. The obese Type II diabetic with blood sugar level of 350 mg/dl at diagnosis may well control his disorder by a reducing diet alone within a few months' time. One should not panic and prescribe insulin or tablets until it is sure that the glucose level will not decrease if the patient follows a reducing meal plan conscientiously.

The first step is to prescribe a diabetic meal plan appropriate to the attainment and/or maintenance of the patient's ideal weight, strength, and working capacity. One hopes that a dietitian knowledgeable about low-cholesterol and low-saturated-fat diets will be available. Patients should be instructed in urine-testing techniques and a diabetic diary (see Chap. 7).

The physician should follow the progress of these patients on diet alone for 2 to 4 months unless hyperglycemia is severe and persistent (over 300 mg/dl). If diabetic control is excellent on diet alone, there is no need to change. If diabetic control is fair to poor, do these patients need oral hypoglycemic drugs or do they need insulin? This is one of the important decisions to make in the second part of the treatment program. One should remember that Type II diabetics are not prone to ketosis and that insulin is used in cases of hyperglycemia or neuropathy. In other words, the use of insulin in these persons is not critical, so there is time to think about it and to discuss it with the patient. Exceptional Type II patients can convert to Type I diabetes and become prone to acidosis. No one has an explanation for this phenomenon.

If obese Type II patients are following a weight-reducing plan and are truly losing weight, most likely there will be a dramatic drop in blood sugar levels early in the program. Frequently, blood sugar levels drop before any perceptible weight loss occurs, if the patient is adhering strictly to the diet. However, this group comprises only 10% of obese patients, so what should be done with the other 90% who do not lose weight? The next step is to consider prescribing an oral antidiabetes agent. A fair trial for oral agents is 3 months (see Chap. 6). If there is no response either to diet or to oral agents, what then? The arguments in favor of and against the use of insulin in obese Type II diabetics are thoroughly discussed in Chapter 14.

At every office visit, patients should bring a sample of a midstream-voided urine specimen, and a complete analysis should be done, including microscopic examination of the sediment. The physician should look for protein and evidence of pyuria, since asymptomatic pyuria is frequent, particularly in female diabetic patients.

The physician should give patients full and honest reports on laboratory tests. He should not say, "Your blood sugar was OK," but should give them the amount in milligrams. Patients should record this amount in their diabetic diaries for comparison.

All patients should go to a diabetes education center. If this is not possible, the physician should make sure that they have instruction books on diabetes in general and on diet. (See Appendix for list of books.)

## Follow-up

When the newly diagnosed diabetic patient is educated, reassured, and feels confident about the state of his diabetes, office visits every 3 months are usually sufficient for the first year. After that, the frequency depends on the physician and the patients.

One excellent diabetologist I know calls all his diabetic patients once a month to check on their progress. This procedure has tremendous psychologic value for the patients and allows the physician to alter the program, if needed, prior to the patient's next office visit. This successful physician is well respected by his diabetic patients.

## General Advice

Patients must be instructed to call the physician any time they feel that they are having problems. The physician must take these calls as soon as possible because calls from diabetics are frequently urgent. The patient may have impending hypoglycemia or acidosis. Therefore, one must never put off calling diabetic patients until noon or after hours.

The physician should instruct patients to report to him any time their urine tests for sugar undergo a sudden increase—from 0 or trace up to 1 to 2% consistently, not just occasionally. This change usually signals an increase in plasma glucose levels and means that an adjustment in the program is necessary.

He should instruct patients to report immediately any serious hypoglycemic episodes, so that proper adjustments can be made. Patients should also report any illness to the physician, especially if preacidosis threatens.

If patients are generally progressing well, with little glucosuria and no complaints, it is not necessary to have them come in weekly or every 2 weeks for plasma glucose determinations. This expensive and unnecessary procedure reflects an insecurity on the part of the physician.

## Special Procedures

The physician should do these special checks about twice yearly in asymptomatic patients.

1. He should examine the fundi of the patients' eyes carefully for evidence of beginning retinopathy. If he does not feel competent to do such an examination, than an ophthalmologist should check these patients at least yearly.
2. He should check the arterial pulses, particularly in the lower extremities in older patients, and record his findings.
3. He should check vibratory sensations in the feet and record the findings. Knee jerk and ankle reflexes should also be checked and recorded.
4. He should carefully examine the feet of all older patients and, if need be, refer them to a competent podiatrist or orthopedist for necessary treatment.

### Consultations

The smartest of all physicians know what they don't know. Good physicians in all fields use consultants frequently. One should not hesitate to call for help with any problems one may have with diabetic patients, whether in relation to metabolic control or to complications. I always think of the words of the Hebrew physician of the thirteenth century, Joseph Zabara, who said, "Before the trouble comes, advice obtain; after it has come, advice is vain." If obtaining excellent consultation means sending patients several hundred miles to a good medical center, one should do so.

## HOSPITALIZATION FOR MANAGEMENT

Is it ever necessary to hospitalize the older, newly diagnosed diabetic, either Type I or Type II? Only under the following circumstances is hospitalization necessary:

1. When Type I patients have marked elevation of blood sugar levels and are possibly preacidotic.
2. When Type I patients live alone and/or are unduly apprehensive about mastering their diet, insulin injection technique, and urine testing.
3. Similarly, the occasional Type II patient who lives alone and who is apprehensive does best with hospital care and teaching for a week or so.
4. Both Type I and II patients should be hospitalized if their diabetes is complicated by other illnesses that make early control of the diabetes more difficult or make management at home a problem for the patient.

If hospitalization is necessary, the physician should proceed with treatment as outlined in this chapter for office management. These patients should be ambulatory unless other conditions prevent it. In addition, the physician should check blood sugar levels each day, taken at different times, to obtain a profile of the 24-hour glucose level variations. One should make use of the services of the hospital dietitian from the first day and be sure that there are several instruction sessions with the patient before his going home. One should also make use of the services of a diabetes nurse-instructor. Hospitalization for 6 to 8 days is usually sufficient.

Physicians should get in the habit of calling the hospital at about 10 P.M. to inquire about the day's urine and blood sugar tests. This enables them to leave an insulin order for the next morning. This procedure can usually save the patient a day of hospitalization.

It is a good idea to have standing orders with hospital nurses to call the physician if anything unusual happens with his diabetic patients, and to call at any time of the day or night—metabolic accidents happen rapidly and orders for medication, fluids, or insulin may be needed immediately.

The physician must be sure that the patient's disorder is not controlled so well in the hospital that during the first day at home, with increased physical activity, he has hypoglycemic episodes. This phenomenon is particularly applicable to insulin-dependent older diabetics, but it can happen to the Type II diabetic taking oral hypoglycemic drugs. The patients should be sent home with blood sugar levels in the 175 to 250 mg/dl range; the fine-tuning of insulin or tablet dosage may be done when the physician has had a chance to estimate the effect of the patients' usual daily physical activity on blood sugar levels. In addition, patients may not be so strict with diet as they were forced to be in the hospital, so this possibility must also be taken into consideration. The physician should let patients know that it takes 6 to 8 weeks to coordinate their program of *diet-insulin or tablets-exercise* to provide ideal diabetic control.

### Sliding Scale or "Rainbow" System for Administering Regular Insulin

Insulin orders based on the percentage of glucose in any given urine specimen are generally to be discouraged. First of all, one is treating the elevated sugar level long after it became elevated, whereas physiologically one wants to prevent that elevation, by giving sufficient insulin before it takes place. Second, the great excursions of blood glucose that may occur within a short time give misleading urine information to guide insulin dosage. Finally, the dose of regular insulin given on this basis frequently proves to be excessive, and the patient has a hypoglycemic episode.

It is usually necessary to give a patient regular insulin (the amount based on urine tests) as an extra injection when he is starting his insulin regimen, or when he has hyperglycemia due to a minor illness. If this procedure is done with a newly diagnosed hospitalized patient, it should last for no longer than the first 24 hours, after which the physician should prescribe a base dose of NPH or Lente insulin for his new patient. In the hospital, it is prudent to ascertain blood glucose determinations at various times of the day—the times when one wants the most information about the sugar levels. These results are far more reliable than those for urinary sugar levels.

The patient at home with an illness necessitates a prescription of regular insulin based on urinary glucose levels. The physician should advise extra regular insulin only for 1 or 2% urinary sugar levels, not for less. The usual rule is to give 10% of the base dose in units of regular insulin for 2% and a little less for 1%. Occasionally, more is needed if the patient is threatened with a preacidotic state (see Chap. 12).

## ELDERLY DIABETICS

The patient who first has diabetes after age 70 or so poses thought-provoking problems that deserve discussion. The newest diagnostic criteria set forth in Chapter 2 do not take into consideration the allowance of a 10 mg/dl higher glucose level per decade after 50 years of age. Nonetheless, I think that this increase must be considered, lest diabetes be diagnosed when it is simply carbohydrate intolerance of the aged.

If in a newly diagnosed elderly Type II patient the elevations of glucose levels are minimal or almost questionable, one should tread lightly when it comes to treatment. These patients do not live long enough to suffer the consequences of diabetic vascular complications, in most instances. In addition, they frequently live alone, and adherence to a strict diabetic diet may be almost impossible. It is best to give them a list of foods to avoid along with another list of classes of food to include in their diet, to assure them of a nutritionally adequate intake. Even then, the diet may be supplemented with a daily multivitamin tablet. The foods to avoid are those with raw sugars such as jellies, jams, syrups, honey, candy bars, heavy frostings, and the like. I am not sure one is always justified in eliminating some of those goodies.

Since many elderly diabetics have a renal threshold much higher than normal, frequently 250 to 350 mg/dl, it is impossible to judge the level of blood sugar from urine tests. Consequently, one must check blood glucose levels more often if there is concern about marked hyperglycemia.

If the restriction of raw sugars alone from the diet does not succeed in keeping blood sugar levels below 200 mg/dl, then one should consider a calculated meal plan and administration of oral antidiabetes agents in the alert and active elderly patient. For details, see Chapters 3 and 6.

### Nursing Home Care

In many cases, it becomes necessary for an elderly diabetic patient to enter a nursing home, usually for reasons other than the diabetes. However, the patient's diabetes must still be treated, and the success of treatment seems to be in direct proportion to the professional reputation of the nursing home. One hopes that the nursing home staff understands the care of diabetes. At this point, the physician must decide whether his patient can be adequately cared for by diet alone, by diet and tablets, or by diet and insulin. The patient probably is maintained with insulin rather than tablets if diet alone does not give adequate diabetic control. With a chronic illness of any kind, unusual stresses occur that change the metabolic picture frequently. Renal or hepatic decompensation can result in a marked increase in blood concentrations of the sulfonylurea drugs with resulting hypoglycemia, which may be serious in elderly patients. Prolonged and severe hypoglycemia can precipitate a stroke.

When a diabetic patient enters a nursing home, it is prudent for the physician to discuss the diabetic care with the chief nurse and to emphasize that diabetic patients in general require closer supervision than do nondiabetics. The physician should discuss diet, urine testing and record-keeping, and administration of insulin or tablets. Good nursing homes can give adequate and satisfactory care.

# 10

# Exercise

The popularity of exercise has increased manyfold in the past few years, as witnessed by the thousands who have taken up jogging. Since unusual and unexpected situations may arise in the diabetic who embarks on an exercise program, the physician should be acquainted with these possibilities. A short review of energy sources and utilization is therefore in order.

## ENERGY SOURCES

Energy stores are mainly those of glucose, glycogen, and triglycerides. In terms of the calories produced, there is a relatively small store of glucose and glycogen. The blood glucose pool is probably around 20 g; the liver glycogen 80 to 120 g; muscle glycogen in the average 70-kg adult is between 300 and 400 g. Total calories from these sources average around 2000 kcal. Triglycerides, which are really another storage form of carbohydrate (labeled "oily candy" by Dr. Rachmel Levine), are in more plentiful supply; 15 kg or so in the average 70-kg person are theoretically capable of furnishing 135,000 kcal. Muscle glycogen cannot contribute to the blood glucose pool because it does not have the enzyme glucose-6-phosphatase (G-6-P) for conversion. Therefore, it contributes fuel to muscle fibers in which it is contained, and its help in maintaining blood glucose levels comes only through the Cori cycle.

Diabetics have less glycogen stored in both liver and muscle than have nondiabetics, and the degree of glycogen depletion seems closely linked to insulin deficiency. In the resting postabsorptive state, free fatty acids (from the triglyceride pool) furnish most of the fuel for muscle metabolism, whereas the major site of glucose consumption is the brain. Following meals, a small amount of glucose energy is derived from aerobic glucose oxidation.

### Fuel Sources and Requirements During Exercise in the Nondiabetic

During short-term exercise, the uptake of glucose by the exercising muscle increases from seven- to twentyfold, depending on the intensity of the exercise. Hepatic glycogen furnishes the required glucose, and hence the blood glucose level generally remains in balance, perhaps falling only slightly.

When exercise lasts more than 2 hours, free fatty acids furnish the energy required. Muscle uptake of these free fatty acids increases markedly, and at the same time, glucose utilization decreases by 20 to 40%. This change prevents rapid falls in blood glucose levels, since after a few hours of exercise, the source of new glucose is from hepatic gluconeogenesis.

## EFFECT OF EXERCISE ON DIABETICS

The exact role that insulin plays in the metabolic response to exercise depends on the amount of insulin available. Too much insulin curtails hepatic glucose output and decreases lipolysis, thus reducing the available fuel supply.

If insulin requirements are adequate or only slightly deficient, exercise produces a fall in blood glucose levels due to use as well as better control of hepatic glycogenolysis. Thus, the overall result of exercise is beneficial.

It has been recently shown that in the uncontrolled insulin-dependent diabetic, exercise produces *increases* in blood glucose levels, in lipolysis, and therefore in ketone bodies, with ensuing ketogenesis and the possibility of precipitating true diabetic ketoacidosis. It seems reasonable that the excess output of hepatic glucose is not used, and the increased fatty acids and ketones are not consumed accordingly, so ketosis is enhanced. In addition, in any exercising body, the output of stress hormones is increased slightly, but in the insulin-deficient diabetic, this output is increased 4 to 8 times.

### Exercise and Blood Lipids

Perhaps even more beneficial than the glucose-lowering effect of exercise is its effect on the blood lipids. Regular exercise programs have been shown to decrease patients' serum triglyceride levels as well as very low-density lipoprotein (VLDL) and low-density lipoprotein (LDL) cholesterol levels. Equally, if not more, important is that exercise produces a rise in HDL (high-density lipoprotein) cholesterol, the so-called "good-guy" cholesterol. In long distance runners, it has been shown that there is a twofold increase in lipoprotein lipase (LPL) that may explain to some extent the beneficial effects of exercise on VLDL.

Since no extensive testing has been done on a large diabetic population, we can only assume that the beneficial effects of exercise on lipids are comparable to those in nondiabetic subjects.

Dr. David Costill and his co-workers at the Human Performance Laboratory of Ball State University have studied Type II diabetics and have found that these patients usually lower their triglyceride levels to normal if the total energy expenditure is moderate to heavy, which means running 4 to 8 miles per day. This level of exercise is greater than the average Type II diabetic maintains for long periods. Other studies have shown some reduction with less vigorous exercise programs. More studies involving both Type I and Type II diabetics are needed.

### Other Benefits of Exercise

Another possible benefit of programmed exercise for diabetics is an increase of insulin binding to receptors and increased insulin sensitivity. The increase in insulin sensitivity is almost proportional to increased physical fitness, as measured by the $\dot{V}O_2$ maximum, according to the results of a study by Dr. Philip Felig and colleagues at Yale University. The results of this experiment give further credence to encouraging the Type II obese diabetic to exercise.

Dr. Peter Forsham and colleagues at the University of California Medical Center, San Francisco, stated that exercise helps to lower platelet adhesiveness in diabetics to a level approaching that of the nondiabetic. This decrease may reduce the danger of thrombotic phenomena in diabetics, particularly as related to retinopathy.

## HYPOGLYCEMIA IN THE EXERCISING DIABETIC

What should athletic diabetics know about preventing hypoglycemia during exercise periods? Many observations have been made on young diabetics in summer camps. In general, their insulin requirements are reduced by 10 to 50% over a period of 7 to 10 days. This beneficial effect is lost after the child returns home unless his exercise program is equally intensive. In most instances, extra food is given at camp rather than attempting to reduce insulin over a short period of time, although both routes are taken.

The school athlete must be informed regarding extra food before practice sessions and before competition. Generally, food intake should be timed so that the peak benefit occurs prior to any possible hypoglycemia. This means taking a sandwich (or 2) an hour before the start of the exercise period. Fast-acting carbohydrates, preferably in liquid form such as soft drinks, should be available during exercise or during games, in case of threatened hypoglycemia. Most young diabetic athletes rapidly learn their requirements for a given period of exercise and rarely suffer severe hypoglycemic episodes. However, they must inform coaches and team members of the nature and treatment of hypoglycemia.

The adult Type I diabetic who exercises 2 to 3 times weekly must also know how much extra food to eat to cover extra exercise. If he is a jogger, it is important that he not jog in the morning before breakfast, but rather after meals, to ensure adequate blood glucose levels. He should carry sugar in the form of hard candies or semiliquid glucose, or any other rapidly absorbed source of sugar. For long-distance or prolonged exercise, food should be taken every 45 to 60 minutes, preferably some form of sugar.

Type I diabetics over age 25 are mainly "week-end exercisers," and they rapidly learn their caloric requirements to prevent hypoglycemia. These requirements are individual, since none of us expend exactly the same number of calories by exercising a given amount. Many do mild exercise for most of a Saturday or Sunday, and in such cases, a midmorning snack of cheese and crackers or a protein-containing sandwich and the same snack midafternoon usually suffice. In addition, some patients need extra food at bedtime, to cover any possible delayed hypoglycemic effect.

The Type II diabetic who is controlled by diet alone or by diet and oral drugs generally need not be concerned about hypoglycemia with mild to moderate exercise. Unusually vigorous exercise in the Type II diabetic who takes a sulfonylurea and whose diabetes is closely controlled might induce enough of a drop in blood glucose levels to warrant a midmorning or midafternoon snack, as in the Type I patient.

## INSULIN INJECTION SITES

Many controlled studies have shown that absorption of insulin from the subcutaneous site of injection is enhanced when the muscle underlying the site undergoes vigorous exercise. For that reason, the diabetic who undertakes exercise using his legs primarily should avoid injecting insulin into his thigh. He should preferably use the anterior abdominal wall. This group of patients includes all joggers and runners.

## EXERCISE PRESCRIPTION

For those patients who have no planned exercise program, the family physician can help to give them a simple, progressive schedule. The following is what I advise for the average middle-aged or older diabetics whose physician has determined that they are able to undergo such a program.

**What Kind of Exercise?** The best and easiest exercise is a walking, or for some a walking-jogging, program. Bicycle riding is fine for the more agile, and an indoor stationary bicycle is excellent unless the older patient has too much arthritis in his hips and knees. Swimming is excellent, and some older persons join groups who swim at clubs, YMCA, YWCA, and such. For the younger diabetics, the racket games are fine, and indeed some patients beyond middle age enjoy a game of tennis.

**How Often?** Three to 5 times per week is preferable, with no more than 2 days' rest between exercise days.

**How Long?** Fifteen to 60 minutes is advised, depending on the person's capability and the type of exercise.

**Pulse Rate.** I ordinarily do not advise the older patients about raising their pulse rates to the maximum for their age, but if one wishes to do so, the following information is valuable. Roughly, 220 minus one's age gives the maximum pulse rate for the person with a healthy cardiovascular system. Those under 50 years of age should aim for 70 to 75% of maximum, and those over 50 should aim for 55 to 65% of maximum. Pulse rates should be checked every 3 minutes during the exercise period.

**Walking.** A suggested prescription for walking for the older patient is as follows:

First week—1 mile in 30 minutes (½ mile out and ½ mile back)
Second week—2 miles in 40 minutes
Third week—1 mile in 15 minutes
Fourth week—2 miles in 30 minutes
Fifth week—3 miles in 45 minutes
Sixth week—4 miles in 60 minutes

## PRECAUTIONS FOR THE EXERCISING DIABETIC

Diabetics should take the following precautions when exercising:

1. One should never start exercising when blood sugar levels are low, such as just before meals.
2. Good shoes are a must, since the diabetic foot must be protected from injury—even the smallest blister can start a pathologic process.
3. One should always exercise with a "buddy" who understands hypoglycemia.
4. Diabetics should carry some sugar with them, in the form of Life Savers or similar hard candy.
5. One should wear an identification bracelet or dog tag.

6. Feet should be examined carefully after each walking or running session, and any slight skin breaks or blisters should be taken care of.

## OBESITY AND EXERCISE

It is generally accepted that when energy intake exceeds energy output, obesity occurs. When treating obesity, most programs strive to decrease the energy intake, but pay little attention to increasing energy expenditure. The medical profession has underemphasized physical activity and its role in weight reduction. Obese children as well as obese adults are generally physically inactive. When a detailed caloric intake study was done, some obese children were found to eat less than the control subjects of normal weight.

A recent study on the effect of exercise alone on the weight of obese women was published in the Archives of Internal Medicine in May of 1975. The author was Dr. Grant Gwinup and the study was done at the University of California at Irvine. All of the 11 obese women studied had given up restricting caloric intake because they did not lose weight. The exercise chosen by all the subjects was walking, and this meant walking as rapidly as was comfortable. Every subject lost a considerable amount of weight and maintained this loss during a period of a year or longer. The weight loss paralleled the amount of exercise, and those who had the greatest loss exercised for about 3 hours daily. No weight loss occurred until walking exceeded 30 minutes daily. Two patients had to discontinue the exercise temporarily, and during this time, gained weight rapidly. During the study, all the subjects were instructed to eat the same kind of food as before entering the exercise program. The quantity of food was to be determined by desire alone.

Brisk walking produces an energy expenditure of around 300 calories per hour. In order to lose 1 pound of fat, there must be an energy expenditure of about 3500 calories. The patient who walks 2 hours per day is expected to lose about 1.25 pounds per week. Those who walk 3 hours daily expect to lose about 2 pounds per week. However, the actual weight loss in this study rarely exceeded half a pound per week. Some of the subjects' body areas may have undergone an increase in muscle mass due to exercising. It was apparent that most of the weight loss was fat loss. Three of the subjects of this study had been obese since early childhood, and they all lost weight, 2 of them being among those who lost the greatest amount of weight during the study period. Although this study involved obese, nondiabetic women, there is no reason to believe that similar results could not be achieved in the Type II obese diabetic.

For further reading, the following articles are excellent.

## FURTHER READINGS

Skyler, S.J.: Diabetes and exercise: clinical implications. Diabetes Care, *2*:307, 1979.
Vranig, M., Horvath, S., and Wahren, J. (Eds.): Proceedings of a conference on diabetes and exercise. Diabetes Care, *28*, Suppl. 1, 1979.

# 11

# Hypoglycemia

Hypoglycemia or "insulin-reactions" occur mainly in the insulin-dependent diabetic, although hypoglycemia can occur in the patient taking oral antidiabetes drugs. There are conflicting opinions about the potential dangers of hypoglycemia. Many physicians unfortunately alarm their patients unduly by stating that hypoglycemia should be avoided at all costs, even if it means having 1 to 2% glucosuria. I think that such a statement is doing an injustice to the patient, and I do not agree. If a Type I diabetic of more than 6 to 12 months' duration has never experienced even a minor hypoglycemic reaction, that patient's diabetes has probably never been well controlled; one can almost always be sure that the patient's blood glucose levels are unacceptably high.

## EFFECT OF HYPOGLYCEMIA ON THE BRAIN

Mild to moderate hypoglycemia leaves no indelible mark on either the brain or the nervous system in general. Hypoglycemia accompanied by unconsciousness of short duration apparently does no obvious long-term brain damage, whereas repeated and prolonged periods of unconsciousness can do permanent brain damage. A former patient of mine, still living and well after 57 years of insulin therapy, has experienced hundreds of hypoglycemic episodes during his lifetime, many of them to the point of unconsciousness and convulsions. At the age of 75, he is still mentally sharp, plays golf almost daily (weather permitting), and enjoys life immensely. Incidentally, he has no microvascular complications and minimal macrovascular complications and has taken 2 doses of insulin every day of his diabetic life. I have never seen a case of severe brain damage from repeated hypoglycemic episodes.

The greatest danger from hypoglycemia is that the patient may be overtaken by hypoglycemia when he is in a situation in which cerebral and muscular coordination is pertinent to survival, such as operating an automobile or other moving machinery or pursuing a sport such as skiing or swimming.

Prolonged hypoglycemia with unconsciousness in the older patient has been reported to precipitate a cerebrovascular accident on rare occasions.

## CAUSES OF HYPOGLYCEMIA

1. Obviously, too much insulin.
2. Generally, unusual amounts of exercise without adequate food coverage.
3. Vigorous exercise just before mealtime. School children should have physical education classes scheduled right after meals, not before.
4. Injection of insulin in thighs on days when active physical exercise is anticipated, especially running.
5. Missing or delay of a meal. Meals should be on schedule, with not more than 30 to 40 minute's variation allowed.
6. Skipping a calculated between-meal snack. One should watch for this in younger patients. If their bedtime urine tests show high sugar levels, they may decide on their own to skip their bedtime snack, so that the urine will "be clear" by morning. In the middle of the night, they may become hypoglycemic.
7. Reduction of caloric intake without reduction of insulin dosage.

## SIGNS AND SYMPTOMS OF HYPOGLYCEMIA

These signs and symptoms are probably determined both by the rate of fall of the blood sugar level and by its total decline. Generally, symptoms and signs can be divided into 2 stages. The first is the adrenal stage, with release of epinephrine, and the second is the cerebral stage, owing to decreased use of glucose by the brain. Fatigue and/or headache may be warning symptoms of ensuing hypoglycemia even before the adrenal stage.

### Adrenal Stage—Autonomic Nervous System Symptoms

These symptoms are as follows:

1. Sweating—occurs in almost 100% of patients.
2. Hunger.
3. Tremor and tachycardia.
4. Anxiety and nervousness.
5. Weakness.
6. Occasional nausea and vomiting.

This stage, usually recognizable by the patient or his parents, is easily treated with sugar in almost any form. However, not all diabetics experience the symptoms produced by the release of epinephrine, particularly those patients whose diabetes has been present for many years. These symptoms may also be masked in patients taking propranolol.

### Cerebral Stage

Central nervous system cells are most sensitive to inadequate levels of blood glucose. The drop in blood sugar levels may be rapid. The transition from the first sweating and shakiness to the point at which adequate cerebration disappears and confusion begins can all happen within 3 to 6 minutes.

What are the signs and symptoms of the cerebral stage of hypoglycemia? These are not necessarily given in order of appearance, but the patient generally goes from muscular incoordination and cerebral inadequacy to a semicomatose stage, and then to convulsions and complete unconsciousness.

1. Perioral paresthesia.
2. Possible headache with visual disturbances.
3. Mental confusion and inability to speak intelligently.
4. Speech slurred; gait ataxic.
5. Unusual neurologic symptoms or signs, including diplopia.
6. Frequent personality changes with bizarre moods, belligerence, depression, or psychotic behavior.
7. Semicoma with muscular twitching and then convulsions.
8. Complete unconsciousness.

Nocturnal hypoglycemic episodes during sleep, especially in young patients, are frequently accompanied by restlessness, rolling, moaning, and, not infrequently, falling out of bed.

An ambulatory person displaying symptoms of the cerebral stage of hypoglycemia can easily be mistaken for an inebriated person, if in public places or driving an automobile that may be involved in an accident. Then, even more serious, the diabetic may be taken by an uneducated police officer to jail, where treatment is withheld. It is thus obvious that the diabetic must have visible and easily found identification, either a bracelet or a necklace.

## HYPOGLYCEMIA IN CHILDREN

Although the symptoms and signs of hypoglycemia in children frequently do not differ from those seen in older diabetics, there are a few that parents learn to recognize early in a hypoglycemic episode.

1. Sudden change in behavior, with irritability, crying, inattention.
2. "Peculiar stare" or "glassy-eyed look," or occasional strabismus.
3. Unusual lethargy or sleepiness.
4. Extreme hunger.
5. Sweating, usually, but not always (The back of the child's neck is cold and clammy).
6. Frequent nocturnal reactions. (Parents should be aware of a simple test to help differentiate restless sleep from hypoglycemic neurologic symptoms. This is the so-called squint reflex. A bright flashlight is held within an inch or so of the sleeping or comatose child's closed eye. If the child is in normal sleep, the eyelids squeeze together by reflex as a result of the bright light. If the child is in a hypoglycemic coma, the reflex is absent.)

## BLOOD GLUCOSE DETERMINATIONS

The physician should draw a blood sample for glucose at once and proceed with treatment. If there is undue delay in drawing the blood sample, the physician should proceed with treatment. If he is confident of the diagnosis, the laboratory test is not needed, and the patient can be spared the unnecessary expense. If there is a question of differential diagnosis, then the physician had best obtain the blood sample before treating the patient, but this question does not mean that one must wait for the laboratory results before beginning treatment.

## TREATMENT OF HYPOGLYCEMIA

If the patient is conscious or semiconscious, but is still able to swallow, he should be given sugar in any convenient and available form. One should remember that it takes about 15 g sugar to relieve hypoglycemia. There are 15 g sugar in 3 sugar cubes, in 3 teaspoons of granulated sugar, honey, pancake syrup, corn syrup, jelly, or jam, and in 6 ounces of soft drinks or fruit juices. If concentrated carbohydrates are not available, one should give the patient any available food—it will relieve the hypoglycemia in due time.

If the patient is unconscious and is unable to swallow, the physician should give him 30 ml of 50% dextrose solution by IV bolus. The patient is usually awake before the injection is completed. This injection furnishes 15 g sugar directly to the blood and is usually sufficient to restore normoglycemia rapidly. If the patient is not awake after receiving 15 g IV, one should inject another 10 g.

If IV glucose solution is not available, then the patient should be given 1 mg glucagon subcutaneously or intramuscularly (IM). He will be awake within 15 to 25 minutes. One should give the full 1-mg dose to all diabetics over 4 years of age and 0.5 mg to children under

4. Glucagon is supplied in a 2-vial kit, one containing 1 mg glucagon and the other 1 ml diluent. It is stable for 5 years in this form.

All insulin-dependent patients should be instructed in the use of glucagon, and other persons in the household should learn how to inject it. It is best for household members to give the diabetic patient his insulin injections a couple of times each month in order to become familiar with injection technique, so that when a crisis requires glucagon, the one who administers it will feel comfortable in so doing. Physicians should advise all their patients who take insulin to have glucagon on hand. Glucagon's immediate action is to stimulate glycogenolysis and thus to elevate blood glucose levels.

When the patient regains consciousness, he should eat some food within the next few minutes, or he should eat his next meal, if the episode happens just before mealtime. This procedure is important if consciousness is restored with glucagon, since its action in adding to the available total glucose is inadequate for prolonged euglycemia. If treatment has taken place in an emergency room of a hospital or in the physician's office, it is usually safe to let the patient go home if he appears well an hour after treatment. It should be made certain that someone else is driving him home.

Children occasionally have prolonged vomiting on awakening from a hypoglycemic episode, and it may be necessary to administer an intravenous drip of 10% glucose for several hours until the vomiting subsides. Sips of cola drinks sometimes help. The vomiting child should not be sent home—he may well suffer further hypoglycemia.

There is no need to hospitalize the treated hypoglycemic patient who is fully recovered, is not vomiting, and is well oriented and ambulatory. The patient should be sent home with an escort.

### Nonresponders

Rarely, a hypoglycemic patient awakens initially in response to IV glucose, but in spite of oral feedings, does not regain normal function. This phenomenon happens more often in older patients and may be related to an associated cerebrovascular insufficiency; his symptoms may resemble a mild, transient ischemic attack. It is best to hospitalize the patient and to order an IV infusion of 10% glucose in water, to run at a rate that maintains blood glucose levels between 100 and 200 mg/dl. As the patients' function is regained, oral feedings can gradually replace the IV infusion.

If the occasional patient does not regain consciousness after receiving IV glucose, his comatose state is due to other causes, which must be found. The other metabolic comatose states in the diabetic are usually not difficult to recognize, and these should be included in the differential diagnosis—ketoacidosis, lactic acidosis, and hyperosmolar coma. The usual differential diagnosis of all other comatose states applies to diabetics as well as to nondiabetics. When the diagnosis is in doubt and the physician is without laboratory help for a diabetic who is unconscious, an immediate infusion of 50 ml 50% glucose should be given as a therapeutic trial. If the patient does not regain consciousness, one must look for causes other than hypoglycemia. No harm is done to any pathologic condition by an infusion of glucose.

## DEATH FROM HYPOGLYCEMIA

Death from hypoglycemia is rare. Most cases reported have involved diabetics who are inebriated at the time of the episode and who are frequently comatose for many hours before beginning treatment. Alcohol diminishes all the physiologic reactions that normally take place to elevate blood glucose levels. In addition, the alcoholic frequently omits food for prolonged periods.

Accidental deaths do occur when the diabetic is physically or mentally incapable of avoiding critical and lethal situations. Motor vehicle accidents lead the list; drowning is not infrequent.

Rarely does the untreated hypoglycemic patient die, even though he may be comatose for 4 to 8 hours. The counterregulatory hormones—cortisol, growth hormone, glucagon, and epinephrine—all work to restore blood glucose levels by antagonizing the action of insulin and by stimulating glycogenolysis and/or gluconeogenesis.

## HYPOGLYCEMIA WHEN TAKING ORAL ANTIDIABETES TABLETS

Severe hypoglycemia in the patient taking these oral agents is uncommon. Chlorpropamide is probably involved more often because of its relative strength. When hypoglycemia does occur, it is most often mild and easily recognizable unless masked by other disorders. There are a few situations that may predispose a patient to hypoglycemic episodes:

1. Occasionally, patients cannot remember whether they have taken their tablets, so they take another dose to be sure.
2. Overmedication by the physician is a problem that speaks for itself. One should tread gently with older patients.
3. Patients continue taking their medications in spite of a failing or absent appetite. The physician should instruct them to stop taking the tablets if their appetite fails, and to call for further instructions.
4. Patients who fail to return at appointed times for office and laboratory visits may take a given dose for several years that frequently proves to be too high.

5. Patients who drink alcohol heavily may be headed for trouble.
6. Patients take drugs that potentiate the action of the sulfonylurea. These drugs include sulfonamides, chloramphenicol, oxytetracycline, salicylates, phenylbutazone, coumarin derivatives, probenecid, propranolol, guanethidine, and monoamine oxidase inhibitors. If such drugs are indicated in the treatment, one must not hestitate to use them, but should check blood glucose levels several times at 4 to 6 day intervals in the beginning to ascertain their effect. The patient should know what to look for.

## INSTRUCTIONS TO PATIENTS

Until your newly diagnosed Type I patients receive adequate education in the care of their diabetes, the physician has the responsibility of giving them a brief course in avoiding and treating hypoglycemia. The following sections contain instructions that are helpful to patients with regard to hypoglycemia.

### Prevention of Hypoglycemia

1. The patient must always follow his diet and eat meals on schedule.
2. If between-meals snacks are prescribed as part of the dietary program, one must always take these snacks as instructed. They must not be omitted because a urine test shows a high level of sugar.
3. Extra exercise requires extra food, the amount to be determined by trial.
4. Physical labor also requires extra food.
5. If urine tests are always negative, and the patient feels shaky and/or sweaty before meals, he should call his physician for instructions regarding reduction of the insulin dose.
6. If the patient takes a midafternoon nap, he should always take a snack prior to lying down.
7. If he lives alone, he should arrange for a friend or relative to speak to him on the telephone each day.
8. School teachers need instructions about hypoglycemia as a rule, and instruction sheets are available for teachers (see Appendix). College students must have roommates who understand diabetes and hypoglycemia.

### Hazardous Situations for the Diabetic Taking Insulin

Certain situations are dangerous for patients who take insulin unless precautions are taken.

**Driving.** Each year fatal road accidents occur when the driver was a diabetic having hypoglycemia, which in most cases could have been avoided. Diabetics should not drive during the 30 to 45 minutes preceding their next meal or before breakfast. They should not postpone regular mealtimes for any reason if they are driving. Before driving home from work, especially if it has been a "hard day," patients should eat a snack 30 minutes before starting out. If working long hours, as for example, a farmer during harvest, diabetics should eat 3 snacks per day, midmorning, midafternoon, and bedtime, and should be sure regular meals are on time.

**Recreational Activities and Athletics.** Swimming, water or snow skiing, snowmobiling, hunting, fishing, hiking, boating, and backpacking are all activities requiring the utmost in brain-muscle coordination, so the diabetic must be assured of adequate supplies of blood sugar at all times. Consequently, he should never undertake such an activity by himself, without others around who can recognize signs and symptoms of hypoglycemia and are able to treat it. The "buddy system" is a must for diabetics. Athletic participation is encouraged, but extra snacks must be taken prior to practice and games. The patient should discuss his situation with his doctor and/or dietitian. Hypoglycemia impairs both mental and physical abilities.

**Dangerous Occupations.** Most states do not allow diabetics who take insulin to drive public vehicles, freight trucks, and similar heavy equipment. Diabetics should not do this type of driving. Electrical work, especially requiring pole climbing, is hazardous. Construction work, especially high scaffold type, is also to be avoided.

## REACTIVE HYPOGLYCEMIA AS PRECURSOR OF MILD DIABETES MELLITUS

Hypoglycemic symptoms occurring between the third and fifth hour after a meal may occur in persons usually who have a diabetic family history and may be a forerunner of frank, mild, clinical diabetes, Type II. Not all diabetologists agree that such occurrences forecast future diabetes. The syndrome has also been labeled reactive hyperinsulinism, since it is felt that the original beta cell response to a glucose load is sluggish and is followed by an overreaction, with the release of excess insulin which in turn produces hypoglycemia. Fasting blood glucose levels are usually normal, but 1- and 2-hour glucose measurements after an oral glucose tolerance test sometimes show impaired glucose tolerance. The 3- and 4-hour measurements frequently show relative hypoglycemia in the range of 40 mg/dl or less. The glucose tolerance test and the appearance of symptoms later in the postprandial period (3 to 5 hours) usually differentiate this condition from so-called reactive functional hypoglycemia.

# 12

# Diabetic Ketoacidosis

## ETIOLOGY OF DIABETIC KETOACIDOSIS (DKA)

Twenty-five percent of all cases of DKA occur as the initial manifestation of diabetes mellitus.

Anorexia from any cause seems to be the signal to the patient to stop taking insulin unless he has been instructed about the need for some insulin every day. This discontinuance may cause DKA.

Physical stress such as trauma, operations, or illness may bring about DKA when patient and physician do not take proper steps to treat the preacidotic phase.

Occasionally, a mentally disturbed teenager or young adult voluntarily stops taking insulin as a revenge tactic, realizing that he will produce a life-threatening situation.

Some diabetics reduce their insulin dose progressively because of a fear of hypoglycemia, without consulting their physician.

Chronic hyperglycemia (300 to 500 mg/dl) can set the stage for acidosis to take place as a result of minor stress in some individuals.

It is generally accepted that to make the diagnosis of DKA, the patient's bicarbonate level must be less than 15 mEq/L and the pH 7.25 or less.

## SYMPTOMS AND SIGNS OF DKA

The patient is usually symptomatic for 18 to 24 hours before calling his physician, and it is obvious that he is acutely ill. His symptoms are as follows:

1. Polyuria and polydipsia.
2. Nausea and vomiting.
3. Diffuse abdominal pain relieved with treatment of acidosis. (However, the occasional diabetic has ketoacidosis in addition to a

condition such as an acute appendicitis, so the physician must be alert to such a possibility.)
4. Variable symptoms of an accompanying illness, upper respiratory, gastrointestinal, or urinary.

The signs of DKA are:

1. Marked evidence of dehydration, with tachycardia and sometimes orthostatic hypotension, and loss of skin turgor.
2. Acetone odor to breath, characteristic and diagnostic.
3. Kussmaul's breathing; characteristically deep and rapid respirations.
4. Altered state of consciousness, ranging from lethargy to frank coma. (In my experience, only 25% of patients are comatose on admission to the hospital.)

## DIFFERENTIAL DIAGNOSIS

One must remember that diabetics may be comatose from causes other than DKA, including cardiovascular accidents, renal failure with azotemia, skull fractures, meningitis, drug or alcohol consumption, lactic acidosis, hyperosmolar coma, and commonly, hypoglycemia. The differential diagnosis between hypoglycemia and DKA should not be difficult to make, especially when immediate laboratory determinations are available. Differential diagnosis between lactic acidosis, hyperosmolar coma, and DKA is discussed later. In children, aspirin intoxication can mimic DKA.

## EMERGENCY TREATMENT

The physician should

1. Admit the patient to the intensive care unit of a hospital, if possible.
2. Start therapy as soon as the diagnosis is established.
3. Draw blood and request immediate determinations for glucose, electrolytes, venous pH, serum bicarbonate, and creatinine levels. He should ask the laboratory for results on the glucose and bicarbonate test as soon as possible, preferably within 30 minutes.
4. Start a flow sheet. This is most important and helpful. The nurse should record on this sheet, in chronologic order, all results of urine and blood chemistry tests, intake of intravenous fluids and insulin, and the patient's vital signs and progress. (See Fig. 12–1.)
5. Avoid catheterization of the patient whenever possible. If it is necessary, a single catheterization should be done; one should not insert an indwelling catheter, since diabetics are prone to pyuria. If an indwelling catheter is absolutely necessary, urinary antibiotics should be administered.
6. Insert a nasogastric tube at once if a comatose patient has gastric retention.

| TIME | 8 P.M. | 9 P.M. | 10 P.M. | 11 P.M. | 12 P.M. | 1 A.M. | 2 A.M. | 3 A.M. |
|---|---|---|---|---|---|---|---|---|
| FLUIDS<br>IV/Oral<br>ST = Start<br>SP = Stop | #1 1000 ml<br>n. sal. IV<br>ST. 8:25 | #1 SP 9:45<br>#2 1000 ml<br>½ n. sal.<br>with 40 mEq<br>KCl ST 9:45 | | | | | | |
| INSULIN<br>IV–IM–Subcutaneous<br>R = Regular<br>N = NPH<br>L = Lente | 8:10<br>R–20 IV bolus | 9:25<br>R–10 IM | | | | | | |
| BLOOD CHEM.<br>Indicate time blood drawn | 8:05<br>Pl. gluc.<br>750 mg/dl<br>Bicarb 10 mEq/L<br>Na 134 mEq/L<br>K 3.6 mEq/L | | | | | | | |
| BP<br>Pulse<br>Resp.<br>Temp. | 110/72<br>110<br>42-Kussmaul<br>100.2 | | | | | | | |
| URINES<br>Time Voided<br>Glu/Ketones | 8:20<br>2%/Heavy | | | | | | | |
| OTHER RX<br>Shock<br>Infections | | | | | | | | |
| State of<br>Consciousness<br>Remarks: | Semicomatose | | | | | | | |

**Fig. 12–1.** Eight-hour diabetic ketoacidosis treatment flow sheet.

7. Examine the patient for the presence of a precipitating illness when proper treatment of the acidosis is under way.

## LABORATORY FINDINGS

**Elevated Plasma Glucose Levels.** These are 300 to 1500 mg/dl, most frequently in the 500- to 1000-mg/dl range. Speed is of essence in obtaining this measurement, and if the laboratory has a rapid glucose analyzer, one can have results in 5 minutes. A rapid and accurate determination of blood sugar levels can be made with the Ames Dextrometer or the Chemstrip-bG, if other methods are unavailable.

**Glucosuria.** The 2-drop Clinitest is best for this determination, and one should try to obtain a second-voided specimen. Usually, there is a 5% sugar level. Diastix is an inaccurate test in the presence of ketonuria.

**Ketonuria.** One should use either Ketostix or Acetest tablets. Test results are usually strongly positive.

**Venous Blood pH.** This is between 6.8 and 7.2, generally. Results below 7.0 are of prognostic significance.

**Serum Bicarbonate Level.** This is below 15 mEq/dl.

**Anion Gap.** There is an anion gap of over 12 mEq/L. [Anion gap = (Na plus K) − (Cl plus $HCO_3$) − 17.] Normal is 0 to 3 mEq/L. Any reading over 10 mEq/L is clinically significant.

**Hyperosmolality.** Eighty per cent of DKA patients have serum osmolalities greater than 330 mOsm/L. The normal range is 280 to 300 mOsm/L. If the hospital laboratory cannot make the determination by the freezing point depression method, one can quickly estimate the osmolality by this formula:

$$\text{Osmolality} = 2 \times \text{Na in mEq/L} + \frac{\text{glucose in mg/dl}}{18} + \frac{\text{BUN in mg/dl}}{2.8}$$

**Serum Potassium (K).** The test results for K are inversely proportionate to pH, so one must remember this when interpreting K levels. A normal K level on the first determination means a lowered K level, actually.

**Other Laboratory Findings.** If the patient's serum is lactescent because of an elevated triglyceride level, one should check the accuracy of the laboratory reports.

Blood gas determinations are unnecessary and expensive, unless pulmonary disease is present.

**Office Laboratory Diagnosis.** If no laboratory facilities are immediately available, one can still make a diagnosis of DKA by doing the following:

1. Test the patient's blood glucose levels with the Ames Dextrometer or Chemstrip-bG.

2. Test a urine sample for both glucose and ketones.
3. Measure serum ketones utilizing the new improved Ketostix or Keto-Diastix (Ames). Either plasma or serum may be used for this test, and it is well to have a large enough blood sample to make several serial dilutions if indicated by the findings. Wet the testing strip with several drops of serum and read exactly at 15 seconds. The test depends on nitroprusside's reacting with acetoacetate to give a distinct color change. Semiquantitative results are read from the color chart in the package as negative, trace (5 mg/dl), small (15 mg/dl), moderate (40 mg/dl), and large (80 to 160 mg/dl). The Ketostix package insert states, "the speed and intensity of color development are similar in urine, serum and plasma." Therefore, the accuracy in testing serum is comparable to the accuracy in testing urine. The color changes are distinct, ranging from buff-pink to a deep maroon, and can be easily interpreted.

   If large amounts of ketone (up to 160 mg/dl) are found in undiluted serum, it would be prudent to dilute the serum with equal parts of distilled water and test this diluted sample. Similarly, if the test is not clearly positive (trace to small on the color chart) with the undiluted serum, repeat it on the first diluted sample because marked lactescence or slight hemolysis may interfere with clear interpretation of color development.

   If ketosis is clinically significant, color changes indicating ketones in the range of 5 to 40 mg/dl will appear in undiluted serum or in the first dilution as indicated.

   Two advantages accrue by doing serum ketone determinations—they confirm or exclude the diagnosis of ketoacidosis, and they afford a simple method of following the patient's progress.

   Of the 3 ketone bodies, acetone does not contribute to the acid-base imbalance, but does impart the characteristic and diagnostic odor to the patient's exhaled breath. Acetone does not react with the improved Ketostix/Keto-Diastix. $\beta$-hydroxybutyrate is the predominant ketone body in ketoacidosis, but does not react with Ketostix/Keto-Diastix, or Acetest tablets. However, its concentration in serum bears a relationship to that of acetoacetate that is commonly expressed as the BOHB/AcAc ratio. This ratio is generally regarded as around 3 in untreated ketoacidosis, but it can vary between 1 (mild ketosis) and 12 (extreme ketoacidosis).

   Thus, if the Ketostix reading on undiluted serum was 40 mg/dl of acetoacetate (acetoacetic acid), the BOHB would be 3 times this or 120 mg/dl, and the total ketones would be 160 mg/dl. It is obvious that in a situation of severe ketoacidosis when the BOHB serum concentration might be 10 or 12 times that of the acetoacetate, the reading on the color chart might underestimate the severity of the acidosis by a considerable amount.

## KETONURIA WITHOUT KETONEMIA

In the normal metabolic state, about 20 mg of ketones, mainly acetoacetate, are excreted daily in the urine, an amount not detected by the usual tests. However, in many relatively benign conditions, urinary excretion of ketones is sufficient to be detected in trace or small amounts by the usual tests utilizing Ketostix or Acetest tablets. The physician should be aware that this represents ketonuria, but not ketonemia. Situations fitting this picture include unusual and prolonged physical exercise, marked caloric restriction, vomiting and diarrhea, common febrile diseases, thyrotoxicosis, and chronic renal insufficiency. This condition may also occur following anesthesia. Patients recovered from ketoacidosis may show ketonuria for 24 to 36 hours after the blood glucose is normalized.

## TREATMENT OF DKA

The syndrome of DKA is composed of 5 serious abnormalities, all of which must be corrected in a vigorous treatment program. These abnormalities are: (1) water depletion, (2) electrolyte depletion (sodium, potassium, phosphate and magnesium), (3) metabolic acidosis, (4) insulin deficiency, and (5) increased output of stress hormones.

### Correction of Volume Depletion and Hyperosmolality

Some idea of volume depletion can be ascertained by noting the patient's skin turgor, jugular vein pressure, and urine output. The serum osmolality is a guide, as well.

For adults, 1000 ml normal (0.9%) saline solution IV should be prescribed during the first 1 to 2 hours. Subsequent infusions should be given at a rate of 400 to 500 ml/hr.

For children who weigh less than 30 kg, 20 ml/kg normal saline solution should be given in the first hour. Then the patient's deficit should be calculated, in addition to maintenance, using a 0.45% saline solution for all subsequent fluids. The second infusion should be 10 to 12 ml/kg/hr.

The physician must use his judgment concerning the speed of IV infusion as well as the total amount of fluids. In children and older persons, overhydration can be harmful and even fatal if it triggers pulmonary edema. Faster rates of infusion may be indicated if the patient is severely hypotensive and dehydrated. Normal saline or 0.45% saline solution is satisfactory for the next several liters. One should check serum osmolality occasionally to guide fluid replacement.

> Caution: Giving 8 to 12 L IV fluids to an adult in the first 24 hours is dangerous and unnecessary, except in the most unusual situations. Ordinarily, 4 to 5 L are adequate, and the patient should be given oral fluids as soon as nausea subsides.

### Potassium Replacement

The physician should check the patient's urinary output to be sure that it is adequate (1 ml/min). However, since K replacement is always required, one must proceed more cautiously if urinary output is compromised.

In general, K loss is 6 to 10 mEq/kg body weight, and the average adult requires about 100 to 150 mEq in the first 4 to 6 hours. If the patient's serum K is normal and the calculated deficit is less than 10%, then 10 to 20 mEq KCl IV can be infused each hour with the patient's IV fluid. If hypokalemia is severe, e.g., under 2.0 mEq, one can give the patient up to 60 mEq/hr.

Recent studies have shown a phosphate depletion of variable magnitude in DKA. This depletion reflects the concentration of 2-3 diphosphoglycerate, an enzyme that enhances oxygen affinity to hemoglobin. Therefore, it is advised that some phosphate be given for replacement, usually in the form of potassium phosphate. However, an excess of phosphate may stimulate an excess loss of calcium and magnesium. For this reason, the present recommendations are to give equal parts of potassium chloride and potassium phosphate. However, if only potassium chloride is available, it should be used as indicated, and it is unlikely that the patient will show marked signs of a phosphate deficit.

The physician should recheck the patient's serum K levels every 3 hours until normal levels are attained.

The following potassium and phosphate preparations are available: KCl in 20-mEq vials and monobasic potassium phosphate ($KH_2PO_4$) in 60-mEq vials.

With moderate K depletion, I advise 30 mEq/L IV fluid; if depletion is more severe, one may use 60 mEq/L, but no more. The average requirement to maintain K levels in acidotic patients is between 155 and 200 mEq in those who are treated without bicarbonate, but it is between 250 and 325 mEq in those who receive more than 250 mEq of bicarbonate during the course of treatment.

Ordinarily, the first serum K level will be higher than normal. It begins to fall as the fluid balance and acidosis are corrected, since K moves into the cells and is lost in the urine. One should not be alarmed if the second K determination is lower than the first; this decrease is expected. However, if both determinations remain low, one should increase K administration immediately.

### Use of Bicarbonate for Severe Acidosis

It is probably wise to use bicarbonate when the patient's pH is 7.0 or less and he is hypotensive, comatose, and critically ill. Bicarbonate can be given as a bolus from 1 to 4 ampules, each containing 50.0 mEq, or it can be diluted and given as follows: one should add 2 ampules (each 50.0 mEq) to 100 ml of ½-normal (N) saline solution to be given intravenously to titrate pH to 7.0 or so; then one should add 1 ampule to 1000 ml of ½-N saline solution and administer it slowly until pH is 7.2 or above.

An important clinical sign is cessation of Kussmaul's breathing. Opponents of the use of bicarbonate have cited its possible effect on CSF osmolarity, with possible ensuing cerebral edema. It is a rare possibility, however. For further details, see discussion of cerebral edema.

### Insulin Administration

The medical practice has come a long way since the days of giving hundreds of units of insulin. Most clinicians have accepted the low-dose programs, and certainly the results have been satisfactory. Two programs are recommended here, leaving the choice to the physician. Regular insulin is used at all times. The half-life of regular insulin is: plasma, 4 to 5 minutes; muscle, 2 hours; subcutaneous, 4 hours.

**Intravenous Infusion Method (preferred if patient is hypotensive).** The loading dose of insulin is 0.3 U/kg for an adult, 0.15 U/kg for children, to be given as an IV bolus. A continuous infusion follows immediately. For adults, one should add 50 U to 500 ml 0.9% saline solution and infuse it at the rate of 1 ml/min, which gives 6 U/hr. The infusion rate is controlled by the pediatic minidrip attachment and an electronic drop counter apparatus. A fresh insulin solution should be prepared every 6 hours. Some insulin binds to the glass or plastic container, but the amount lost does not affect the results obtained. Albumin in the bottle is not required. For children, the figure of 0.1 U/kg/hr is used. One should adjust the speed of infusion to deliver that amount.

> *Caution:* If the second plasma glucose reading, taken 2 hours after administration of the IV bolus, has not decreased by at least 20%, one should not hesitate to repeat the bolus in the same or greater number of units. The occasional patient requires more than the average amount of insulin. Similarly, if using the IM administration described in the next section, one may need to repeat the original bolus or even to increase the amounts of insulin.

**Intramuscular Method (not to be used if patient is hypotensive).** This is probably the method of choice, since no special apparatus is needed and the administration of insulin is done easily.

The insulin bolus can be given either IV or IM. If given IV, one should use the dosages given in the previous section. If given IM, 15 to 20 U for an adult and 0.25 U/kg for a child are average dosages. Thereafter, hourly IM injections of 6 to 10 U for an adult and 0.1 to .15 U/kg/hr for children should be administered.

**Decreasing Insulin Dose with Recovery.** When the patient's plasma glucose level has fallen to 250 to 300 mg/dl, one should decrease the insulin dose by 50% and administer an IV infusion of 5% glucose in normal saline solution at the rate of around 150 ml/hr for adults, less for children. One can soon give small doses of regular insulin every 6 hours subcutaneously, the amount determined by the plasma glucose and urinary glucose findings and by the size of the patient.

## Subsequent Orders

1. The physician should order urine tests for glucose and ketone bodies every hour, or with children, as urine is available.
2. Tests for plasma sugar, bicarbonate *or* pH, and potassium levels should be repeated every 2 hours.
3. One should not hesitate to double the patient's insulin dose if the blood sugar level is not decreasing and the bicarbonate level is not increasing. Not all patients respond satisfactorily to the low-dosage program.
4. The physician should leave orders for the nurse or house officer to call him every 2 hours for progress reports during the acute stage (first 8 hours) of the treatment.
5. He should leave orders to cover his patient's overnight needs for insulin and fluids. The condition of a postacidotic patient can worsen in the 8 to 10 hours between the physician's evening and morning hospital visits.

## Follow-up Care

The patient's plasma glucose level should be down to 200 to 300 mg/dl in 6 to 8 hours, and he should be out of acidosis within 12 hours of therapy.

1. As soon as the patient's nausea has subsided and the acidotic state is controlled, the physician should prescribe oral feedings, fluids at first and then solids.
2. The physician should then resume preacidotic insulin doses for established diabetic patients and prescribe an insulin program for new patients. For most adults, the dose is around 20 to 30 U Lente or NPH insulin. For children, the requirements may be approximately 0.5 to 1 U/kg. (See Chapter 8 for insulin requirements in children.)

3. For several days, the patient may need small, supplementary doses of regular insulin before meals, depending on premeal urine glucose test results.

## CEREBRAL EDEMA

An occasional case of fatal cerebral edema has been reported in a patient who is apparently recovering well from the metabolic abnormalities associated with ketoacidosis but who develops cerebral edema. The cause of this is not entirely clear, but several factors associated with treatment may be contributory. One theory states that too large and too rapid a reduction in serum osmolality caused by a too rapid decline in blood glucose concentration will create serious osmotic gradients, since the changes in CSF and brain osmolality are slower than the changes in the serum osmolality. For this reason, it is advisable to change the IV infusion to half-normal saline solution with 5% dextrose when the blood glucose declines to around 250 mg/dl.

A second theory associates cerebral edema with sodium bicarbonate administration, since it is possible that dissociated carbon dioxide enters the CSF before adequate amounts of bicarbonate. This process then causes a paradoxical worsening of the CSF acidosis and also may cause fluid shifts into the CSF.

## EDUCATION OF PATIENT

Before the patient leaves the hospital, he should be taught or should review ways to prevent ketoacidosis, in the hope of avoiding further such episodes. In addition, the physician should make arrangements for his patient to attend a reputable diabetes education center, where experts teach the fundamentals of diabetes. The educated patient rarely develops ketoacidosis.

The physician should advise the patient that his urine tests may show ketones 24 to 48 hours after leaving the hospital and that this is nothing to worry about, provided he feels well and his urinary glucose level is minimal.

## STRESS HORMONES AND DKA

Recent studies have emphasized that an excess of stress hormone is necessary for the development of frank DKA. The stress hormones involved are glucagon, cortisol, catecholamines, and growth hormone. Early studies using somatostatin to suppress glucagon and growth hormone provided some evidence of their influence in DKA. The most common precipitating factor in the development of acidosis is some form of stress, most frequently an infection. In recent years, concentrations of stress hormones measured in the laboratory have shown marked increases in patients with acidosis. Similarly, the administration of stress hormones to stable diabetics results in an increase in both plasma glucose levels and ketone concentrations.

How does one control the unusual increase in stress hormones? Small increases in stress hormones are probably beneficial and helpful to patients with acidosis, but large excesses are certainly detrimental. Experimentally, $\beta$-adrenergic blocking agents and metyrapone tartrate have been successfully used, the first to block catecholamines, the second to block cortisol production. Studies continue. To reduce the degree of stress is obviously helpful to these patients. This reduction includes treatment of the stress-inducing condition, elimination of infection, reduction of dehydration, and reduction of fever, which may be more important than formerly realized. Most patients with DKA do not or cannot take food by mouth. It is well known that fasting induces secretion of stress hormones, so it is important to substitute calories parenterally until oral feedings can be resumed.

Further studies on ways to block or to reduce the output of stress hormones should contribute information on treatment of DKA.

## SERIOUS PROGNOSTIC SIGNS

Mortality in the United States from ketoacidosis is now just under 5%, but with early and vigorous treatment it could be much lower. Poor prognostic signs include the presence of shock, a rapidly rising blood urea nitrogen (BUN) during the first few hours of treatment, and deep and prolonged coma, particularly in the young or the elderly patient.

## RECOGNITION AND TREATMENT OF PREACIDOSIS

Preacidosis is the state of hyperglycemia and ketonuria without acidosis, usually brought on by a minor infection, such as respiratory, gastrointestinal, or urinary. This state is easily treated at home by the patient if he understands what is happening and what to do about it. This is where patient-education is so important. The majority of patients who receive adequate education concerning the recognition and emergency treatment of preacidosis are able to avoid developing full-blown ketoacidosis. I devote considerable time to teaching this important aspect of acidosis to the students in the Diabetic Education Center at Deaconess Hospital, Spokane,

Washington. Physicians all should do the same. My instructions to students are summarized in the following paragraphs:

With the advent of a minor illness, such as a respiratory infection, a gastrointestinal upset with nausea and/or diarrhea, or a urinary tract infection, patients may not feel like eating, particularly if nauseated. Lack of appetite does not mean that diabetics can get along without insulin. They need some insulin every day, even though they may not take in many calories. Insulin should never be completely omitted unless one is instructed to do so by the physician.

Diabetics should then check their urine for sugar and ketones; there will probably be 2% sugar and positive ketones. The presence of positive ketones almost always indicates a need for extra insulin.

Patients should call their physician immediately, and he will advise them as to the amount and kind of insulin to take. However, if out of town when this happens, or if for any reason a physician cannot be located, patients should proceed as follows until medical help becomes available.

If patient feel that they will be eating little or no food, starting in the morning, they should take half the usual daily morning dose of insulin. If, however, their appetite is good and they will consume the usual diet, they should take the full dose of morning insulin.

These diabetics should check their urine for sugar and ketones every 3 hours. If the urine still has high sugar levels and positive ketones, patients should take an injection of regular insulin, one-fourth of their total daily dose. Example: A total daily dose is 60 units. However, the patient takes only 40 units in the morning, the remaining 20 in the evening. This morning, since his appetite is gone, he has taken half the usual morning dose, or 20 units. Now, 3 hours later, he takes a dose of regular insulin equal to one-fourth of the total daily dose, i.e., 15 units. The patient should repeat this every 3 hours, giving another injection of 15 units of regular insulin if the urine tests continue to show high sugar levels and positive ketones.

If, after 2 doses of regular insulin, the patient's urine tests are showing no improvement in either sugar or ketones, medical help must be found, even if in a strange city. The reason for this emergency is that the infection may be far more severe than thought. The progression to frank acidosis is a definite possibility.

Patients must hydrate themselves, and it is best to use clear liquids for this. This means liquids containing sugar, such as the real soft drinks, fruit juices, and of course, water. A few ounces taken at frequent intervals are easier to keep down. Patients should drink at least 1 pint per hour and preferably more.

If the administration of extra doses of regular insulin as instructed results in improvement of the symptoms and a decrease in sugar and ketones in the urine tests, then patients can almost be certain that they have avoided frank acidosis. For the next few days, their urine tests may show 1 to 2% sugar levels as well as a small amount of ketones. In such situations, it is prudent to take an extra dose of regular insulin before each meal if the urine tests show 1 to 2% sugar levels. This dose, of course, is in addition to the usual daily dose of insulin. The amount of regular insulin required varies, but an average dose is 10% of the normal total daily dose.

# 13

# Immunologic Reactions to Insulin

## PURIFIED INSULIN

Insulin, a polypeptide hormone currently derived from animal pancreas, is expected to invoke some immune response. For most diabetics, this response is insignificant, but for a few it can become a major and difficult clinical problem. This chapter discusses the recognition and treatment of such immunologic reactions. Mammalian insulins differ in structure, but human and pork insulins are identical, except pork insulin has an alanine at position 30 of the B-chain and human insulin has a threonine. Desalanine-porcine insulin is being investigated experimentally. Pork insulin is the least antigenic, whereas beef insulin is significantly antigenic to most patients.

Until 1972, commercial insulin contained around 7 to 8% noninsulin ingredients, mainly proinsulin, proinsulin intermediates, and C-peptide. Proinsulin is composed of the 33-35 amino-acid C-peptide chain plus the A- and B-chains of insulin connected by their disulfide bridges. The final step in the release of insulin takes place when the C-peptide chain splits off in the beta cell granule and is released into the circulation in concentration equimolar to insulin. (The laboratory method for determining levels of endogenous insulin in the presence of exogenous insulin uses C-peptide measurement.)

In discussing allergic reactions to insulin, one must realize that the most common are related to the purity as well as to the immunogenic property of a given insulin. Pork insulin is less antigenic than beef insulin for most persons, since at positions 8, 9, and 10 in the A-chain (highly immunogenic sites), pork and human insulin are identical. Beef insulin differs at positions 8 and 10. It has been recently reported that no cases of allergy, fat hypertrophy, or fat atrophy have been reported in patients treated with purified pork insulin.

Several hormones other than insulin are implicated as "impurities" in the commercial preparation of insulin. Proinsulin is the main indicator of insulin purity, although glucagon, somatostatin, and pancreatic polypeptide are also extracted from the islet cells. In order to remove such substances, 2 procedures are now employed. The first is gel-filtration, which separates proteins according to molecular size, and the second is ionic exchange, which separates proteins according to ionic charge. The "single-peak" insulin marketed in 1972 was subjected to gel-filtration chromatography only. This insulin had a proinsulin content of 300 to 3000 parts per million. Since April of 1980, all insulin marketed by Eli Lilly and Company is subjected to purification by both gel-filtration and ionic exchange, resulting in "improved single peak" and "purified" insulins. The proinsulin content of the mixed beef-pork single peak insulin is less than 50 parts per million, and the purified pork and purified beef insulins both have fewer than 10 parts per million. Novo and Nordisk of Denmark also market similarly purified pork and beef insulins in the United States.

There is some evidence that neutral regular insulin is less antigenic than NPH or Lente insulins. NPH contains the protein protamine, whereas the Lente family contains no foreign proteins. There is little clinical evidence that protamine itself is antigenic in man.

Recent studies suggest that the immune response to insulin may be genetic, and several investigations are being pursued. Early reports indicate that a strong human response to insulin may be associated with HLA B15 and Cw 3, but that B8 and another unidentified HLA locus are associated with a weak immune response to insulin.

## CUTANEOUS REACTIONS

Almost all diabetics who take exogenous insulin at the beginning have variable degrees of skin reactions at the injection site that last from a few hours to several months. Some reactions appear immediately following injection, while others are delayed for 6 to 8 hours. Some subside within a few minutes; others last 24 to 48 hours or longer. Almost 50% of patients who have an insulin allergy have allergies to other drugs. The severity of the local reaction varies from almost none to stinging, burning, and itching, with swelling, erythema, and even induration. Treatment usually relieves the symptoms and minimizes the local reactions.

The following are recommendations for treatment of cutaneous reactions to insulin:

1. Well over 50% of such reactions subside spontaneously within 30 to 60 days because they desensitize themselves. If discomfort at the site of injection is not severe, nothing further need be done.
2. One should check the patient's injection technique, making sure that the injection is subcutaneous and not intradermal.
3. One should be sure that the patient is using isopropyl alcohol and not rubbing alcohol, since an ingredient of the latter may be sensitizing.
4. With a switch to purified pork insulin, about 75% of such patients improve.
5. If the patient does not improve with purified pork insulin, he may respond to purified beef insulin, especially if the patient is a child.
6. One should mix small doses of dexamethasone with the insulin, starting with 0.04 mg in each injection. An alternative mixture is chlorpheniramine maleate (Chlortrimeton), using 0.1 ml of the 100 mg/ml strength, which gives a dose of 10 mg and shows as 10 units on the U-100 insulin syringe.
7. A rare patient may require desensitization—see discussion of systemic reactions in this chapter.
8. It has been suggested that in rare cases of skin allergy, the offending substance might be zinc, since all insulin preparations contain zinc. A skin test can be done for zinc allergy. If confirmed, the Eli Lilly Laboratory will supply zinc-free sodium insulin by request.

## SYSTEMIC ALLERGIC REACTIONS

Systemic allergic reactions to insulin are rare, but can elicit general bodily responses, including serum sickness, purpura, angioedema, and an Arthus phenomenon. There is often a history of having taken insulin in the past, with a lapse of months to years before resuming insulin injections.

The treatment of the acute stage of a systemic reaction is the same as for any other acute allergic reaction. Then, if the patient must have insulin to survive, the first step is to determine which insulin is the least antigenic for this patient. This usually proves to be pork insulin. In all cases of systemic allergy, the simplest and most satisfactory procedure is to use the Insulin Allergy Desensitization Kit furnished free on request by Eli Lilly and Company. A telephone call to the clinical research director is the appropriate first step. The primary care physician may want to consult a diabetologist when confronted with such a patient. Complete directions accompany the

Lilly kit and are not repeated here. About 90% of patients with severe systemic allergy to insulin can be desensitized by this method. Some of the remaining 10% may respond to low-dose steroid treatment, on a long-term basis.

## INSULIN RESISTANCE

The 24-hour endogenous insulin requirement for a healthy, 70-kg man is probably around 25 to 40 units. There is no fixed maximum exogenous insulin requirement for Type I diabetics over which they are classified as "insulin resistant." However, the generally accepted figure is over 200 U daily for the adult and over 2.5 U/kg body weight for the child. There is no complete satisfactory explanation for insulin resistance. One may speculate about a circulating insulin-binding antibody or perhaps a reduced cellular sensitivity. Recent studies have demonstrated a reduction in the number of cellular receptors and perhaps a decreased affinity for insulin in patients termed "insulin resistant." Further reports have suggested insulin degradation by an unidentified cellular hormone. True insulin resistance caused by a high titer of anti-insulin antibodies occurs rarely. The Joslin Clinic studied all patients seen between 1940 and 1960 and reported that 0.01% demonstrated true insulin resistance, i.e., 1 in every 10,000 diabetic patients. Again, as in insulin allergy, there is a history of intermittent insulin treatment in more than 50% of these patients.

It is astounding to realize that, in a high percentage of insulin-resistant patients, more than 1000 U/day are required to establish any degree of normoglycemia. Patients requiring up to 25,000 U/day have been reported, but it is unlikely that this phenomenon represents the effects of insulin antibodies alone. One must always keep in mind some rare clinical states associated with insulin resistance, such as hyperfunction of the anterior pituitary or the adrenal cortex, resulting in excessive production of growth hormone and cortisol. Liver disease, leukemia, and lipoatrophic diabetes are included in the differential diagnosis. Quantitative measurement of anti-insulin antibodies is easily done and confirms the diagnosis. In most cases, increased titers of IgG antibody to beef insulin are found, and a reading of 50 mU/ml or greater is generally felt to indicate immunologic insulin resistance.

The treatment of insulin resistance is successful. First, one should be aware that in more than half these patients, spontaneous recovery takes place within 6 months. However, there is no way to predict which patients will undergo spontaneous recovery, so steps should be taken, the first of which is to prescribe purified pork insulin. Because antibodies sometimes bind insulin at the injection site and prolong its action, it is preferable to start with 2 doses per day of regular insulin, and in 4 to 6 weeks one can switch to intermediate-acting insulins. Ordinarily, if the patient's diabetic control has been poor with the previous insulin, with blood sugar levels of over 250 mg/dl, one should use the same amount of pork insulin. If blood sugar levels have been under 200 mg/dl, then one should prescribe only half the previous dose of insulin and adjust as indicated by degree of control. This process results in a decrease in insulin requirements in about 50% of these patients. The physician should make certain to reduce the patient's total dose as indicated by blood glucose levels, urine tests, and early evidence of hypoglycemic episodes. Experimentally, other less antigenic insulins are being tried, such as fish and desalanine-pork insulin and an encouraging preparation known as sulfated insulin, which appears to be less antigenic than either beef or pork insulin. Reports in the literature indicate that the average insulin-resistant patient who changes to sulfated insulin requires about 15% of his former insulin dose for diabetic control. The primary care physician should consult with a specialist before entering into a treatment program for his insulin-resistant patients. If all else fails, one can use glucocorticoid agents on a short-term basis. One should start with high doses, 60 to 80 mg, of prednisone per day, lowering the dosage as rapidly as possible, certainly within 2 to 3 weeks. The drug should be discontinued when most evidence of insulin resistance has disappeared. Caution is needed, since individual response is not predictable, and all side effects are prominent. A complete discussion of such therapy with the patient is certainly in order before starting.

Two unusual forms of insulin resistance are worth noting. One type is due to destruction of insulin at the subcutaneous or intramuscular injection site. Patients so affected respond to intravenous insulin. Aprotinin, a pancreatic protease inhibitor, can be added to insulin for such patients. The second type is due to a defect in insulin's relation to cell receptors. A response has been documented, using several thousand units given intravenously.

## LIPOATROPHY

Loss of subcutaneous fat at the site of insulin injection, mainly in young female patients, has been observed for many years. Numerous theories of its cause have been proposed. The condition is probably due to impurities in commercial insulin preparations, since the use of purified insulins relieves most cases of lipoatrophy. In about 15% of these patients, a local cutaneous allergy is also present, and this must be alleviated before the lipatrophy is arrested. This relationship gives rise to the theory that abnormal immune response is an etiologic factor. At any rate, the physician should prescribe purified pork insulin and should tell the patient to inject it in the perimeter of the atrophic area. Filling in of subcutaneous fat may be noticeable in the first few weeks, but severe areas may not be restored completely for 6 months or more. It has been reported that this procedure is efficacious for over 95% of patients with lipoatrophy. Once the area is filled in, one must be sure to advise patients to continue to rotate sites of injection, so that fat hypertrophy is avoided.

## LIPOHYPERTROPHY

This is the occurrence of fatty tumors at the site of insulin injection and is probably not an immune response, but is simply the physiologic magnification of the function of insulin to stimulate lipogenesis. It develops most often in patients who fail to rotate injection sites. Lipohypertrophy is usually relieved by the simple procedure of rotating injection sites, but there apparently is some further advantage to using purified pork insulin. The hypertrophic areas eventually disappear if the patient avoids injecting insulin into them.

# 14

# Obesity

Hundreds of books and thousands of reports have been written on the problem of obesity, both in diabetes and in general. Prevention and treatment of obesity are almost insurmountable problems for the average primary care physician. Obesity is defined as a weight for height, age, and build that is 20% above normal. The risks associated with obesity become far more severe when a person exceeds normal weight by 25% or more.

## RISK OF OBESITY

Obesity alone is not as great a risk factor as was formerly believed, but it rarely occurs alone. Most often, obesity is accompanied by high blood pressure, hyperlipidemia, gout, and diabetes. Then, it becomes an important risk factor, and mortality from almost all causes is greater in these persons. Furthermore, the greater the obesity, the greater the risk.

Obesity cannot be accurately measured by weight alone, since a 250-lb football player may not have any excess fat. Sophisticated methods are used in research programs to determine fat excess accurately, but for most patients, charts work well. The experienced physician has little problem in determining whether or not obesity exists. A simple rule to remember for average normal weights for persons of medium build is as follows:

> Female—100 lb for 60″, plus 5 lb/inch above 60″
> Male—106 lb for 60″, plus 6 lb/inch above 60″
> If light frame, deduct 10%; if heavy frame, add 10%.

In the United States, 35% of the population between ages 50 and 70 are overweight (not all obese), but 50% of women in this age group are overweight. Persons who weigh 25 to 30% above normal have a 130 to 150% mortality rate, according to insurance statistics. The risk, greater for men, is greatest when obesity occurs at a younger age. Obesity has a profound effect on cardiac and pulmonary function, among other things.

### Risk of Diabetes

Obesity is the *main cause* of diabetes. Between 60 and 75% of all Type II diabetics are obese at the onset of diabetes. Obesity is another body stress, which the metabolic system cannot handle above a given level. Since about 70% of all diabetes appears after age 45, it is easy to see why the physician's main job in treating these patients is to see that they lose weight.

One does not have to be severely obese to be at high risk for diabetes. Moderately obese persons are 5 times more likely to have diabetes, and the risk increases with the degree of obesity. In a study of a large group of middle-aged men in Norway some years ago, researchers did not find a single case of diabetes in men who were underweight. In almost all the races of the world, a high incidence of diabetes occurs with obesity; incidentally, the same is true of pet dogs.

The physician should ask all his new, older, obese patients whether they have diabetes. If they do not, he should look for it anyway because there is a high chance of it.

## PATHOGENESIS OF DIABETES IN OBESE PERSONS

The newly diagnosed obese diabetic has a normal concentration of endogenous insulin; in some cases, even an excess. The obese nondiabetic adult often produces more than the normal amount of insulin. What factors produce diabetes in one but not in another? The answers are not entirely known. There is now ample evidence that the obese Type II diabetic has a decrease in the number of cell receptors for insulin, and in addition, a probable decreased affinity for insulin. A theory of possible insulin degradation at the cell level has been proposed, but there is little evidence to prove it. Undiscovered hormone factors could play a part. It is obvious that receptors are sensitive to loss of excess fat, since weight reduction almost always restores cell receptors to normal numbers.

Excess production of insulin by the beta cells may continue for 10 to 20 years in obese diabetics. However, at some time, if the patient lives that long, the beta cells may become exhausted and may not be able to produce the amount of insulin necessary, so that exogenous insulin must be given. Studies being done on obese diabetics, by measuring serum insulin levels, will answer some of these questions in the future.

## TREATMENT OF OBESE DIABETICS

The most difficult task facing the physician in the treatment of obese diabetics is making sure that they lose weight. Even partial weight loss reverses the diabetic state. In many patients, diabetes completely disappears (is "cured") and rarely returns unless the patient becomes obese again. Studies have shown drops in blood glucose levels within 10 to 14 days of severe caloric restriction, even though weight loss in pounds was minor.

### Diet Therapy

Diet therapy is the only sensible therapy for the obese diabetic. How easy it is to write that simple sentence—reduce the patient and cure the diabetes! After 26 years of practice with hundreds of fat diabetics, no one knows better than I how difficult it is. My success ratio over the years is about 6 to 8%, and if I counted the long-range follow-up, it is closer to 4%.

The physician should not be overenthusiastic about the restriction of calories when first prescribing a diet plan for obese diabetics. The physician and the dietitian should sit down with the patient and find out how much food this person can "live with." In other words, will he adhere to this diet and be content? If the calorie level is such that the patient loses only 1 pound every 2 weeks, that is all right—after all, 2 pounds a month is about 25 pounds per year. Reinforcement is important. The patient should have brief chats with the dietitian every 6 weeks or so. Encouragement and praise from the physician is also of psychologic benefit. In addition, one must elicit the help of the other members of the patient's family.

Other aids are also available. First, group therapy is helpful, just as it is for alcoholics. Weight Watchers and similar organizations can be useful to a motivated patient. Weight-loss clinics, with reputable personnel, also do a good, but usually expensive, job. Exercise can be helpful when done on a regular basis. For details of exercise planning for the obese patient, see Chapter 10. Behavior modification classes have their share of success. I mention surgical intestinal by-pass procedures only to condemn them. I do not feel that they have any place in the management of the obese diabetic.

The physician must explain thoroughly to his obese patients the consequences of continued obesity. Elevated blood sugar levels alone are the least of their worries, since patients are generally unaware of unpleasant symptoms from a blood sugar level of 250 to

350 mg/dl. However, they should know the mortality risk and the risk of cardiovascular diseases, and that they are not immune from microvascular complications—Type II diabetics frequently lose their sight from retinopathy. They also can have severe neuropathy. When associated with hypertension, the risk of cerebrovascular accidents is high.

### Oral Antidiabetes Agents

Should one prescribe oral antidiabetes tablets? I think so, when diet obviously is not going to work. One should give the patient a trial of 3 months on diet alone and then suggest a sulfonylurea for help. Before 1977, phenformin was a great aid in reducing blood sugar levels in obese diabetics, but the life-threatening possibility of lactic acidosis caused the drug to be banned in the United States. If diet and sulfonylureas together do not work, and the patient has a midday blood sugar level of 350 mg/dl but still feels well, insulin may be considered.

### Insulin

Should one prescribe insulin? This is a moot question. Some of the best diabetologists in the country give insulin and others would not hear of it. It is disturbing to have a patient with a blood sugar level of 350 mg/dl, which might damage his vascular system, his large nerve trunks, or even his retina. It is known that insulin does have 2 disadvantages for the fat diabetic: it stimulates appetite and it helps to lay down fat, i.e., it is lipogenic. Many fat persons are resistant to insulin, and in order to lower their high blood sugar levels, 100 U or more of insulin are needed. The rare older obese diabetic, for some unknown reason, can suddenly lose the ability to secrete insulin, and in essence, becomes a Type I diabetic. This patient may even develop diabetic ketoacidosis. Large amounts of insulin given to obese Type II diabetes may cause an increase in triglyceride concentrations. So, although the answer is unknown, I feel that if a patient has complications of diabetes, he must be given insulin when all else has failed. Moreover, if the physician feels more secure with the patient who takes insulin, he should prescribe it.

## MOTIVATION

Generally, motivation is the key to success or failure. Does the patient think that he should lose weight, or is it his spouse or children who think so? If the patient is not motivated, all is lost, and one might as well forget any attempts at a weight-loss program.

Some persons enjoy being fat, and that enjoyment overpowers their fear of the complications of obesity. We probably should say that some persons enjoy doing the things that make them fat.

Certain older diabetics, for whom eating may be their only remaining pleasure, do not care about losing weight for the sake of living a few years longer. I can appreciate their philosophy, since it becomes philosophy rather than science at that point. So, I sit down with my obese older patients, most often women, and ask them whether they are interested in living a few extra years in trade for an austere dietary regimen. In a surprising number of patients, the answer is straightforward—they would rather continue their present eating habits and take the consequences. This decision relieves the patient of frustration over not being able to please the physician, and it relieves the physician of worrying about how to make the patient stay on a diet of 800 or 1000 calories. The physician should give the patient a diet that seems workable, even though he knows that the patient will follow her own dietary rules. At any rate, the physician has done his part in explaining the risks to the patient, and the patient has made the decision.

I am astounded that all obese patients are not motivated enough to reduce their weight at least partially, knowing that this loss could well result in (1) "cure" of the diabetes, (2) reduction of hypertension, (3) reduction of elevated cholesterol and/or triglyceride levels, (4) reduction of elevated uric acid (if present), (5) their feeling better when they look in the mirror, and (6) a longer life.

In summary, obesity is the main cause of diabetes. Over 70% of all diabetics are Type II, and over 60% of all such diabetics are overweight at the onset of their diabetes. Obesity by itself does not carry as great a risk as when it is combined with other factors, including hyperlipidemia, hypertension, hyperuricemia, and of course, diabetes. All obese individuals are at greater risk for cardiovascular events and early death. Weight loss reverses most of the pathologic effects and reduces the patient's risk, but in spite of these benefits, enforcing a weight-loss program is one of the most difficult tasks facing the physician. Nonprofessional persons who supervise group therapy are the most successful, and one should enlist their help. One should not overlook the benefit of a regular exercise program, and walking is one of the easiest forms of exercise.

# 15

# Surgery

Diabetic patients who are maintained in good control can undergo any type of surgical procedures. There is a slight increase for diabetics in overall mortality rates for all types of operations—3.4%, as compared with 2.5% for nondiabetic patients. Special attention must be directed to certain areas of importance to diabetics' altered physiology and metabolism, such as (1) insulin or oral antidiabetes agents, (2) maintenance of water and electrolyte balance, (3) choice of and duration of anesthesia, (4) avoidance of anoxia because of added cardiovascular risk, and (5) control of infection.

As with nondiabetic patients, the stress of surgical procedures stimulates secretion of those stress hormones that act either as insulin antagonists or as hyperglycemic stimulants. Included in this group are corticosteroids, catecholamines, glucagon, and growth hormone. Any steps that the physician can take to minimize this stress are helpful to the patient.

## PREOPERATIVE PREPARATION FOR ELECTIVE SURGICAL PROCEDURES

The physician's job in the preoperative preparation of the diabetic patient is much simpler if the operation is planned for a given time and if the physician has seen the patient at frequent intervals during the week before to fine tune his diabetic control and to make sure that he is in the best of metabolic balance. One warning—the patient's diabetes should not be controlled too closely, since it is generally better for his blood sugar level to be a bit hyperglycemic than hypoglycemic. Urine test results that show up to ½% sugar and FBS levels in the order of 160 mg/dl, with postprandial levels slightly higher, satisfy the patient's metabolic needs. Hypoglycemia during any surgical procedure is physiologically harmful. In some surgical procedures, hypoglycemia can stimulate bleeding from the surgical site, as in eye operations, so it must be avoided.

The physician should try to have his diabetic patient scheduled as the first surgical case in the morning, since this timing simplifies the control of the patient's metabolism during the day. However, if an infection is present, and the procedure is scheduled for last, then one must program insulin and IV fluids to meet the patient's needs.

The physician should never allow anesthesiologists to write insulin orders for his patients. They are not generally familiar with patients' requirements and, what is more important, they are not generally familiar with the management of diabetes, and we do not expect them to be. It is usually prudent to discuss IV fluid requirements for the patient with the anesthesiologist. At that time, the physician can indicate that he plans to handle the patient's insulin orders.

## MINOR SURGICAL PROCEDURES

For most diabetics undergoing minor surgical procedures, when oral feedings will be resumed at lunchtime, one should simply omit the patient's morning insulin or oral agents. Then one should give the patient about half to two-thirds the usual dose after the noon meal, when one can be sure the patient has eaten all or most of the meal. Sometimes, lingering nausea causes him to lose his appetite, so he must then be given an even smaller amount of insulin or oral agents. Occasionally, an IV infusion of 5% glucose is needed to allay the nausea and to hydrate the patient.

## MAJOR ELECTIVE SURGICAL PROCEDURES

Different procedures apply to Type I and Type II diabetics who are undergoing major operations.

### Type II Diabetics

**Admission to Hospital.** The patient should be admitted the evening before the operation. One should obtain a blood glucose determination before supper and a fasting glucose reading the next morning.

**Oral Antidiabetes Agents.** These drugs should be discontinued. On the morning of the operation, one should administer 5% glucose IV in saline solution. Depending on the level of the fasting blood glucose, regular insulin is added to the IV infusion. If the patient is well controlled by diet alone and his diabetes is mild, there is probably no need for insulin in the bottle. If the patient takes oral agents and his FBS level is in the 150- to 200-mg/dl range, one should add 5 to 10 U regular insulin to the IV infusion bottle, assuming the rate of infusion is about 150 ml/hr. Subsequent additions of insulin to further IV solutions depend on the results of the blood sugar tests taken during or after the operation. Do not get excited about insulin's sticking to the wall of the bottle and tubing—it does, but only about 10%—so 1 unit out of 10 units would be lost this way, and if it worries you, add 11 units instead of 10. Always use purified pork insulin.

**Blood Glucose Determinations.** If the physician is concerned about the patient's blood sugar response to the added insulin, he should do a blood sugar test while the patient is in the operating room. One must be sure that the technician obtains the blood from the arm that is not connected to the IV equipment. One can allow a 25- to 50-mg/dl additional increment when glucose is being administered, as a rule, so one should remember to subtract this increment from the laboratory figure to give a more accurate approximation. If the operation is major and prolonged, blood sugar levels may need to be checked more frequently.

The physician should always ask for a blood sugar reading about 2 hours after the operation. He must be certain to inform the nurse to call the result to his office. Otherwise, it is easy, in the busy office routine, to forget about the diabetic patient recovering from the operation.

### Diabetics Undergoing Surgical Procedures Who Are Controlled by Insulin (both Type I and Type II)

**Insulin.** There are 2 generally accepted methods of giving insulin on the day of a surgical procedure. One can either give half the usual morning dose subcutaneously prior to the procedure or one can control the glycemia with regular insulin added to the IV infusion. I favor the former, in which half the dose of NPH or Lente or a mixture gives a basis to work from. I hesitate to give more than that, since hypoglycemia should be avoided, and one should not mind if the patient's blood sugar level is between 160 and 260 mg/dl during an operation. However, in patients whose total daily insulin requirement is small, half the usual dose of NPH or Lente insulin may be too much. Therefore, I suggest the following:

If the patient has mild Type I diabetes, requires fewer than 30 U/day of insulin for diabetic control, and his FBS is not more than 50 mg/dl above normal on the morning of the operation, he should not have any depot insulin, but should control his diabetes entirely with regular insulin in IV infusions, relying on interval blood sugar checks to determine the amount needed.

If the patient takes over 40 U/day of insulin, then he should have half his usual morning dose of NPH or Lente subcutaneously prior to the surgical procedure.

If an operation will not be done until afternoon, one should not give the patient half his usual morning dose subcutaneously in the morning, but about 45 minutes prior to the start of the operation. Since 5% glucose IV is running slowly (q8h) while the patient awaits the operation, one can add regular insulin to this first bottle, in the amount of 10 to 15 U, again depending on the patient's usual daily dose. In addition, a blood sugar test should be ordered approximately 45 minutes before the patient is called to the operating room. This test is a valuable help in determining the patient's insulin dose. The output of stress hormones usually starts with the operation, and this is the reason for giving the half dose beforehand.

**IV Fluids.** Every diabetic needs 50 g glucose every 8 hours for energy and to avoid ketosis, so this means at least 1000 ml 5% glucose to be given every 8 hours. The first infusion of 5% glucose IV during an operation generally does not have insulin added to the bottle except as outlined. However, if the surgical procedure lasts longer than 60 to 90 minutes, one should draw blood for a glucose test at the 90-minute point. One should make certain that the laboratory knows it must be done immediately. If the result is over 280 mg/dl, one should add 10 to 15 U regular insulin per 1000 ml IV fluid, the exact amount depending on the patient's usual daily dose. Generally, if his total daily requirements are under 30 U, one should add 10 U regular insulin; if his daily requirements are over 40 U, one should add 15 U regular insulin. Susequent additions again must be determined by blood sugar levels, determined as often as necessary to ensure the patient's welfare.

**Urine Tests.** These are generally an unreliable guide to insulin dosage during or immediately after an operation. I rely on them only if blood sugar tests cannot be done. Some hospitals have instruments for immediate glucose checks on the surgical floor with a nurse or aide who is instructed to run blood sugar tests. Thus, one can obtain a result in under 10 minutes from the time the blood sample is taken.

## Follow-up Care

If the patient is to receive IV fluids for several days, insulin requirements will probably remain at half the usual dose or less, barring complications or infections. One can continue to administer regular insulin in the IV infusion bottle, or one may control the patient's diabetes with his morning subcutaneous dose of insulin, the amount depending on daily FBS levels. Each postoperative day, one should obtain both fasting and 4 P.M. blood sugar levels.

In the unusual patient whose insulin requirements are high and for whom the stress of a surgical procedure has been marked, it may be necessary to give supplemental doses of regular insulin in addition to the IV insulin. The need for this supplement is indicated by a progressive rise in blood sugar levels to above 300 mg/dl.

The patient should resume eating as soon as possible. Since he will probably start with a limited caloric intake, the depot insulin dose had best be cut back to half of the usual dose or less. One can supplement this with small doses of regular insulin before lunch and supper, guided now by urine glucose tests done q.i.d.

## EMERGENCY SURGICAL PATIENTS

In the case of an acute appendicitis, or a ruptured viscus, or an accident, when immediate surgical intervention is indicated, one must handle the patient's diabetic state by careful and repeated observations concerning fluids, electrolytes, and insulin. There is no rule of thumb for such cases. One must not hesitate to use the laboratory for frequent and repeated determinations of blood glucose levels, electrolytes, bicarbonate, and/or pH, if impending ketosis is suspected. Control of blood glucose levels in such cases is best done with repeated doses of regular insulin, either subcutaneous, IM, or IV. The physician can follow a protocol similar to that found in this book for treatment of diabetic ketoacidosis. Most patients do well when supplied with adequate fluid, electrolytes, oxygen, and insulin. One must remember that such a patient needs his physician's attention or that of a reliable house officer almost continuously for the first critical hours. This need may necessitate an all-night vigil, to minister to the metabolic requirements of a diabetic undergoing an emergency and perhaps lifesaving operation. Maybe soon we shall be able to neutralize medically the excess secretion of stress hormones that antagonize the diabetic state, but are needed by the body to bolster its defenses. There must be a neutral ground somewhere.

## RESUMING ORAL ANTIDIABETES TABLETS

There is a tendency for the attending physician to continue to prescribe insulin for the diabetic patient indefinitely after an operation, even though control was excellent preoperatively with sulfonylurea tablets. Surgical procedures do not worsen the diabetic state beyond the first 10 to 14 postoperative days (without complications), so there is no reason that the patient cannot return to his former program, provided it controlled the diabetes satisfactorily.

## MISCELLANEOUS REMINDERS

The following should be kept in mind with regard to diabetic patients who are undergoing operations.

1. Regional or spinal anesthesia is preferred whenever possible.
2. If the patient has cerebral sclerosis or nephropathy, doses of sedatives must be reduced.
3. Hypoxemia, shock, and similar disorders generally reduce the patient's insulin requirements.
4. One should not try to attain strict control of the patient's diabetes during and right after an operation. Blood sugar levels between 150 and 250 mg/dl are best.
5. The charge nurse should be reminded that the postoperative patient has diabetes and requires the usual extra nursing observation, particularly during the first 48 postoperative hours. In addition, the physician should leave a written order on the patient's chart to be called should any unusual change take place in the condition of the patient or in the amount of sugar showing in the urine tests. Postoperative diabetics have been known to develop ketoacidosis, which is inexcusable.
6. When the physician resumes the full preoperative prescription of insulin or oral agents, he should make certain that the patient is eating all the food on his tray.

# 16

# Infections and Skin Disorders

## INFECTIONS

It is the general opinion of practicing physicians that diabetics are predisposed to infections, despite statistical studies that indicate that only urinary tract infections occur with significantly greater frequency. However, one must remember that certain unusual and frequently fatal infections are known to occur only in diabetics. In addition, foot infections are far more frequent in diabetics. No doubt the state of control of the patient's glycemia has a direct bearing on the course of infection and recovery. Infections account for about 25% of the deaths associated with ketoacidosis.

### Miscellaneous Infections

Some of the infections that occur to a greater extent in diabetics are discussed in the following sections.

**Malignant External Otitis.** This usually occurs in elderly diabetics. Symptoms and signs are ear pain and drainage and swelling of the soft tissues about the ear. Granulation tissue is abundant in the ear canal at the osseus-cartilage junction. Half these patients suffer a facial nerve palsy. The primary care physician should consult an otolaryngologist. *Pseudomonas aeruginosa* is the most common infecting organism.

**Rhinocerebral Mucormycosis.** This rare infection is caused by fungi of the genera mucor, rhizopus, and absidia and usually occurs in acidotic patients. Two-thirds of all patients with this disease have diabetes. Although the infection occurs rarely, the physician should recognize it early, since it responds to treatment with amphotericin B. Patients have sudden periorbital pain with nasal discharge that is bloody at first, but later may be black, owing to necrosis of the nasal turbinates. Signs of extension to the meninges and brain may be present. Untreated patients frequently die within 6 to 8 days.

**Tuberculosis.** At one time, this disease was a serious problem for diabetic patients, but, as with the nondiabetic population, its incidence is low, and it is no higher in diabetics. However, periodic skin testing in diabetics known to be tuberculin-negative is advisable.

**Bacterial Pneumonia.** Pneumonia contributes to fatalities in cases of ketoacidosis. Underlying bacteria are frequently *Klebsiella pneumoniae, Staphylococcus aureus,* and *Escherichia coli*; few are of pneumococcal origin. Why diabetic patients have more infections with gram-negative or staphylococcal organisms is unknown.

**Emphysematous Cholecystitis.** This is a rare infection, but over one-third of such cases occur in diabetics. It is a mixed aerobic and anaerobic infection, with evidence of gas around the gallbladder. Symptoms are similar to those of acute cholecystitis. Complications, including gangrene of the gallbladder and perforations, are not uncommon. Mortality is 15 to 25% higher than in acute cholecystitis. Treatment includes cholecystectomy and broad-spectrum antibiotic therapy.

**Skin and Soft-Tissue Infections.** Although not proven in any long-range statistical studies, it is apparent to the physician who treats diabetes that staphylococcal skin infections are not unusual, including furuncles and carbuncles. There is well-substantiated evidence that diabetes predisposes patients to staphylococcal colonization of the skin and nasopharynx. It has been stated that one-third of insulin-dependent diabetics are staphylococcus carriers, compared with 10% of the nondiabetic population. Postoperative clean-wound infections may be more frequent in diabetics.

**Bacteremia.** Gram-negative sepsis occurs more frequently in diabetics. In one series of studies, *E. coli* from the urinary tract was the source of infection in 86% of the cases of bacteremia. The mortality rate is higher than in nondiabetics. In addition to gram-negative sepsis, diabetes seems to predispose patients to group B streptococcal bacteremia.

**Necrotizing Soft-Tissue Infections.** Seventy-five per cent of patients with necrotizing cellulitis have Type II diabetes, are middle-aged, and are obese. Such infections are characterized by necrosis of the skin and subcutaneous tissue and frequently by cellulitis of the underlying muscle caused by mixed aerobic-anaerobic organisms. The lower extremities and the perineum are favorite sites. Small skin ulcers may drain a reddish-brown, foul-smelling fluid, and subcutaneous emphysema occurs in about 25% of patients. Organisms isolated from patients include anaerobic streptococci, bacteroides, and aerobic or facultative gram-negative bacilli, including pseudomonas and enterococci. Bacteremia occurs in 50% of the patients. Treatment requires parenteral antibiotics as well as indicated surgical intervention and drainage. Mortality approaches 60% in diabetics with necrotizing cellulitis, in spite of therapy.

**Nonclostridial Gas Gangrene.** This is a rare but rapidly fatal disease in diabetics if not diagnosed and treated early. It is frequently secondary to a Bartholin cyst infection or anal or perineal involvement, such as an anal fistula. Half such infections occur in patients with diabetes. These infections are usually caused by a mixture of aerobic and anaerobic organisms. Response to early antibiotic therapy, combined with surgical incision and debridement, is frequently lifesaving.

**Group B Streptococcal Infection in Pregnancy.** Neonates of diabetic mothers are at an increased risk of acquiring a group B streptococcal infection in the first 10 days of life, particularly if the mother has a low level of antibodies. Meningitis or pulmonary infection may result from such infection. One must watch the newborn carefully for any signs of such infection.

**Fungal Infections (Vaginal).** Mucocutaneous candida is frequently found in the young female diabetic who has continuous glucosuria. When a patient complains of burning, itching, and probably vaginal discharge, one can almost always be certain to find *Candida albicans* as the culprit. This infection is a leading sign and symptom in new and untreated diabetes. The available antimycotic preparations work well, although recurring infections may fail to respond. Other mycotic infections frequently found are caused by *Coccidioides immitis* and *Malassezia furfur*.

**Foot Infections.** These are discussed in Chapter 17.

There is evidence that the increased incidence of certain infections in diabetics may be related to the decrease in chemotaxis of the polymorphonuclear leukocytes as well as decreased phagocytosis. Other factors that affect host resistance need further study in the diabetic population.

## Urinary Tract Infections

Urinary tract infections, common in female diabetics, are frequently overlooked since they are often initially asymptomatic. It is important that such infections be recognized and treated immediately to prevent ascending infection, with its potentially serious involvement of the renal parenchyma. There is evidence that repeated urinary tract infections may accelerate the nephropathy that results in renal decompensation and ultimate failure.

Every diabetic patient should bring a clean, midstream urine specimen for complete analysis, including careful microscopic examination, at each office visit. Two of the most important findings are proteinuria and bacteriuria. For years, the question has been asked whether to treat asymptomatic bacteriuria vigorously in the diabetic. The general agreement is that if the urine has 100,000 or more bacteria per ml on quantitative culture, treatment is indicated. In a recent study of 230 female diabetic patients, almost 20% were found to have urinary tract infections as compared with 5% of a control group. No difference was found in diabetic men.

How can one tell whether the infection is limited to the bladder or whether the renal parenchyma has been invaded? A new diagnostic technique makes this differentiation in almost all cases. Antibody coating of bacteria is determined by an immunofluorescence test. The presence of antibody-coated bacteria indicates an infection of renal origin, whereas the absence of antibody coating means that the bladder is the probable site of infection. In the previously mentioned study, 79% of the women with urinary tract infections were found to have antibody-coated bacteria, thus suggesting ascending infections.

The consequences of renal parenchymal infection may range from a mild and treatable acute pyelonephritis to a severe and sometimes fatal renal abscess. In between, one may see emphysematous pyelonephritis, characterized by gas production in and around the kidneys. (Emphysematous cystitis is recognized by the patient's passing gas with urination.) In addition, a more serious involvement is that of papillary necrosis, which presumably is the result of both infection and ischemia. Perinephric abscesses occur infrequently, but may be serious in the diabetic.

In addition to bacterial infections, diabetics are predisposed to fungal infections of the urinary tract, particularly candida, but occasionally also infections caused by *Torulopsis glabrata*. However, most fungal infections of the urinary tract are clinically insignificant. Fungal infections may rarely result in cystitis, pyelonephritis, renal or perinephric abscesses, and occasionally a clinical picture that resembles a gram-negative sepsis. For diagnosis of a significant fungal infection, urologists generally feel that a fungal count of 10,000/ml urine is significant, although higher fungal concentrations frequently do not produce symptomatic infections. One should consult a competent urologist if a serious fungal infection threatens a patient.

What course of action should be taken by the primary care physician in handling urinary tract infections in his diabetic patients?

1. He should do a complete urinalysis, including careful microscopic examination, on a clean, midstream urine specimen at each office visit.
2. If obvious and symptomatic lower urinary tract infection is present, treatment is the same as for any other patient with supposedly simple acute cystitis. If the infection does not clear within 10 to 14 days, the physician should seek urologic consultation, since a complete renal study may be indicated.
3. If the patient has symptoms of renal parenchyma involvement, which might include fever, chills, flank pain, and abdominal pain, one should not hesitate to enlist the help of a urologist.
4. If bacteriuria only is seen on microscopic examination and the patient is asymptomatic (this occurs frequently), further study depends on the judgment of the physician. So much depends on the technician who examines the slide of urinary sediment; he may report the presence of bacteria in small, moderate, or heavy concentrations. Many physicians look at the slides and make their own decisions.

   Many laboratories report bacteria as follows:

   Trace—0 to 2/H.P.F. (high-powered field)
   1+—3 to 10
   2+—11 to 20
   3+—20 to 150
   4+—packed field

   A 3+ or 4+ finding warrants a second urinalysis, and if consistent, then a quantitative culture.
5. Does the presence of glucosuria play a part in urinary tract infections? In one study, the number of patients with positive cultures in the presence of 1 to 2% glucosuria was identical to the number of patients with negative cultures, also showing 1 to 2% glucosuria. One would feel that urinary sugar provides nutriment for bacteria, but this may not be significant.
6. When treatment is completed, the physician should pay particular attention to urinary findings at weekly intervals for several weeks, since recurrences and relapses are common. Relapses mean reinfection with the same organism, whereas recurrences may be infections by the same or new organisms. It may be wise to extend the course of treatment in many diabetics beyond the usually accepted 10 to 14 days, in order to prevent recurrences.

## SKIN DISORDERS

### Necrobiosis Lipoidica Diabeticorum (NLD)

One occasionally sees this skin lesion on the pretibial area, mainly in young female diabetics. The lesions are best described as circumscribed, shiny, atrophic plaques with an erythematous border and sometimes a yellowish central area. Telangiectatic vessels course through the lesion. Occasionally, a smaller plaque spontaneously disappears. The etiology of this disorder is unknown, but it is probably related to a diminished blood supply in the involved areas. The lesions may precede the onset of clinical diabetes by several years, but generally they occur in patients who have had diabetes for years. There is no relation to the degree of diabetic control. Young women are embarrassed by the appearance of the lesions, which are difficult to hide with cover-up makeup. However, a waterproof leg makeup is sold under the name of Ultima II.

Treatment is not universally successful in curing the lesions, but is worth a trial. Intralesional injection of steroids every 3 to 4 weeks sometimes elicits a good response. Occlusive dressings with steroid ointments have helped in some cases. The latest treatment being investigated is the administration of aspirin and dipyridamole, apparently with encouraging results, although more studies are needed. The primary care physician should refer the patient to a dermatologist for continued treatment.

This skin lesion also occurs in persons who are not diabetic and who have normal glucose tolerance. Perhaps as many cases occur in nondiabetics as in diabetics. Many patients have been tested for up to 10 years without showing any evidence of glucose intolerance.

### Recurrent Bullae on Extremities

Diabetics occasionally experience recurrent outbreaks of tense bullae, filled with serosanguinous fluid that is bacteriologically sterile. These lesions appear mainly on toes, fingers, and forearms and vary in size from several millimeters to several centimeters. They are most often seen in persons who have had diabetes for more than 5 years. Generally, they dry and heal without scarring. The etiology is unknown, and there is no relation to the degree of control of blood sugar levels.

# 17

# Impaired Diabetic Limbs

Gangrene occurs with greater frequency in diabetic men and women than in the nondiabetic population. Approximately 50% of lower extremity amputations in diabetics are due to uncontrolled infections in the presence of adequate blood supply, whereas the rest are due to occlusive vascular disease, frequently complicated by spreading infection and gangrene. The important consideration is that many amputations can be avoided if the physician is familiar with extrinsic factors leading to infection and tissue breakdown. Etiologic factors include damage by external forces and pressures, thermal injuries, chronic edema, obesity, and fungal or bacterial invasion.

## NEUROPATHIC FOOT

It is important to remember that the foot is frequently involved with motor as well as sensory neuropathy. When this happens, the intrinsic muscles lose their strength, which in turn upsets the balance between deep toe flexors and long extensors. The foot deformity that results causes a protrusion of the balls of the foot (metatarsophalangeal joints), hammer toes, and arch elevation (pes cavus). The abnormal weight-bearing surfaces break down, and calluses and trophic ulcerations result. The coexisting sensory loss allows these changes to occur without the patient's realizing it. In extreme cases, sensory deprivation that results in fractures of the bones of the foot and/or ankle gives rise to Charcot's joint. All this is usually preventable or correctable. In addition to wearing proper footwear and to limiting foot pressures by other means, outlined in the final section of this chapter, one must teach the patient the importance of daily self-observation of his feet. He must be taught to look for calluses, small cracks, fissures, hot spots, small suppurations, and ingrowing toenails.

### Sympathetic Nerve Impairment

Loss of normal sweating results in a dry foot that is subject to scaling, cracking, and fissuring. The physician should advise the patient to have a daily foot bath in lukewarm water, followed by application of a water-soluble fat such as lanolin, olive oil, or Nivea cream.

New procedures in thermography techniques enable one to recognize neuropathic changes earlier.

## MICROANGIOPATHY

Although one does not usually associate arteriolar change with foot disorders, the fine arterioles supplying the skin of the foot do frequently occlude, resulting in painful and indolent ulcerations. Lesions are seen mainly on the tips of the toes, the posterior surface of the heel, and occasionally, on the lateral aspect of the leg. The ultimate in patience is needed for healing these lesions. Meanwhile, the lesions should be kept meticulously clean and protected from bacterial invasion.

## INTENSIVE TREATMENT OF FOOT ULCERS

Early and definitive treatment of foot ulcers is vitally important in saving the foot. The key to healing is to make the patient stay off his feet. This recommendation may mean an original period of hospitalization, since the patient may have painless neuropathic ulcers. One must remember to use heel protectors for the diabetic during bed rest. Intensive antibiotic treatment is a must, and anaerobic organisms are frequently found in these ulcers. Consultations with appropriate subspecialists are usually necessary to provide complete treatment.

## PERIPHERAL VASCULAR DISEASE

Peripheral vascular disease (PVD) can involve the large vessels, the medium to small vessels, or the microcirculation. Large vessel disease is not as frequent in diabetics as it is in nondiabetics, but when it does occur, it requires immediate diagnosis and treatment. Small vessel disease involves small arteries and arterioles, and the result of occlusion is patchy gangrene of the foot or toes. There may be fair pulsations in the dorsalis pedis or tibialis posterior arteries, even though small vessel gangrene is present. Microangiopathy is the result of capillary basement membrane thickening, which is greatest in the most dependent parts of the body.

The evaluation of risk factors varies with investigators, but cigarette smoking, hypertension, elevated cholesterol and/or triglyceride levels, and questionably hyperglycemia have all been implicated. Age over 50 and duration of diabetes are important factors. In addition to the intimal changes, a marked amount of medial calcification most often accompanies PVD in the diabetic. Vascular insufficiency often develops at an earlier age in diabetics, sometimes in those under age 40. Small vessel disease of the lower extremities may affect the patient's ultimate prognosis. The older diabetic is at greater risk of morbidity and mortality, so it is important for the physician to evaluate the degree of involvement and to formulate a plan for therapy as soon as it is obvious that the peripheral arterial circulation is compromised.

Diagnostic procedures are no different from those of nondiabetics, so only a brief review is included here:

1. Intermittent claudication is by far the outstanding complaint. Its location gives some clue to the area of the occlusive disease.
2. Rest pain after a period of exercise pain usually means increasing severity.
3. The patient should be examined carefully for bruits over large vessels.
4. An examination of the affected limb shows tight, shiny skin, with loss of hair, hypertrophy of toenails, and delayed return of capillary blush.
5. One should palpate for pulsations in the tibialis posterior, dorsalis pedis, and poplitea arteries.
6. Elevation pallor and delayed venous filling on lowering leg should be observed. Rubor on dependency of feet is present frequently.
7. Noninvasive tests include: Doppler's ultrasonography, for measurement of segmental pressures and analysis of pulse wave forms; plethysmography, to measure volume changes.
8. Since arteriography involves considerable morbidity and a 0.05% mortality risk, it is usually reserved for candidates for surgical reconstruction.

Medical treatment generally gives these patients little permanent relief from their symptoms. The following points should be kept in mind, however.

1. Walking shorter distances, using a shuffling gait, and taking frequent rest periods when walking may alleviate some of the pain.

2. Burger's exercises probably have more psychotherapeutic than physiologic value. If desired, the physician should instruct the patient to lie in bed, to elevate his legs for 1 minute (supported by the padded back of a chair), to let his legs hang down from the bed for 3 minutes, and to rest them horizontally on the bed for 6 minutes. The exercise should be repeated 3 times daily.
3. Immaculate foot care is a must to avoid ulceration and gangrene. The physician should instruct the patient in proper foot care.
4. Vasodilator drugs are worthless in the treatment of this disorder, as is sympathectomy.
5. Two aspirins taken at bedtime will decrease platelet aggregation, unless there are contraindications.
6. Revascularization operations, i.e., bypassing the occluded segment, have given remarkable results and relief to the patient. Indications include claudication that completely incapacitates the patient, impending complete occlusion, and stubborn healing of a necrotic extremity lesion. Initial limb salvage is achieved in about 75% of the cases, falling to 50% in 5 years, and to about 40% in 10 years.
7. When all else has failed, or when the patient has a cold and dying limb beyond hope of revascularization, then amputation is the only solution.

In summary, the most important contribution the primary care physician can make in an effort to decrease the number of amputations in his diabetic patients is the constant teaching of preventive techniques outlined in this chapter. The principal requirements are regular and periodic self-observation of the feet, well-fitting shoes, and proper skin care.

## CARE OF THE FEET (ADVICE FOR PATIENTS)

The older patient with diabetes who has impaired blood circulation in the lower extremities is in some danger of developing infections and gangrene of the feet or toes. Foot complications may be prevented by adequate control of the diabetes and by strict adherence to the following points, which should be reviewed with all diabetic patients over 35 years of age.

1. Cleanliness of the feet and avoidance of "athlete's foot" (tinea pedis).
2. Avoidance of bruises, cuts, and skin irritations and proper attention given to toenails, corns, and footgear.
3. Avoidance of burning or freezing the skin of the feet and avoidance of strong soaps and antiseptics.
4. Avoidance of constricting the circulation with tight garters or socks.
5. Abstention from tobacco.

6. Use of measures to improve circulation.
7. Selection of a podiatrist for present or future foot care.

Adherence to these admonitions and to the directions that follow obviates the necessity for many amputations and helps to prevent cramps on walking and numbness and pains in the legs at night.

**Cleanliness.** One should wash the feet daily, using a mild soap or a skin detergent. One should blot the skin, not rub with a rough towel. Cleansing tissue should be used between the toes. Drawing the towel between the toes or spreading the toes too far apart may cause breaks in tender skin. After the bath, one should apply a hand lotion or a cream with a lanolin base. Dusting the feet with a mild foot powder before putting on footgear helps to control perspiration.

Tinea pedis is to be suspected if tiny blisters are found between the toes or if cracking and weeping of the skin occurs. Many nonprescription drugs are too irritating and too strong. Infection can be avoided by using shower slippers or bathing slippers when in a public shower or pool. In case of suspicious blisters or itching, one should see one's physician, who should start proper treatment early.

**Cuts and Skin Irritations.** Walking in bare feet should be avoided at all times, since stepping on sharp objects or stubbing the toes may lead to serious complications. When not wearing shoes, one should always wear well-fitted bedroom slippers. One should not arise from bed without putting on slippers, and one should always turn on a light when arising at night, to avoid bruising the feet or stumbling.

**Care of Toenails.** Toenails should be cut straight across, never curved in like fingernails. One should not cut the toenail shorter than the fleshy part of the toe, nor should one use a sharp-pointed file to clean around the nail fold, but an orange stick with cotton saturated with hydrogen peroxide is satisfactory. If one's toenails tend to grow inward, a small piece of cotton inserted under the corners of the nails may help. Podiatrists should be consulted for instructions pertaining to individual nail conditions.

**Corns.** These are no more than pressure sores. Callus formation on the bottom of the feet indicates arch strain or improper foot balance. Diabetics should not cut or file corns or calluses. If they suffer from corns or calluses, then they should see a podiatrist and should inform the podiatrist of their diabetes. Patients should not use medicated corn pads or other strong corn remedies.

**Stockings.** Short socks may cause as much trouble as ill-fitting shoes. Socks should fit so as to leave room at the end of the foot when one is standing. Socks should be put on clean each day, and new socks should be laundered before wearing.

**Shoes.** The first requirement of a well-fitting shoe is its shape. A shoe must be the shape of the foot it is expected to fit and it must fit the arch length and the overall length of the foot. A shoe must fit snugly at the heel and at the waist of the foot. The heel height must be consistent with the use and comfort of the shoe. One should not wear high heels for walking, shopping, or housework. Soft leathers and flexible shoes are preferred. One should wear new shoes for 2 or 3 hours at a time for the first few days to avoid irritation.

**Burning or Freezing of the Skin.** When the circulation of blood is poor, the skin of the feet is less sensitive than normal. Thus, extremes of temperature may be felt, and the skin of the feet may be injured by heat or cold that might not harm other parts of the body. One must take great care to avoid burning or freezing the feet. The greatest danger is from hot water bottles or heating pads, so one should never use a hot heating pad or a hot water bottle below the knee. It is safer to use woollen socks to keep the feet warm at night. One should test the temperature of the bath water with the elbow, not the foot.

**Drugs and Antiseptics.** All corn medicines are composed of some form of acid and should not be used on diabetic feet. Strong antiseptics such as tincture of iodine, solution of bichloride of mercury, carbolic acid, and medicated salves should also be avoided, unless specifically prescribed by the physician.

Simple cuts, burns, and blisters are best treated with a dry, sterile dressing. Patients should not break blisters because the unbroken skin is the best natural protection. If blisters do break, they should be covered with an antibiotic ointment and a sterile gauze dressing. If there is any question about infection, patients should consult the physician.

**Constriction of the Circulation.** Diabetics should never wear tight garters or tight bandages around the leg. If they need to wear elastic stockings, they must be checked by the physician. Patients should not sit with their legs crossed because it constricts the circulation and promotes nerve pressure.

**Tobacco.** Diabetics should avoid the use of tobacco entirely. Nicotine constricts the small blood vessels and this constriction results in a diminished blood supply.

**Massage.** Light massage of the feet and limbs with a lanolin-based cream improves circulation.

**Podiatrists.** All diabetics who do not already have a podiatrist should be examined to determine the extent of professional care needed for their feet. Many painless conditions that are not apparently serious may cause future problems. Control of these conditions before trouble ensues prevents many hours of discomfort. A podiatrist advises patients as to footwear and individual problems not covered in this chapter. Diabetics should not complicate their condition with an infection that can be avoided.

## SAVING THE DIABETIC FOOT*

Diabetes is the commonest cause of amputation of the leg in civilian life. Yet it is not the disease itself which causes the amputation, and only in a minority of cases is it directly due to the ischemia that is a vascular complication of the disease. The common sequence of events is that the foot becomes partially insensitive from diabetic neuropathy. It is then liable to damage from unnoticed pressures and trauma. Once the skin is broken, the foot becomes infected. The infection spreads because the patient continues to walk on the painless, infected limb. The patient then goes to a surgeon with gross spreading infection. The surgeon may recognize that the limited blood supply is overtaxed by the demands of the infection, and he amputates to avoid spreading gangrene.

In many cases, perhaps in most cases, the blood supply in such cases is adequate for maintenance of normal activity. It is inadequate only for controlling gross infection.

Thus, for practical purposes, most amputations could be prevented if only infection could be prevented. For this purpose, we need to understand how and why the skin breaks down in a foot which has diminished sensation.

The most important factor in tissue breakdown is not any internal weakness or "trophic" change. It is the amount and timing of external force and pressure.

There are four levels of pressure on the foot that should be considered dangerous under certain circumstances. Each of the four is linked to specific conditions which render the forces safe or unsafe.

1. Sustained pressures that result in ischemic necrosis.
2. High pressures that break or penetrate the skin.
3. Moderate repetitive stress which results in autolysis of the tissues.
4. Forces that press on infected tissue and spread the infection.

1. Low pressures, between 0.5 lb/inch$^2$ and 5 lb/inch$^2$, may be dangerous by causing ischemia of the tissues under pressure. These low pressures may occur inside a moderately tight shoe or even a sock. They are dangerous only if they are maintained constantly for many hours. The damage that occurs from prolonged ischemia may be frank gangrene, or may be a change in the fatty tissues whereby fat is replaced by fibrous tissue.

*This section is included courtesy of its author, Dr. Paul W. Brand, F.R.C.S., Chief Rehabilitation Branch, United States Public Health Service Hospital, Carville, La., and Clinical Professor of Surgery and Orthopedic Surgery, Louisiana State University Medical School. It was a paper read at the twenty-sixth postgraduate course of the American Diabetes Association in Dallas in 1979.

Since almost all *sustained* pressures on the foot occur because of tight shoes, this involves careful fitting of all footwear. However, it is difficult to measure pressures inside shoes, and we find it is really much more practical to monitor the time factor. No new shoes should be worn for more than two hours at a time for the first day or two. A red flush at the border of the foot after the shoe is removed suggests there has been a problem. Even old shoes are best changed after four or five hours. We recommend that all diabetics and other patients with problem feet keep two pairs of shoes in current use and one pair of slippers. One pair of shoes is worn to work and for the morning. The second pair of shoes (kept in the office or workshop) is worn for the afternoon and the journey home. The slippers are worn in the house. In this regime the feet are safe from ischemic necrosis.

2. High pressures, between 600 and 1,000 lb/inch$^2$ and above may crush or tear or cut the tissues in a single application of force. These forces may occur when a patient stands or walks barefoot on a small projection such as a sharp stone or broken glass. The damage is mechanical rather than biological.

To be safe from high pressure all that is needed is to avoid walking barefoot, even in the house. Barefoot walking is good for normal feet, but dangerous for insensitive feet.

3. Moderate pressures, between 25 and 65 lb/inch$^2$ are typical of ordinary walking on the sole of the foot in a shoe. They are neither painful or harmful but may be dangerous if they are repeated constantly on the same piece of tissue thousands of times a day for many days in succession. The damage occurs because of a sequence of events. The first few thousand steps may result in mild inflammation. The next few thousand occur on inflamed tissue which is less compliant and which results in spillage of lysosomal enzymes from the inflammatory cells. Finally with more repetitive moderate stress, the tissue breaks down and ulcerates. This is an autolytic tissue destruction.

To avoid damage from repetitive stress, it is necessary (a) to spread the forces of weightbearing as widely as possible over the foot. For this a total-contact molded insole of Plastazote in an extra-depth shoe is one good method; (b) to limit the number of steps per day. The better the shoe the better the spread of pressure. The better the spread of pressure the safer it is to walk longer distances. It is good also to inspect the feet every evening to look for red areas and hot spots as these may indicate impending ulceration and the need for rest.

4. Finally, if the skin is once broken by any one of the previous three types of force, secondary infection may enter the foot. On an infected foot any pressure may result in spread of the infection and

more serious involvement that may lead to osteomyelitis and then to amputation.

Every wound or ulcer must be taken very seriously. Early rest and antibiotics followed by a plaster cast until the ulcer heals will keep the foot safe from spreading infection.

### Surgical Management

High localized pressures are often caused by irregular projections of bone or by partial paralysis that results in foot drop, claw toes, or inversion of the foot. If these conditions are corrected surgically so that the foot become plantigrade, then it becomes much easier to provide a simple shoe and insole to prevent localized pressure.

Insensitive feet in a diabetic can easily last a lifetime in most cases, but the price of safety is vigilance and care.

# 18

# Pregnancy

The ultimate in care is required for the pregnant diabetic, and this care includes both recognition and therapy of any problems that may arise. Many of these problems, subtle from the maternal standpoint, may be fatal to the fetus.

## CLASSIFICATION OF PREGNANT DIABETICS

Table 18–1, White's classification of diabetes in pregnancy, gives important information for anticipation of problems. Class A and B patients present few problems, and if sufficient attention is paid to those problems, there should be a fetal survival rate, without congenital defects, of close to 100%.

However, all other patients (Classes C through T) should be treated by a team of specialists, if fetal survival and normal fetal development are to be ensured. This team of specialists should include an internist diabetologist, an obstetrician with experience in diabetic care and delivery, and a pediatrician knowledgeable about the problems of infants of diabetic mothers. The primary care physician who practices in small communities has a responsibility to send such pregnant diabetics to the closest appropriate facility for care, even though it may mean traveling several hundred miles for each visit. In many foreign countries, this practice is routine. It is simply impossible for the average primary care physician or obstetrician to gain enough experience with such cases. One in every 500 pregnancies occurs in a known diabetic, and 2½% of pregnant women develop gestational diabetes. This means that if a physician delivers 200 children per year, only 3 or 4 of their mothers may be diabetic. If referring high-risk pregnant diabetics to such a center is impossible, then the physician must become familiar with these problems and their solutions, discussed in this chapter, and he must be prepared to

Table 18–1. White's Classification of Diabetes in Pregnancy

| Class | Characteristics |
|---|---|
| A | glucose tolerance test abnormal; no symptoms; euglycemia maintained with treatment by appropriate diet, but without insulin |
| B | adult onset (age 20 or older) and short duration of diabetes (less than 10 years); no evidence of vascular disease |
| C | relatively young onset (ages 1 to 19) or relatively long duration (10 to 19 years); no evidence of vascular disease |
| D | young onset (age less than 10) *or* long duration (20 years or more) *or* evidence of minimal vascular disease (e. g., background retinopathy) |
| E | pelvic vascular disease (calcification of blood vessels determined by roentgenogram) (note: this category is no longer used) |
| F | nephropathy |
| R | proliferative retinopathy |
| RF | both nephropathy and proliferative retinopathy |
| G | multiple failures in pregnancy |
| H | arteriosclerotic heart disease |
| T | pregnancy after renal transplantation |

(Modified from Marble, A., et al. (Eds.): Joslin's Diabetes Mellitus, 11th Ed. Philadelphia, Lea & Febiger, 1971.)

spend at least 4 to 5 times his usual number of hours in care and management of these patients.

Patients classified beyond Class D are at high risk for fetal death or malformation, and it would be prudent to discuss in depth with the patient and her husband the wisdom of continuing or discontinuing the pregnancy, especially if microvascular complications are severe.

Experiences at diabetic specialty centers reveal that favorable outcomes are expected in over 90% of all diabetic pregnancies.

When we speak of outcomes, we refer to the delivery and subsequent survival of a normal infant, since the survival rate of these mothers is essentially 100%. In gestational diabetes, with normal fasting glucose levels and adequate care, one can expect a fetal survival rate of almost 100%, whereas the woman with pregestational Type I diabetes with microvascular complications can expect a 20% fetal loss, of which almost 75% is due to congenital fetal deformities. Thus, if one could prevent fatal fetal congenital conditions, overall the survival rate would approach 95%. Overall, 40% of perinatal mortality is due to congenital fetal deformities, and extensive studies are being done in an effort to determine the exact factors that might contribute to the problem.

There is positive evidence that most congenital deformities begin sometime in the first 7 gestational weeks. Therefore, diabetes must be controlled from the first day of pregnancy. So often, patients do not see their physicians until they have missed 1 and possibly 2 menstrual periods. Valuable time is lost. It is wise for the primary care physician to discuss this important factor with young female diabetic patients who are potential mothers and to suggest that pregnancies be planned only after 6 to 8 months of meticulous diabetic control.

## GESTATIONAL DIABETES

Gestational diabetes is defined as diabetes occurring only during a pregnancy. It may occur in pregnant women at any age. Patients may display varying degrees of glucose intolerance and may have no clinical evidence of vascular disorders; some require insulin injections for adequate diabetic control. Many physicians are confused concerning the difference between gestational diabetes and White's Class A diabetes of pregnancy. Actually, the milder gestational diabetics who have only elevated postprandial glucose levels, but not elevated fasting levels, fall into the category of Class A. These patients show little if any increase in perinatal mortality over the nondiabetic pregnant person and require only minimal dietary regulation. However, frequent fasting glucose determinations should be made, in case these patients develop overt diabetes.

Other gestational diabetics may be at higher risk for perinatal loss if they have a positive history (as outlined) and show elevated fasting plasma glucose levels (greater than 105 mg/dl). These patients require a program of diet and frequently insulin in addition to the usual antepartum observations.

The stress of pregnancy in all cases calls for the beta cells to secrete more insulin because of the increased concentration of hormones that have contrainsulin effects, namely human placental lactogen (HPL), cortisol, estrogen, and progesterone. At full term, the nondiabetic pregnant woman is secreting about 3 times the normal amount of insulin. If the beta cells cannot meet this demand, then gestational diabetes occurs.

Since unrecognized and thus untreated gestational diabetes carries an added risk of fetal death and fetal malformation, the physician must be aware of this possibility. The first opportunity to recognize suspicious factors is when recording the family medical and obstetric history.

### Significant Factors

Several factors indicate a predisposition to gestational diabetes.

1. Previous stillbirth—this is important.
2. Previous macrosomic infant, namely over 4000 g.
3. Previous babies with congenital abnormalities.
4. Family history of diabetes.
5. Age of patient—some observers report increased perinatal mortality in patients over 25 years of age.
6. Obesity—may be a minor factor.

### Screening for Gestational Diabetes

Various screening techniques have been reported, including a simple, 1-hour postprandial plasma glucose test, a 2-hour postprandial plasma glucose test, or a complete oral glucose tolerance test (OGTT). All have their advocates and all methods are satisfactory. However, many patients do not require the full OGTT, and if the physician is planning to screen all pregnant women, he should use a simple and low-cost plan.

Because the onset of gestational diabetes most often is during the second or third trimester, the most propitious time to screen patients is between the twenty-fourth and twenty-eighth week in the normally progressing pregnancy.

**Screening of All Pregnant Patients.** The physician should evaluate the history of diabetic risk factors of all new patients on their first visit. If history is positive, and the patient is in a high-risk category, a random blood glucose test should be ordered, either fasting or at least 2 hours postprandial. If the fasting blood sugar level is over 105 mg/dl, or if the postprandial blood sugar level is over 130 mg/dl, one should proceed with a 3-hour oral glucose tolerance test (OGTT). If the patient's random blood sugar level is normal, one should repeat a 2-hour postprandial test at 24 to 28 weeks; if it is still normal, it should be repeated once more at 32 weeks. For these tests, one should give 100 g glucose at 9 A.M. and take the blood sample at 11 A.M.

For pregnant women with no risk factors for diabetes in their history, one should order a 2-hour screening between 24 and 28 weeks, using the 100 g glucose load as discussed. As an alternate, some clinics do a 2-hour screening on the first visit, and if negative, repeat same at 24 to 28 weeks. Again, a 2-hour blood glucose level of 130 mg/dl or more calls for a 3-hour OGTT.

For patients with a positive screening test but a normal OGTT, one should repeat the OGTT at 28 weeks.

Is there an advantage to a 2-hour post-glucose screening over a 1-hour test? It seems so, from studies recently reported. Many reports indicate that the 1-hour test is adequate and accurately defines possible gestational diabetic patients. This method uses 50 g glucose given midmorning or afternoon, with a blood sample drawn exactly 1 hour later. Plasma glucose levels exceeding 140 mg/dl indicate the need for a complete OGTT. An alternate method uses a simple lunch containing 50 g carbohydrate. This lunch could consist of a sandwich (2 slices of bread) with any meat or cheese filling and a liquid, which would be 1 c orange juice, ⅔ c apple juice, or 12 oz regular cola.

The community-based screening program in Cleveland, recently studied by Merkatz and colleagues, uses the 2-hour glucose test following a 75-g glucose challenge. The researchers point out that the 1-hour test shows a high number of false-positive results that do not appear in the 2-hour. In addition, almost 25% of patients with negative results with the 1-hour test have positive results with the 2-hour test. The researchers designated 120 mg/dl capillary blood as the top range for normal. This procedure resulted in an OGTT for 12% of all those screened, and 25% of these patients were positive for gestational diabetes, giving an overall positive figure of 3%.

An excellent review of screening procedures and other factors in gestational diabetes is found in Diabetes Care (3:399, 1980).

## ORAL GLUCOSE TOLERANCE TEST (OGTT)

To perform the test, one should follow the procedure outlined in Chapter 2, except that one should give 100 g glucose to the pregnant person instead of the standard 75 g. The standards of interpretation are different from those for nonpregnant women, since we know that normally the FBS is lower in pregnancy, and the elevation following ingestion of glucose is normally more prolonged.

When a physician orders an OGTT, he should ask the laboratory to tell him the the results of the fasting glucose test before proceeding with the rest of the test; if the patient's fasting glucose level is elevated above 135 mg/dl (plasma) there is no need to do the 1- and 2-hour determinations.

An OGTT is positive when 2 or more of the following values are met or exceeded:

> Fasting—105 mg/dl (all values given are for plasma; they are 15% less for whole blood determinations)
> 1-hour—190 mg/dl
> 2-hour—165 mg/dl
> 3-hour—145 mg/dl
> (Based on criteria of O'Sullivan using Somogyi-Nelson method and converted from whole blood results to plasma. Adjustments may be necessary when using other laboratory methods.)

Since a patient with a positive OGTT in the first trimester may develop frank, overt, gestational diabetes as the pregnancy progresses, it is important that a program of control be started at once.

## FACTORS DETRIMENTAL TO FETAL SURVIVAL AND PERHAPS CONTRIBUTORY TO CONGENITAL ANOMALIES

### Hyperglycemia

The fetus in the nondiabetic uterus has an immature mechanism of glucose regulation, and the plasma levels of both insulin and glucagon do not vary greatly. Glucose readily passes through the placenta into the fetal circulation, but insulin does not pass in either direction. Thus, if the maternal circulation presents hyperglycemia to the fetal circulation continuously, fetal hyperinsulinism will result, which can be detrimental by virtue of (1) increased body fat (macrosomia), (2) possible inhibition of the pulmonary maturation processes, resulting in the respiratory distress syndrome (RDS), (3) neonatal hypoglycemia, (4) possible cause of congenital anomalies(?), and (5) chronic hyperglycemia, which can result in larger placentas, which in turn can produce larger amounts of anti-insulin hormone, human placental lactogen.

An impressive study by Karlsson and Kjellman from Sweden showed that perinatal mortality is proportional to maternal blood sugar levels during the last weeks of pregnancy. Their figures are as follows:

| mean sugar levels | perinatal mortality |
|---|---|
| over 150 mg/dl | 24% |
| 100–150 mg/dl | 15% |
| below 100 mg/dl | 4% |

### Morning Vomiting and Ketonuria

The effect on the developing fetus of even mild ketonuria may be far more important than is presently realized. In a recent study, it was reported that ketonuria during pregnancy resulted in children with significantly depressed IQs. Similar results were shown in children of nondiabetic mothers who had ketonuria during pregnancy.

### Pederson's Prognostically Bad Signs during Pregnancy (PPBSP)

**Clinical Pyelonephritis.** This is a urinary tract infection (culture-positive) with a temperature elevation exceeding 39° C.

**Precoma or Severe Acidosis.** Precoma is diabetic acidosis with a venous bicarbonate level below 10 mEq/L. Patients with severe acidosis have venous bicarbonate levels of 10 to 17 mEq/L.

**Pregnancy-Induced Hypertension.**

**"Neglecters."** This term includes pregnant, diabetic women who are in labor when first admitted, who are psychopathic or of low intelligence, or who are in poor social circumstances and seek treatment fewer than 60 days before term.

The prevention of some of these critical complications is the responsibility of the attending physician, with the cooperation of the patient.

Urinary tract infections must be recognized and treated promptly. Complete urinalysis is a must at every visit. The patient should bring a clean, midstream specimen.

The physician must give the patient adequate instructions concerning the prevention of acidosis and home treatment in episodes of possible preacidosis. Acidosis during pregnancy is the outstanding factor accounting for perinatal fetal death. Susceptibility to acidosis seems to be the greatest during the second trimester, since insulin requirements may be increased during this period. Ketoacidosis occurring during the second trimester may be lethal to the fetus, whereas acidosis occurring in the last trimester is not always lethal to the fetus.

Hypertension first appearing during pregnancy is readily recognized during routine office checks.

"Neglecters" are a problem, and only education of diabetic women long before pregnancy occurs has favorable results.

## MANAGEMENT OF PREGNANT DIABETICS

### Diet

At the present time, one must take a look at the old ideas regarding diet in pregnancy and discard most of them. The Committee on

Maternal Nutrition of the National Research Council recommends an average weight gain of 24 pounds during the course of pregnancy. This suggested weight gain, which is associated with a low incidence of hypertension, prematurity, and perinatal mortality, applies to both diabetics and nondiabetics.

**Composition.** A diet consisting of 40 to 50 kcal/kg is recommended. This is about 300 kcal/day higher than requirements for nonpregnant women, to meet the extra nutritional demands of pregnancy. The composition of the diet generally is: carbohydrates, 45% of total calories and protein, 20 to 25%. Because of the additional protein required to produce new tissue, 30 g/day of additional protein over the usual nonpregnant requirements is felt to be adequate. In the mature female, 1.3 g/kg body weight is adequate, whereas for adolescent pregnancy, 1.5 to 1.7 g/kg is recommended.

The remaining caloric requirements are met by fats, with emphasis on polyunsaturated fats. If there is a large loss of sugar from renal glucosuria, one may have to supplement the diet with additional carbohydrate.

**Supplements.** The pregnant patient can meet her 50% increase in calcium requirements (1.2 g/day) with 3 to 4 cups of milk or milk product equivalents daily. An iron supplement is needed, but with a well-balanced diet, a vitamin supplement is not.

**Sodium Intake.** Recent studies have altered our thoughts about the need for sodium restriction during pregnancy. It now appears that the alterations in the renin-angiotensin-aldosterone system that result in increased aldosterone production and renal sodium retention are normal, pregnancy-induced physiologic alterations to preserve the necessarily increased circulating blood volume. Sodium restriction, therefore, is not indicated in the patient's routine management, and the presence of dependent edema is no indication to prescribe heroic doses of diuretics. Indeed, diuretics may be dangerous to both mother and fetus.

## Weight Reduction During Pregnancy

Commonly, gestational diabetics are overweight before pregnancy begins. One's first thought is to begin a reducing program, primarily to reduce the severity of the diabetes. One should not do this. Severe caloric restriction most often results in mild ketonemia and ketonuria, a result of burning excessive amounts of fat. There is accumulating evidence that maternal ketonemia may be damaging to the central nervous system of the fetus. Therefore, the physician should prescribe a diet that provides the acceptable pattern of weight gain and aims to avoid excessive gain.

## Underweight Pregnant Diabetics

The diabetic who does not gain enough weight during pregnancy apparently is at greater risk for hypertension, antepartum hemorrhage, and low-birth-weight infants. Some of these patients require monthly dietary counseling and encouragement. One assumes that inadequate weight gain is due to inadequate caloric intake, not to excessive urinary loss of glucose.

## Pattern of Weight Gain

The acceptable pattern of weight gain in pregnant diabetics is: a minimal gain in the first trimester and a progressive gain in the next 6 months of half to three-quarters of a pound per week. It seems logical that the second trimester weight gain is mainly maternal, whereas the last trimester weight gain is mainly fetal and placental.

## Insulin Therapy

Nondiabetic pregnant women are glucose intolerant when compared to the nongravid state. Fasting glucose levels are lower (65 to 85 mg/dl) than in nonpregnant women (90 to 120 mg/dl) and the postprandial levels are slower in returning to normal because the glucose disposal rate is prolonged.

Insulin therapy, when indicated, must be adequate to maintain blood sugar levels as close as possible to nondiabetic pregnancy levels. Excellent control would mean that fasting plasma glucose levels should not exceed 100 mg/dl; 1 hr postprandial not over 130 mg/dl; 2 hr postprandial not over 120 mg/dl; and 3 to 4 hr postprandial not over 105 mg/dl.

Usually, in the first trimester the insulin requirement decreases, in part owing to the use of large amounts of glucose by the developing fetus. The physician should discuss this phenomenon with the patient and should instruct her accordingly, since hypoglycemia can occur without the usual warning symptoms. Morning sickness with vomiting and loss of food can also contribute to hypoglycemia. Hypoglycemia itself does not adversely affect the fetus.

About the fourth month of pregnancy, insulin requirements increase, and this continues until delivery. One can readily understand why this happens, since the titers of cortisol, estrogen, progesterone, and placental lactogen are continuously increasing. In some patients, total daily insulin requirements may be almost twice those before pregnancy. One must remember that hyperglycemia in the last month of pregnancy can be dangerous to the fetus.

Occasionally, in the last few weeks of pregnancy, the patient's insulin requirement decreases. However, if there is a decrease of 50% or more, one should look for placental insufficiency or fetal distress.

One hopes that the pregestational pregnant diabetic has her disorder well controlled prior to becoming pregnant and that she takes 2 doses of insulin daily. If not, it is prudent to prescribe 2 doses throughout pregnancy, since control of diabetes is usually much better and adjustments are easier to make, particularly when daily insulin requirements exceed 20 U. When giving 2 doses per day, best results are attained by using mixtures of short- and intermediate-acting insulins. Two-thirds of the total dose can be given before breakfast, using a mixture of one-third short-acting and two-thirds intermediate-acting insulin; the other one-third is given before supper, using a mixture of equal parts of short-acting and intermediate insulin. Variations will be needed to meet individual requirements.

## Outpatient Care

Physicians should see these patients more often than they see nonpregnant diabetics. The primary care physician should consult the obstetrician about particular exams and laboratory determinations that each will do regularly, to avoid an overlap. In general, the primary physician should be in charge of the patient's diabetic care and control, including guarding against the development of unexpected complications. The following outline represents a satisfactory program:

1. The physician should plan to see the patient twice monthly in the first trimester and probably weekly thereafter, but the frequency of visits is best determined by the physician's judgment.
2. During early office visits, the physician should educate the patient about the problems associated with diabetes and pregnancy, impressing on her the need for the most meticulous control throughout the pregnancy. Educational material should be given to her to study.
3. Unless home monitoring of blood glucose is being done, plasma glucose levels should be determined at each office visit.
4. The physician should carefully review the record of the patient's urine tests and insist that she do q.i.d. tests. He should evaluate the patient's renal threshold as well as possible.
5. The physician should stress the importance of testing the urine for ketones, as discussed later in this chapter.
6. A complete urinalysis on a clean, midstream specimen should be done at every office visit, with emphasis on the presence of any pyuria and/or proteinuria. If pyuria is present, it should be treated until eradicated. (See Chap. 16.)

7. The physician should weigh the patient and make dietary changes if indicated.
8. A brief ophthalmoscopic examination of the retina should be done at least monthly in the first trimester and at each office visit thereafter. On rare occasions, rapidly advancing retinopathy occurs during pregnancy.
9. If the patient is in Class D or beyond and has proteinuria, it is best to do quantitative urine protein and serum creatinine tests at the start of pregnancy and repeat these tests of renal function at least monthly. Increasing renal decompensation frequently correlates with increasing placental decompensation, and this complication should alert the physician to a guarded prognosis for the fetus. In addition, if preexisting nephropathy becomes more severe, the pregnancy may have to be terminated to ensure maternal survival.
10. Basing judgment on the results of urine and blood glucose tests, the physician should make the necessary adjustments in the patient's insulin dosage.

## Home Glucose Monitoring

The overwhelming advantage of frequent home monitoring of blood glucose levels in pregnancy has been adequately demonstrated in many reported cases; it appears to be almost a requirement of adequate diabetic control. For details on methods and equipment, one should see Chapter 26.

The frequency of checking blood sugar levels depends to some extent on the problems one has in attaining excellent control of diabetes. In a reported series, patients were asked to monitor their glucose levels 7 times a day once a week, before and after each meal (2 hours postprandial) and before the bedtime snack. On all other days, 2 to 4 determinations were required. The objective is to maintain blood sugar levels at all times in the 60- to 110-mg/dl range.

## Gestational Diabetics

The gestational diabetic who has only slight elevations of blood sugar levels may control her diabetes well with a moderate dietary program, particularly during the first trimester. As pregnancy progresses, especially in the third trimester, she may need a small morning dose of either NPH or Lente insulin, with adjustments indicated by blood and urine sugar levels.

How high should the patient's fasting blood sugar level be before resorting to insulin? Anytime it exceeds 110 mg/dl, insulin should be administered. One should remember that nondiabetic pregnant women have fasting blood sugar levels between 65 and 85 mg/dl. Ordinarily, one should start with small doses, 10 to 20 units of NPH or Lente, and do the fine tuning based on plasma glucose levels. The patient may later require 2 daily doses, a mixture of NPH or Lente and regular insulin in the morning and a small dose of either NPH or Lente at bedtime, to sustain adequate insulin levels throughout the night. Ordinarily, these women do not have difficulty in controlling their blood glucose levels. Permanent diabetes occurs in only 2% to 3% immediately or soon after delivery, but 75% of gestational diabetics develop permanent diabetes during their lifetime.

### Oral Antidiabetes Agents

There has not been sufficient study to ascertain the effects of the oral agents on the fetus, and the Food and Drug Administration does not approve of their use in pregnancy. Occasionally, a Type II patient controlled by oral antidiabetes drugs becomes pregnant. The physician must discontinue the oral agent at once and give the patient insulin if dietary measures do not control her diabetes.

### Ketonuria and Ketoacidosis

It is important that the patient understands how to test her urine for ketones. The test can be done either with a separate reagent or with the combined glucose-ketone stick. Ketosis is a significant risk factor for the fetus, since it may cause irreparable damage to the fetal nervous system. A recent study suggested that ketosis in pregnancy in both diabetic and nondiabetic women resulted in lowered infant IQs. Starvation ketosis must be avoided as well as diabetic ketoacidosis.

The physician should instruct the patient to test her urine for ketones in the following situations:

1. Whenever 3 or 4 consecutive urine tests show 2% glucose.
2. During any illness, especially when accompanied by fever.
3. If vomiting occurs from any cause.
4. If the patient is undergoing any unusual, stressful situation.

If the patient reports ketonuria, one must act promptly and investigate the cause. A blood glucose level under 100 mg/dl indicates starvation ketonuria and may occur with severe morning sickness or a gastrointestinal upset from any cause. She may require a day or so of hospitalization for IV feeding of 5% glucose with 40 mEq/L potassium. A blood glucose level exceeding 150 mg/dl suggests the possibility of early diabetic ketosis, and small doses of extra regular insulin with an ultimate increase in the total daily dose may be the only treatment necessary. If the patient is developing frank ketoacidosis, she must be hospitalized and treated vigorously (see Chap. 12).

Again, the physician must stress the importance of testing for ketones whenever urine tests for glucose show levels of 1 to 2% for 3 to 4 consecutive tests, whenever she is ill from any cause, whenever she has nausea and vomiting from any cause, and in any stressful situation.

## ASSESSING FETAL HEALTH

Several accurate and reliable methods for assessing fetal health are available, and the physician in charge must be familiar with such tests. Under ordinary circumstances, one does not use all of them. With uncomplicated Class A and B and gestational diabetes, there may be no need to assess fetal health. However, most obstetricians feel more comfortable on determining the state of fetal health.

### Simple Tape Measurements

The physician measures and records in graph form the fundal height and maternal girth on each visit after the first trimester. These measurements give important information regarding the size of the fetus and/or the development of hydramnios.

### Ultrasonography

One can undertake serial sonography, starting in first trimester, to chart the rate of fetal growth, to estimate fetal weight, to locate the placenta, and to disclose gross congenital abnormalities. Sonography is most frequently done at midtrimester, to ascertain fetal age as well as size. The size of the thorax and the intrauterine volume are good indices.

### Amniocentesis

This procedure determines the amniotic fluid's phospholipid nature, specifically the lecithin-sphingomyelin ratio (L/S), which is an index of fetal pulmonary maturity. Amniocentesis is often done weekly, beginning around the thirty-second week, and requires only 5 ml amniotic fluid.

When lecithin is present in the amniotic fluid in twice the concentration of sphingomyelin, it means that the fetal lung has begun to manufacture surfactant in sufficient amounts to prevent the development of the respiratory distress syndrome (RDS). This usually occurs about the thirty-fifth week. A safe value is usually a 2 to 1 ratio, but a safer value is a 3 to 1 or 4 to 1 ratio. Any ratio under 2 to 1 must be carefully monitored.

### Estriol Excretion Measurements

It has been known for many years that low estrogen and progesterone levels may occur in complicated diabetic pregnancies. The bulk of estrogenic hormone excreted in pregnancy is estriol, and usually a fall in estriol levels occurs with the onset of fetal distress. The fetal adrenal glands contain enzymes required for the 16a-hydroxylation of dehydroepiandrosterone, a precursor derived from the maternal adrenal glands and circulated through the placenta to the fetus. Thus, estriol levels serve as a marker for fetal-placental integrity.

However, many studies have shown that the test is not entirely reliable. A recent report from the University of Southern California Medical Center by Dr. Goebelsmann and colleagues stated that the measurement of unconjugated plasma estriol was more reliable than the measurement of either the total plasma estriol (conjugated and unconjugated) or the urinary estriol levels. The researchers followed 70 diabetic pregnancies and presented evidence that the daily plasma unconjugated estriol measurements were a reliable index of fetal status and, further, that a drop of 40% from the highest mean values of the 3 preceding days indicates fetal distress when substantiated by a positive nonstress test and a positive contraction stress test. In this series, a significant drop of plasma unconjugated estriol levels occurred in 12 of the 70 patients, but fetal distress was documented in only 2 of these 12, both of whom had a positive nonstress test and a positive contraction test. From the studies it seems obvious that false abnormal results occur frequently and that it is mandatory to substantiate the estriol test with the other tests of fetal distress.

Another important consideration is access to sophisticated laboratories, in which a blood specimen can be drawn at 8 A.M. and a report can be given the same day. Since both the nonstress test and the contraction test are as reliable as the estriol test, are less expensive, and can be done easily, these tests might be the acceptable alternative to the estriol test.

### Nonstress Test (NST)

This simple test gives a gross indication of fetal distress, if positive. The procedure is as follows: When the patient feels fetal movements, the external monitor is started and runs for 20 minutes. Five accelerations of pulse rate of 10 to 12 beats per minute are considered to be a normal response. If there are fewer than 5 acceleration periods, the test is repeated for another 20 minutes. If again there are fewer than 5 accelerations, one should proceed to the contraction stress test. It is good practice to do the NST twice weekly from the thirty-second to the thirty-sixth week and daily thereafter until delivery.

### Contraction Stress Test (CST)

This newer test is helpful in evaluating fetal status. A small dose of IV oxytocin is followed by uterine contractions, thus slowing blood flow to the fetus, with transient fetal hypoxia. A healthy fetus shows no change in heart rate; this response gives a negative test result, which almost always assures the physician that the fetus is healthy. A slowing of the fetal heart rate after a uterine contraction is a positive test result. Such a result probably indicates the need for delivery, especially if associated with a significant fall in the patient's estriol level.

## PREDELIVERY ROUTINE

On the day of the anticipated delivery, whether by induction or by cesarean section, the patient who has required insulin during the course of her pregnancy should receive 5% glucose IV containing 10 to 15 U regular insulin. The rate of infusion should be about 200 ml/hr, thus delivering 10 g glucose and 2 to 3 U insulin/hr. If the anticipated delivery is prolonged, additional fluids and insulin may be needed. At the time of delivery, one can stop the insulin infusion and replace the bottle with 5% glucose without insulin. This procedure avoids postpartum hypoglycemia.

## TIMING OF DELIVERY

All patients who are other than Class A or gestational diabetics should be hospitalized a few days prior to their anticipated delivery date. This allows time for improving diabetic control and for assessing fetal health by the methods outlined. The ideal is to carry the pregnancy to the furthest time that will ensure a minimal risk of respiratory distress syndrome. At the same time one should not postpone delivery to the point of increasing the chance of fetal loss. There is a general rule that states, "the longer the mother has had diabetes, the earlier the delivery." At this point, the physician's judgment is matched against the high chance of death either in utero or in the nursery from prematurity. With the introduction of reliable tests for assessing fetal health, delivery time is being carried closer to full term than formerly. Instead of delivering diabetic infants around 36 weeks of gestation, most deliveries take place between 37 and 39 weeks unless there is evidence of fetal distress.

High-risk patients, some of whom may show borderline abnormalities on tests of fetal health, may need to be hospitalized for several weeks prior to the expected delivery time, so that daily fetal-health monitoring can be done and immediate delivery can take place if indicated by deteriorating fetal health.

Problems exist on both sides. As pregnancy advances, so does the incidence of stillbirths. On the other hand, an early delivery, particularly before the thirty-seventh week, is accompanied by a higher incidence of hyaline membrane disease and the resultant respiratory distress syndrome. However, in patients with a prior history of stillbirth, one may think in terms of an earlier delivery. The decision is often a matter of judgment based on the results of one or more of the tests of fetal health, some of which indicate the need for immediate delivery.

## INDUCTION OF LABOR OR CESAREAN SECTION?

Uncomplicated pregestational and gestational diabetics usually do well when labor is induced, unless definite indications for cesarean section exist. For patients with complicated diabetes or with obstetric indications, or other factors described in this section, a cesarean section is indicated. An experienced team of specialists can best determine the optimum time of delivery.

Recent reports indicate that monitoring of fetal pH, using fetal scalp blood samples, may be of help in making a decision about immediate delivery. This monitoring is done when fetal stress tests show some form of deceleration. Fetal acidosis is considered to be mild when pH is 7.24 and severe when less than 7.20. Most of these studies have taken place in university medical centers.

### Possible Indications for Cesarean Section

1. Diabetes—any diabetic patient with microvascular disease of significance or with ketoacidosis near term (''neglecters'').
2. Systemic indications—toxemia, hydramnios, uncontrolled hypertension.
3. Obstetric problems—abnormal presentations, disproportion, placenta previa, failure of induction, prolonged labor, previous cesarean sections.
4. Fetal distress—any indications from the assessment tests as outlined previously.

## IMMEDIATE POSTPARTUM CARE

Almost as soon as the infant and placenta are delivered, there is a marked reduction in the patient's insulin requirements. For the gestational diabetic who has required exogenous insulin, injections should be stopped immediately. If she has had a dose of insulin 6 to 10 hours preceding delivery, it may be necessary to provide extra carbohydrates for a few hours. Similarly, the pregestational diabetic shows a marked reduction in her insulin requirements. In many cases, this reduction removes the need for an insulin injection for the first 24 postpartum hours; injection of insulin is gradually resumed during the next few days.

## PROBLEMS OF THE NEONATE

Neonatal conditions that are more than transient should be managed by a pediatrician familiar with such problems. It is well to solicit the cooperation of such a pediatrician before delivery.

To obviate hypoglycemia of the newborn, some investigators have advised against giving IV glucose during delivery, since maternal hyperglycemia results in fetal hyperglycemia, triggering fetal hyperinsulinism, with resulting neonatal hypoglycemia. However, administering small doses of insulin for metabolism of the IV glucose results in small increases in maternal glucose levels. If the delivery is prolonged, the maternal glucose is needed and is readily used. It is important to check maternal glucose levels every 3 to 4 hours during delivery, in order to maintain a state as close to euglycemia as possible.

**Transient Metabolic Abnormalities.** These may include hypoglycemia related to fetal hyperinsulinism as a result of persistent maternal hyperglycemia, hypocalcemia, and hyperbilirubinemia.

**Changes Due to Prematurity.** Respiratory distress syndrome (RDS) results from insufficient amounts of surfactant causing variable degrees of hyaline (fibrinous) membrane formation in the lung that causes alveolar collapse and other changes interfering with proper oxygen and carbon dioxide exchange.

**Changes Probably Due to Inefficient Placental Function—Microsomia.** Long-standing diabetics with vascular disease often give birth to small and underweight babies. This factor increases the mortality risk.

**Changes Due to Fetal Hyperinsulinism, Secondary to Maternal Hyperglycemia.** Macrosomia, frequent in Classes A, B, and C, slightly increases the risk of neonatal mortality. Its incidence can be decreased by better control of maternal hyperglycemia in the third trimester of pregnancy.

**Changes Due to Congenital Malformations.** These are the most serious problems. It is generally felt that there is a twofold increase in major and minor congenital deformities in infants of diabetic mothers. Pedersen and Yssing recently reported a series in which there was a threefold increase. Skeletal defects and congenital heart disease were the outstanding major malformations. Pedersen and Yssing correlated major malformations with diabetics in Classes D and F (White's), with complications during pregnancy, and with low birth weight. Women with uncomplicated pregnancies had no major malformations. There was also an indication that excellent blood sugar control in the first trimester resulted in fewer major malformations.

## CONTRACEPTION FOR DIABETICS

There is general agreement that 2 pregnancies are sufficient for the diabetic. This limitation means that a satisfactory method of contraception is a must. It is prudent to advise diabetic women who wish to have children to try to have them early, when diabetes has been present for a shorter time.

Many physicians have reservations about oral contraceptives. Dr. John Ensinck and colleagues at the University of Washington have shown that synthetic estrogens and progestational agents interfere with lipid metabolism, since all women who take oral contraceptives have a slight increase in triglyceride levels. If some diabetic women already have a defect in their ability to clear lipids, the hormones may have an additive effect. However, the researchers feel that it is probably safe to take oral contraceptives for 2 years. We must always weigh the dangers of oral contraceptives against the dangers of pregnancy in the diabetic.

The gestational diabetic who reverts to normal carbohydrate tolerance postpartum is at a greater risk of developing impaired glucose tolerance or overt diabetes when given oral contraceptives. In a report summarizing studies done on 32 gestational diabetics, Kalkhoff stated that 14 or 44% of these patients developed diabetes while taking combined estrogen-progestin oral contraceptives (Diabetes Care, 3:421, 1980).

The diaphragm, probably the first choice for the diabetic woman, when properly fitted and used with a spermicidal agent, affords average protection without unwanted side effects. The condom-sheath is still a reliable form of contraception if used properly and if acceptable by both partners. The intrauterine device is generally contraindicated for the diabetic, since its effectiveness in preventing pregnancy is poor. In one report, 8 out of 22 diabetic patients using intrauterine devices became pregnant within a year.

Tubal ligation should be considered when the family is complete. Vasectomy for the husband is a second choice, and consideration must be given to the possibility of a second marriage if the wife's diabetes is of long duration and if serious complications are beginning, particularly renal involvement.

In summary, if a family practitioner manages pregnant diabetics, he should generally limit himself to White's Class A and B patients or to gestational diabetics. For all others, it is prudent to refer them to a larger center, where experts manage their progress. The physician should see the pregnant diabetic twice monthly in the first trimester and probably weekly thereafter. Early in the pregnancy, he should evaluate evidence of microangiopathy by checking the optic fundi and by doing simple tests of renal function. The tests should be repeated as indicated, but he should look at the optic fundi at every visit.

Through diet, insulin, and exercise, the patient must keep blood glucose levels as close to nondiabetic pregnant levels as possible, remembering that these levels are considerably lower than in the nonpregnant woman. The physician should check blood glucose levels at every visit, some fasting and others 2 hours postprandial.

Insulin requirements usually decrease in the first trimester and increase progressively after that. There is strong evidence that hyperglycemia in the last 4 weeks of pregnancy can affect fetal survival.

The patient should understand the need for accurate q.i.d. urine testing for glucose and ketones when indicated. The physician must impress on her the seriousness of ketosis and the need to call him immediately if her urine shows ketones.

With all patients except Class A and gestational diabetics, home monitoring of blood glucose is indicated.

Plans should be made ahead to monitor fetal health. The physician should discuss them with the patient, as well as approximate delivery time and type of delivery.

After delivery, the physician should discuss contraception with the patient.

Finally, one must discuss the total costs of pregnancy, from conception to postpartum, especially for diabetics in Class C and beyond. A reasonable estimate is in the region of $10,000, and most likely more if extended periods of hospitalization are needed prior to delivery.

# 19

# Relation of Diabetic Control to Degenerative Complications

## IMPORTANCE OF DIABETIC CONTROL

The majority of diabetics die from the degenerative complications of diabetes. Only 7 to 10% of diabetic deaths result directly from diabetes, such as death from ketoacidosis and hypoglycemia. For many years, it was felt that hyperglycemia was not related to complications, and consequently, strict control of diabetes was not considered to be important. This theory was taught in some of our medical schools. We hope that such teaching has "gone out of style" by this date.

In the past 10 to 15 years, numerous studies have shown a clear relation between hyperglycemia and microvascular complications, as well as neuropathy. The frequent occurrence of retinopathy in conjunction with nephropathy and neuropathy has led to the term "triopathy," which seems appropriate. Premature cataracts in diabetics should probably be included in this group, since evidence links their occurrence with chronic hyperglycemia.

The factors that determine the risk of degenerative complications seem to be the *duration* and the *intensity* of diabetes, particularly hyperglycemia. It is generally agreed that the macrovascular complications, that is, those affecting the larger vessels of heart, brain, and extremities, are probably not so closely related to chronic hyperglycemia.

Although the triopathy of complications applies more to Type I diabetics who develop diabetes in childhood or youth, similar changes are not uncommon in the Type II diabetic. However, neuropathy can be both frequent and serious in the adult-onset diabetic who has chronic hyperglycemia. By the same reasoning, the atheromatous changes that one looks for in the older diabetic are frequently present prematurely in the Type I diabetic who developed the disease in childhood or youth. Therefore, it is important that we direct our efforts toward establishing normoglycemia in all diabetics and that we attempt to avoid hyperlipidemia in diabetics of all ages. One cannot divorce abnormalities of fat metabolism from hyperglycemia; this relationship is discussed later. It is difficult to relate all microvascular and neuropathic changes to chronic hyperglycemia, since evidence from many clinics throughout the world suggests that approximately one-third of insulin-dependent diabetics who have had various degrees of glycemic control for 20 to 40 years do not have evidence of triopathy and indeed have a minimum of macrovascular disease. Perhaps there is a genetic difference in tissue vulnerability to hyperglycemia, hyperlipidemia, and various hormonal concentrations. However, there are still two-thirds of insulin-dependent diabetics who may benefit from the establishment and maintenance of "physiologic control."

The main degenerative changes in diabetes occur in cells of tissues in which insulin is *not* required to effect glucose entry. Thus, hyperglycemia as a result of insulinopenia or cell-receptor insufficiency allows pathologic changes to take place. In 1976, Drs. Cahill, Etzwiler, and Freinkel, speaking for the American Diabetes Association, had the following to say in the editorial pages of the New England Journal of Medicine (*294*:104, 1976):

> ". . . the burden of proof is upon those who maintain diabetes control is without effect. The goals of appropriate therapy should include a serious effort to achieve levels of blood glucose as close to those of nondiabetics as feasible—the contention that microvascular complications occur independently of hyperglycemia and insulin deficiency and that control of metabolic events is not a factor in their progress does not appear tenable any longer—the weight of evidence supports the concept that the microvascular complications of diabetes are decreased by reduction of blood glucose concentrations."

Diabetologists now generally agree on the importance of immaculate chemical control as a means of minimizing or perhaps avoiding both microangiopathy and neuropathy. In addition, the well-being of a diabetic depends on his maintaining normal metabolic functions through diabetic control. Numerous studies have been reported on this subject, and many long-term studies are in progress. The last section of the chapter describes briefly some of the most important investigations relating to this subject and the pathophysiology involved.

## GLYCOSYLATION AND CAPILLARY BASEMENT MEMBRANE THICKENING (CBMT)

Ample evidence supports the theory that CBMT results from chronic hyperglycemia and its associated metabolic abnormalities, and thus CBMT is the underlying disorder responsible for microangiopathy, affecting primarily the retina and the kidneys, but other tissues as well.

Spiro was the first investigator to note that hyperglycemia stimulated the attachment of glucose molecules to proteins, a process known as *glycosylation*. The protein of capillary basement membranes is one of the few proteins in the body that contains glucose. Spiro and others found that the enzyme that facilitates glycosylation, glucosyltransferase, is increased in the presence of insulinopenia and consequent hyperglycemia in diabetics. Restoring normal levels of insulin, with the resulting normoglycemia, reduces the levels of this enzyme. Glycoproteins are normally part of cell membranes, and only in the atmosphere of hyperglycemia does excessive glycosylation of proteins take place, with resultant membrane thickening and functional impairment.

One of the outstanding examples of glycosylation of proteins occurs in hemoglobin A-1c in the presence of hyperglycemia, and there is a direct correlation with the degree of elevation of blood glucose levels. For further details, see Chapter 28.

Renal glomeruli are filters serving to remove certain substances presented by the blood. Impairment of this filtering mechanism occurs as a result of basement membrane thickening, which apparently increases the porosity of the filter, so that the first evidence of the disorder is a loss of protein in the urine. Many other types of cells in the body possess cell-membrane deposits of glycoproteins, some of which serve important functions, both helpful and harmful. Insulin-secreting beta cells have glycoproteins that act as viral receptors, glucose sensors, or antigens. Cell receptors for insulin on fat and muscle cells are glycoproteins. Cell membranes of red blood cells, white blood cells, and platelets may contain excess glycoproteins that interfere with proper function. Increased platelet adhesiveness, excess "rigidity" of RBCs, and decreased phagocytosis of

WBCs have all been documented in the diabetic with chronic hyperglycemia.

In the crystalline lens, glycosylation of lysine occurs, and this process may contribute to the development of premature cataracts in the diabetic. Similarly, glycosylation has been seen in the proteins of the myelin sheath of nerves; it probably contributes to impaired nerve function.

## SORBITOL PATHWAY

Another etiologic factor in degenerative diabetic complications may be the persistence of sorbitol in target tissues. Again, this pathway is not dependent on insulin, but on an enzyme, aldose reductase. During periods of hyperglycemia, large amounts of glucose enter the cell in those tissues that do not depend on insulin for glucose entry. The aldose reductase in the cell converts excess glucose into sorbitol, a nonmetabolizable sugar that remains as a soluble detritus within the cell and increases osmotic tonicity. Such cells, therefore, pick up water and become swollen, a physical impediment to efficient function. It has been reported that sorbitol also interferes with the ability of protein to reduce disulfide bonds that affect aggregation of protein molecules. Many investigators regard the sorbitol pathway as the key to degenerative diabetic complications. One will hear much about sorbitol in the future.

Dr. Kenneth Gabbay of Harvard Medical School has done pioneering research on the role of sorbitol in diabetes. His research group has found the aldose reductase enzyme in the lens and practically all parts of the human eye, including cornea, retina, choroid, and optic nerve. In addition, the enzyme has been found in the beta cell, peripheral nerves, renal papillae, brain, seminal vesicles, placenta, and possibly in the endothelium of the aorta. Gabbay's group has worked with drugs that inhibit this enzyme and apparently have no metabolic or adverse effects. Some drugs have been tried experimentally in human diabetic neuropathy with some success, but clinical experience is too limited to evaluate it at this point.

Dr. Chylack of Harvard Medical School has presented data showing that one such drug prevents swelling and opacification of the human lens in vitro when the lens is bathed in a high-glucose environment. Additionally, Dr. Ken Oshita of the National Eye Institute, National Institutes of Health, has shown the key role of sorbitol in cataract formation. He has demonstrated that the first step in the development of a diabetic cataract is the accumulation of sorbitol from glucose and galactitol (dulcitol) from galactose in the lens fiber, thus drawing in water. He has demonstrated that cataract formation can be prevented by a variety of aldose reductase inhibitors. Dr. Peterson of Pfizer Center Research reported that one drug inhibitor was effective in preventing sorbitol accumulation, neuropathy, and cataracts in experimental diabetic, galactosemic animals. Thus, there is hope that some of these drugs will help to prevent degenerative complications in both eyes and the nerves and that they will be of value to diabetics with nephropathy and macroangiopathy.

## CHANGES IN PLATELET FUNCTION

The relationship of change in platelet function to microangiopathy is becoming more obvious as new studies are reported. There is strong evidence of increased platelet adhesiveness and aggregation in the presence of sustained hyperglycemia. Additionally, there is evidence of changes in several humoral cofactors of coagulation that affect platelet function, including increases in 2 plasma glycoproteins, fibrinogen and von Willebrand factor, which derives from endothelial cells. All these changes revert to normal when hyperglycemia is brought under control. Recent studies show that increased production of prostaglandin precursors increases platelet aggregation. Aspirin, which has been shown to block the increase in prostaglandin precursors, may be the simple answer to one element of occlusive vascular disease.

## STUDIES RELATING POOR DIABETIC CONTROL TO COMPLICATIONS

Many studies in the past decade have related the degree of diabetic control to the incidence and severity of complications. Only a few reports are summarized here.

> A report from the Joslin Clinic in 1975 covering 73 Type I diabetics who were alive and well after an average of 42.9 years of insulin administration states: "We don't know precisely the reason for this long survival. Multiple factors are probably involved, but a *meticulous day-by-day care of their illness* might have been an important one." Insulin-induced hypoglycemia was the most common complication and is indicative of meticulous control.
>
> Dr. George Goodkin, in analyzing the Equitable Life Assurance Company's well-researched study of more than 10,500 diabetics over 20 years, stated that the diabetics who demonstrated generally poor control of blood sugar levels showed a mortality rate 2½ times greater than a comparable group of well-controlled diabetics. Even when the onset of diabetes was after age 30, risk was twice as great.
>
> A pioneer advocate of meticulous diabetic control, Dr. James W. Sherrill of the Scripps Metabolic Clinic, published a report on

diabetic retinitis in 1951. He reported on 26 diabetics under his care for variable periods, all of whom had been maintained with excellent diabetic control. The duration of diabetes ranged from 21 to 38 years; some patients had been under Dr. Sherrill's supervision for more than 30 years. All these patients had normal vision, and only 6 of them had retinopathy more advanced than the occasional "berry aneurysm."

Drs. Esterly, Jackson, and Guthrie (of the Universities of Missouri and Kansas) have studied the capillary basement membrane of muscles in many diabetic and nondiabetic children. In general, their conclusions were that normal capillary basement membrane thickness was seen from 5 to 20 years from the onset of diabetes in patients whose disorder was well controlled and from 5 to 15 years from the onset in most patients whose diabetes was controlled moderately well. Patients whose diabetic control was poor showed increased membrane thickness in under 5 years. The researchers also recently reported that when poor diabetic control is improved, a definite decrease in basement membrane thickening can be seen in 8 to 24 months.

Dr. Osterby did a meticulous study on the thickness of glomerular capillary basement membranes in both nondiabetic and diabetic children. Her conclusion was that children receiving single doses of intermediate-acting insulin, and thus having varying degrees of glucosuria, developed progressive thickening of their glomerular basement membranes 2 to 5 years from the onset of diabetes. In the same clinic, Dr. Lundbaek observed normal glomerular capillary basement membrane thickness in a few patients who remained essentially aglycosuric with multiple doses of insulin for up to 5 years from the onset of diabetes.

A report from Paris on a study of retinopathy by Dr. Job and colleagues showed that patients with adequate diabetic control had the least progression of retinal changes. The 42 patients were divided into 2 groups, 1 taking multiple daily injections of insulin and the other taking a single daily dose. Retinal changes were quantitatively estimated by counting the microaneurysms and by noting their progression over a period of approximately 3 years. The mean yearly progression in the number of microaneurysms was less in the multiple-injection than in the single-injection group.

Drs. Bloodworth and Engerman, studying dogs made diabetic with growth hormone or alloxan, showed conclusively that the degree of diabetic control determines the rate of development of microangiopathy.

Dr. Bloodworth also reported that poor control for 5 to 6 years produced severe retinal and renal changes in diabetic dogs. The group of dogs maintained in good diabetic control for the same period had no evidence of kidney changes.

Drs. Bloodworth, Mauer, and others have shown definitely that an affected kidney from a diabetic rat, when transplanted to a normal rat, gradually returns to normal. Similarly, when a normal kidney is transplanted into a diabetic rat, the kidney shows nephropathy in 8 to 24 months. Human kidney transplants frequently show arteriolar hyalinosis within 2 to 3 years.

An outstanding report, by Dr. Jean Pirart of Brussels, appeared in the journal Diabetes Care (1, 168, 252, 1978) and is entitled "Diabetes mellitus and its degenerative complications: a prospective study of 4,400 patients observed between 1947 and 1973." It is important reading for the student of diabetes. Briefly, Dr. Pirart's conclusions were as follows: Peripheral and coronary atherosclerosis increases strongly in prevalence and in incidence with age, whatever the duration of diabetes. Arteriopathy increases with the duration of diabetes, but slowly. There seems to be no direct relation between chronic hyperglycemia and atheromatous changes. Diabetic triopathy (retinopathy, nephropathy, neuropathy) is a function of the duration and intensity of diabetes and more precisely of hyperglycemia. This abnormality can be lessened by treatment.

Dr. Harry Keen and co-workers at Guy's Hospital in London reported a 6-year retinopathy study. In the group whose blood sugar levels never exceeded 199 mg/dl, there was an increased incidence of retinopathy from 1.3% at the start of the study to 3.3% in the sixth year. In the group whose blood sugar levels exceeded 200 mg/dl, 6.8% of patients had retinopathy at the start of the study, and this figure increased to 23.5% of patients after 6 years.

A study reported by Guthrie showed stunting of growth in children who had persistent hyperglycemia. By age 18, male diabetics in this category were 6 inches shorter and females 3 inches shorter than their counterparts who had maintained excellent diabetic control.

The Joslin Clinic reported a study involving 451 diabetic patients whose diabetes began when they were under 20 years of age; the duration was from 10 to 36 years. Of 101 patients with nephropathy, only 1 came from the excellent diabetic control group. Concerning retinopathy, there were few severe cases in the good and excellent diabetic control group, but 31% came from the fair to poor diabetic control group.

Many similar studies are being undertaken, and the interested reader will find reports in the medical literature. The evidence is certainly in favor of making every attempt to normalize the metabolic functions of the diabetic as well as possible with the tools available.

# 20

# Diabetic Retinopathy and Other Eye Disorders

## DIABETIC RETINOPATHY

Diabetic retinopathy is the second leading cause of new blindness in the United States and the leading cause in persons under age 65. Meticulous diabetic control and early retinal treatment will improve these statistics. Most diabetics with early retinopathy have no visual impairment and are unaware that anything is wrong with their eyes until informed by their physician. The prevalence of retinopathy is related to the duration of diabetes, but it is seen sooner in older patients. Only 10% of diabetics who are under age 30 at the time of diagnosis have retinal involvement in the first 10 years of their diabetes, whereas 25 to 35% of patients over age 60 at the time of diagnosis have retinopathy in the first 10 years. However, the prevalence seems to merge in both age groups after 15 years' duration of diabetes, at which point 60 to 70% of diabetic patients have retinopathy. After 25 years of diabetes, approximately 90% have some degree of retinopathy. However, 80% of these patients have no visual impairment because they have minimal involvement. Only 2% of all diabetics in the United States are totally blind as the result of diabetic retinopathy.

### Ophthalmoscopic Findings

The physician who takes care of diabetic patients must be trained to recognize all stages of diabetic retinopathy and to know when to refer a patient to an ophthalmologist. Routine fundoscopic examinations should be done twice yearly in the office on a routine basis for all diabetic patients. One should remember that Type II older diabetics are not immune to retinopathy, and they require the same careful examination. Most physicians do not have time to dilate the patient's pupils before an examination, but a careful scanning of both fundi almost always reveals some evidence of changes when present. A thorough fundoscopic examination requires dilatation of the pupils and is best done by the specialist. Such a referral is in order every few years for all diabetics, even though nothing disturbing is seen by the family physician. When the fundoscopic examination is completed, the physician should examine the patient's lens, since diabetics develop cataracts much more often than do nondiabetics.

Because of the availability of early therapy with photocoagulation, the diabetic who has anything more severe than minimal background retinopathy should be seen regularly by a competent ophthalmologist, preferably one who is capable of carrying out treatment if necessary. The progress of retinopathy is characteristically slow and is not alarming. Indeed, some patients have continued to show nothing but a few small aneurysms for 20 to 30 years. However, some retinopathy, particularly in the 20- to 30-year age group, may progress rapidly, hence the need for the specialist's opinion.

Involvement of the retina can occur in 2 stages, background and proliferative retinopathy. As stated previously, about 80% of patients who have retinopathy have background retinopathy only, with satisfactory vision. Background retinopathy consists mainly of microaneurysms that look like red dots, sometimes called "berry" aneurysms. Occasionally, an aneurysm is surrounded by a ring of retinal hemorrhage, and others may show some hard exudates. The most common form of hemorrhage in background retinopathy is the punctate (or dot) hemorrhage, which frequently looks like a microaneurysm. The other hemorrhages one may see are flame-shaped, and the larger ones are easily identified. The hard exudates are usually yellow-to-white dot-like particles scattered around the microaneurysms, and they are apparently the result of leakage of extracellular fluids from the aneurysm. Dilated veins, sometimes segmental or "sausage-link type," are easily identified.

Fluorescein angiography is a relatively new procedure that has proved to be useful in studying retinopathy. An injection of 10% sodium fluorescein is given intravenously while the fundus is studied through a monochromatic filter that transmits only the wavelength of the dye. This water-soluble dye diffuses through the damaged vessels and appears at the sites of leakage.

Although background diabetic retinopathy usually remains relatively benign for many years, about 5% of these eyes unfortunately will have macular involvement, with a loss of central visual acuity. Peripheral vision is usually well maintained, and the person thus can manage without help. This type of maculopathy occurs more often in Type II diabetes and can progress to legal blindness.

### Proliferative Diabetic Retinopathy

Probably fewer than 10% of diabetic patients develop proliferative retinopathy. This condition is manifested by neovascularization or new vessels showing on the inner surface of the retina, and some may adhere to the posterior layer of the vitreous. This neovascularization consists of many tortuous blood vessels of all sizes, some almost as large as the retinal arteries. The vessels are most abundant in the posterior fundus close to the disc. When the vitreous begins to detach and to separate from the retina, traction on the fragile vessels causes hemorrhage into the vitreous or into the preretinal space. This hemorrhage may result in partial retinal detachment. All these changes pose an imminent threat to vision.

Careful examination of the fundus may show important early changes, such as cotton-wool exudates in the absence of hypertension, clusters of both dot and flame hemorrhages, venous beading, silvery lines replacing peripheral retinal venules and arterioles, and a dark-appearing retina. Any such evidence on fundoscopic examination calls for an immediate ophthalmic consultation. Diabetics with proliferative retinopathy may become legally and even totally blind. However, in some cases of proliferative diabetic retinopathy, adequate visual function may remain, particularly if the neovascularization involves only the periphery and not the macular area.

### Florid Retinopathy

A few unfortunate patients undergo rapid progression (within 12 to 18 months) of proliferative retinopathy, with marked hemorrhage and ensuing blindness. It has been observed that most of these patients are young adults who have had poor diabetic control for most of their life. It occasionally is seen during pregnancy.

### Pathogenesis

No one understands the exact etiology and pathogenesis of diabetic retinopathy, but most authorities agree that there must be a hypoxic retina. Recent studies have shown lactic acid accumulation in diabetic retinopathy, especially when glucose concentrations are high. Several RBC changes that have been observed in poorly controlled diabetes directly contribute to hypoxia. These are decreased erythrocyte 2,3-diphosphoglycerate (2,3-DPG) levels and increased concentration of HbA-1c. Mural cells (pericytes) may be involved because they regulate the tone and luminal size of the retinal capillaries, the loss or damage of which may be due to the accumulation of sorbitol. Other findings in retinopathy include increased capillary permeability, thickening of the capillary basement membranes, and capillary occlusions. Further study will clarify the role of each pathologic change in diabetic retinopathy.

### Rubeosis Iridis and Neovascular Glaucoma

About 50% of patients with proliferative retinopathy show proliferation of a fibrovascular membrane on the anterior surface of the iris that is known as rubeosis iridis. Eventually, the membrane may cover the filtering portion of the angle. This process results in aqueous outflow obstruction with increased intraocular pressure, resulting in a form of secondary glaucoma termed neovascular glaucoma. In addition, the abnormal vessels in this membrane bleed easily, resulting in hyphema.

The early stages of this disorder may be treated with laser photocoagulation of the abnormal vessels in the filtering structures of the chamber angle, which may keep the angle partially open. Panretinal photocoagulation may be helpful in preventing rubeosis. The prognosis for useful vision is doubtful in most cases.

### Prevention

Before considering treatment, we should discuss prophylaxis, which brings us to the question of the effect of blood sugar control on microvascular complications. Studies now show a distinct correlation between good diabetic control and a reduction in the frequency, severity, and rate of progression of diabetic retinopathy. An outstanding 5-year study demonstrated an increase in retinopathy in dogs with poorly controlled diabetes, as compared with almost an absence of retinopathy in dogs with well-controlled diabetes. Most diabetologists definitely feel that control of blood sugar levels is related to diabetic retinopathy, but there are exceptions, e.g., some patients with poorly controlled diabetes have no problems, and an occasional patient with well-controlled diabetes has severe retinopathy. Until further studies are completed, the clinician should encourage excellent diabetic control in all patients, not only in relation to retinopathy, but also in relation to other microvascular changes. For a more detailed discussion, the reader is referred to Chapter 19.

### Treatment

There is accumulating evidence that the hypertension associated with diabetes has a deleterious effect on retinopathy. Control of hypertension is a must.

Because platelet aggregation may play a role in occluding retinal capillaries, and because aspirin has been shown to be a satisfactory inhibitor of such aggregations, it appears that aspirin may be beneficial in slowing the progression of diabetic retinopathy. Indeed, it has been observed that patients who take aspirin on a long-term basis have a lower incidence of retinopathy. A study is underway in the National Eye Institute's Diabetic Retinopathy Study, Phase II, to evaluate aspirin. This study group is also continuing its evaluation of the value of photocoagulation in diabetic retinopathy. A vigorous program to treat background diabetic retinopathy associated with macular edema is in progress.

Photocoagulation, in the form of argon laser or xenon arc, is the major treatment for proliferative diabetic retinopathy. Argon laser is preferable to ruby laser because argon wavelengths are readily absorbed by hemoglobin, thus allowing vascular obliteration. The argon laser beam is much smaller than the xenon arc and therefore can be used closer to the macula and disc. At the present time, 2 methods of treatment are used, focal and panretinal. Focal treatment is aimed at coagulation of the neovascular tissue, whereas panretinal treatment attempts to coagulate the entire peripheral retina, except in the region of the macula and disc.

The early results of the National Eye Institute's Diabetic Retinopathy Study showed that photocoagulation provides a tremendous benefit in reducing severe visual loss and in preventing progression to more severe stages of retinopathy. Only about 10% of the treated eyes showed progression to severe visual loss (5/200 or less), as compared with 28% of untreated eyes. When Phase II of the Diabetic Retinopathy Study is completed, there will be many more answers.

Pituitary ablation was performed extensively prior to the advent of photocoagulation, but is rarely indicated now. One may still consider it in a case of rapidly progressing florid retinopathy with a likely prognosis of complete blindness. Results in some patients who have undergone pituitary ablation have been satisfactory from the standpoint of arresting progression of the disorder and restoring useful vision. In addition, most patients experience a reduction in insulin requirements, frequently down to one-half or one-third of their former doses. Substitution by the oral route with the other appropriate end-organ hormones is not a major problem.

**Vitrectomy.** Since 1974, an operative procedure has been performed that removes the vitreous and the neovascular proliferation and replaces the vitreous with a saline-like solution. The result in many cases is the restoration of vision. In a recent report by Drs. Blankenship and Skyler on 100 patients, visual improvement took place in about 50. The National Eye Institute is now directing a Diabetic Retinopathy Vitrectomy Study, designed to compare the effects of treatment given early, within 1 to 6 months of the onset of vitreous hemorrhage, with treatment given 1 year after the onset of vitreous hemorrhage.

### Family Physician's Responsibility

Since strong evidence suggests that chronic hyperglycemia contributes to microangiopathy, it is imperative that the family physician impress on patients the importance of maintaining strict control of blood sugar levels.

Fundoscopic examinations should be done at least twice a year. If the family physician does not feel capable of performing such an examination, the patient should be referred to an ophthalmologist at least yearly. In addition, if even minimal retinopathy is detected, the eye specialist should become part of the patient's diabetic management team because the timing of treatment by photocoagulation is vital to the maintenance of normal vision.

## EYE DISORDERS OTHER THAN RETINOPATHY

### Transitory Refractive Changes

Newly diagnosed diabetics, particularly those whose blood glucose levels are elevated when the diagnosis is made, experience rapid changes in visual acuity from hour to hour or from day to day. These changes are more noticeable as treatment is started and as blood glucose levels begin to lower. The cause of this disturbance is most likely a variation in the water content of the lens due to sorbitol content in relation to blood glucose levels. It has been observed that myopia is associated with marked hyperglycemia, whereas hyperopia usually develops as blood sugar levels decline toward normal.

The attending physician must explain to the patient that these changes are not serious, that they completely subside within a few weeks of control of the diabetes. Most important is that the patient should not obtain a new pair of eyeglasses during this period, since ordinarily they do not correct a refractive error that might be present after the diabetes is controlled. The patient should wait for at least 6 weeks of good diabetic control before going for a visual acuity check.

### Cataracts

Persons with diabetes are subject to 2 different types of cataracts, the rare, true "diabetic" cataract and the common senile cataract.

Metabolic cataracts, which occur rarely, may develop at any age, but most often in younger patients, even young children. These cataracts usually disappear spontaneously with 6 to 8 weeks of blood sugar control. However, with persistent hyperglycemia, they may develop into mature cataracts. Juvenile-onset cataracts are usually bilateral and cortical and involve both the anterior and posterior subcapsular regions. The lens shows minute dots of varying sizes, commonly labeled "snowflakes." Study of the lens has shown that, in addition to edema of the lens fibers, there is an influx of sodium and a loss of intracellular potassium, causing a precipitation or macroaggregation of normally translucent lens proteins, with the subsequent development of opacities. The attending physician can reassure the patient with this rare type of cataract that spontaneous recovery generally occurs with blood sugar control.

The ordinary "senile" cataract occurs at an earlier age and with a higher incidence in persons with diabetes. Recent studies have shown that the sorbitol content of the lens in diabetics may be a key factor in producing these cataracts. Treatment is the same as in the nondiabetic. For a further discussion of the sorbitol pathways, the reader is referred to Chapter 19.

# 21

# Diabetic Neuropathy

Not long ago, Dr. Max Ellenberg, for many years an outstanding investigator of diabetic neuropathy, stated, "Diabetic neuropathy presents such a wide range of manifestations that it is taking over the role of syphilis as 'the great imitator'." Neuropathy may be somatic or visceral, and sometimes both types are present. It usually occurs in older patients, frequently in Type II diabetics, but it may occur in Type I patients who have had diabetes for many years. Neuropathy is often found in mild or moderate diabetics who have had months or years of poor or indifferent control. This chapter briefly reviews the most frequent manifestations of diabetic neuropathy.

## PATHOGENESIS

The exact etiology of neuropathy is still undetermined, but 2 theories have been proposed. One suggests that neuropathy occurs primarily because of microangiopathy that diminishes the vascular supply. The second and more popular theory is that of sorbitol formation.

As discussed in Chapter 19, in an atmosphere of hyperglycemia, large amounts of glucose enter the cells of those tissues not dependent on insulin for glucose entry. Nerve cells are in this category. Excess glucose is converted to sorbitol by means of an enzyme called aldose reductase, but because sorbitol is a nonmetabolizable sugar, it remains as a soluble detritus in the cell and increases osmotic tonicity. Therefore, such cells become swollen with fluid and are unable to function efficiently.

Sorbitol has been found in Schwann's cell of the peripheral nerve in nondiabetics, but only in physiologic amounts. In the diabetic, it is speculated that the sorbitol and water content of Schwann's cell increase and cause cell death and segmental loss of myelin. Some doubt this theory, so further study is needed.

The initial structural alteration in human nerves seems to be axonal degeneration, followed by a decrease in the number of axons as well as by evidence of axonal regeneration and segmental loss of myelin that involves the surviving fibers. Thus, the segmental loss of myelin is the etiologic factor.

## PERIPHERAL NEUROPATHY

An acute type of peripheral neuropathy is characterized by aching pains with cramps and tenderness of leg muscles. The disorder, which usually involves the legs, but may involve the arms and the back, has no objective neurologic signs and is worse at night. The patient's diabetes is always found to be out of control. Within 4 to 6 weeks of diabetic control, this type of neuropathy usually disappears. Chronic peripheral neuropathy is usually symmetrical and is characterized by pain and paresthesias. It is also worse at night. The pain in the early morning may be so severe that narcotics are required for relief.

On examination, one finds diminished vibratory sensation, variable findings on sensory testing, and frequent loss of ankle and knee jerk reflexes. Further diagnostic studies should include a lumbosacral spine roentgenogram and a lumbar puncture. CSF pressures are not elevated, but 75% of patients have moderate elevation of spinal fluid proteins to about 60 to 70 mg/dl. Any findings over 100 mg/dl suggest another pathologic condition, such as spinal cord tumor. Frequently, the patient is depressed, loses his appetite, and consequently loses weight. One rarely sees a frank, unilateral, motor paralysis.

In peripheral neuropathy of long duration, one often sees the classic "stocking-glove" distribution, wherein the distal extremity is affected before the proximal extremity. The foot is usually affected before the hand. There is usually a gradient of involvement, with the distal portions of the limb being more severely involved, and when motor function is impaired, it usually follows a similar pattern. Ankle jerks are generally the first deep-tendon reflexes to be lost.

### Diabetic Amyotrophy

This disorder, characterized by weakness and wasting of the muscles of the pelvic girdle and the quadriceps with little sensory involvement, is usually unilateral. It may so incapacitate the patient that he takes to his chair or bed. Diabetic amyotrophy is almost always found in older men with mild diabetes. Within 3 to 6 months, the neuropathy is usually completely healed, with or without treatment.

### Mononeuropathies

These disorders are the result of ischemic nerve infarction and are characterized by a sudden onset of pain, unilateral involvement, and usually spontaneous recovery. Commonly involved are 2 cranial nerves, the oculomotor and the abducent. Peripheral nerves frequently involved are the femoral, the sciatic or one of its branches such as the obturator, which supplies the adductor group of muscles of the thigh, and the peroneal, the involvement of which results in footdrop. Motor involvement is predominant. Spontaneous recovery takes place in 4 to 15 weeks. When footdrop occurs, one must protect the ankle with an appropriate brace.

Extraocular muscle paralysis is usually preceded by 1 to 5 days of severe pain along the ophthalmic branch of the trigeminal nerve. Pupillary function is not disturbed. Unilateral frontal headache in conjunction with extraocular motor paralysis in a diabetic almost always means neuropathy, and unless other neurologic manifestations are present, there is no indication to consider arteriograms. The paralysis invariably disappears within 6 to 12 weeks.

**Truncal Mononeuropathy.** A newly discovered mononeuropathy, recently described by Dr. Ellenberg, is termed "truncal mononeuropathy." Unlike other mononeuropathies, the involvement is primarily sensory instead of motor and is usually unilateral, affecting mainly the thoracic nerves. The disorder, which affects older diabetics more often, is usually of long duration. It follows nerve root distribution, and the pain is worse at night. Differential diagnosis involves all intra-abdominal disorders as well as coronary insufficiency and herpes zoster. The course of the disorder is self-limited; most cases heal in about 3 months.

### Upper Extremity Involvement

Upper extremity involvement with peripheral neuropathy is not unusual. The most common involvement is muscle atrophy that is most noticeable in the first interosseous space. This neuropathy frequently involves all the interosseous muscles of both hands as well as the thenar and hypothenar eminences. Occasionally, the disorder ascends to involve the muscles of the forearm.

Sensory involvement, especially of the finger tips, can result in deep and painless burns from cooking as well as from smoking cigarettes. Another major problem is the incapacity of those patients who make their living with their hands and fingers, e.g., dentists, assemblers of small parts, and persons with similar occupations. In addition, the learning of braille in the case of the blind diabetic becomes difficult or impossible.

## Differential Diagnosis of Diabetic Neuropathy

Neuropathy of nondiabetic origin can occur in the diabetic patient and must be ruled out by proper scrutiny of the patient's medical history, laboratory determinations, and physical findings. The following are some that need to be considered:

1. Neuropathy due to drugs or toxins. The patient's medical history is important.
2. Neuropathy due to connective tissue disease, dysproteinemias, renal failure, and carcinoma. Medical history and findings are usually adequate.
3. Heavy metal poisoning or vitamin deficiency.
4. Infectious agents such as Guillain-Barré syndrome, syphilis, or diphtheria. Usually there is no impaired cutaneous sensation.
5. Alcoholic neuropathy in the diabetic patient. The patient's medical history is useful.
6. Spinal cord lesions. Sensory nerve conduction velocities are usually decreased in diabetic neuropathy, but not in spinal cord lesions.

## Treatment

1. First of all, one must control the diabetes as perfectly as possible and maintain that control.
2. Physical therapy, where there is loss of motor function, is valuable in keeping muscles in tone, just as it is for strokes. However, it does not help the sensory disturbances.
3. For pain relief, codeine or a similar analgesic may be required for a short time. Phenytoin (diphenylhydantoin, Dilantin) is worth a trial, since it has proved beneficial in many cases. The usual dose is 0.1 g t.i.d.; if no relief is seen after 7 days of therapy, it should be discontinued. Two of the tricyclic antidepressants, imipramine and amitriptyline, have been reported to be helpful in some cases.
4. Vitamin $B_{12}$ (cyanocobalamin), 1000 $\mu$g/ml, can be administered by subcutaneous or IM injection. There is no proof that it has any value, but those of us who have prescribed it for years have a "feeling" that it helps. Patients who take insulin can inject their own vitamin $B_{12}$ subcutaneously, using the insulin syringe. The usual program is to take 1 ml (1000 $\mu$g) 3 times a week for 6 weeks. One should not promise the patient anything, but one should be optimistic. If it does not help, neither does it harm.
5. It has been said that the more painful the neuropathy, the better the prognosis for recovery. The clinical course of the disorder usually

is about 3 to 6 months, but it may extend to 18 months before improvement or recovery is evident. In some patients, the changes are permanent and irreversible.

### Neuroarthropathy (Charcot Joint)

One does not often see this form of neuropathy, but when it occurs, there is no question about what has happened. The disorder is characterized by complete sensory loss while motor power is left intact. Joints are thrust beyond their normal range, and ligaments are torn without the patient's feeling a twinge of pain. The foot feels mushy, and the roentgenogram confirms the diagnosis. The physician should send the patient to an orthopedist in order to relieve weight-bearing on this joint, usually by the prolonged use of a walking cast. The involved joint surfaces usually heal by fibrous ankylosis. Some patients heal surprisingly well.

### Neuropathic Ulcers

The patient who develops a neuropathic ulcer has no pain and no temperature sensations in the foot; he may first notice a wet spot on his sock. The ulcer occurs at weight-bearing sites as a result of neuropathic disturbances that cause wasting of the interosseous muscles of the feet. Following the loss of the balancing action of these muscles, the toes are pulled by the long flexors into a claw position, i.e., dorsiflexed at the metatarsophalangeal joint and flexed at the interphalangeal joint. In this position, the protective fat pads are pulled off the heads of the metatarsal bones and the metatarsal bones themselves become misaligned. Thus, the shearing pressure acting on the plantar skin during rapid walking leads to callus formation and then to ulcerous breakdown.

The physician must distinguish such ulcers from ischemic ulcers, although in some cases, both elements may be present. Neuropathic ulcers always occur at weight-bearing sites, usually the heads of the metatarsal bones, but occasionally the toes. Vascular ulcers are situated at random. Neuropathic ulcers have a healthy and granulating base. The foot is usually warm and the pulses are palpable. Vascular ulcers are ischemic.

The patient should be advised to do the following:

1. Eliminate weight-bearing.
2. Have an orthopedic consultation, if indicated.
3. Have the physician carefully trim the callus and treat any infection with antibiotics. (The reader is referred to Chapter 17 for discussion of treatment of foot ulcers.)

4. After healing, have a plastic innersole made that is molded to the foot and that removes weight from the involved area.
5. Finally, if nothing else helps, ask an orthopedist to consider surgical removal of the offending metatarsal head, provided the patient has adequate peripheral circulation.

## VISCERAL NEUROPATHY (AUTONOMIC)

Almost every organ system in the body can be affected.

1. Eye: mainly extraocular muscle palsies (see section on mononeuropathies).
2. Gastrointestinal tract: gastroparesis diabeticorum; gastric retention; atony; and nocturnal diabetic diarrhea. This last is probably the most frequent gastrointestinal neuropathic involvement.
3. Genitourinary tract: neurogenic vesical obstruction of the bladder; impotence in the male; and retrograde ejaculation.
4. Autonomic nervous sytem: anhidrosis, particularly of the feet; trophic skin disturbances; and cardiovascular manifestations.

The pathology of autonomic neuropathy is poorly understood. Some studies have reported loss of myelinated fibers of the vagus nerve and sympathetic trunks and inflammatory changes in the autonomic ganglia.

### Gastroparesis Diabeticorum

This condition, characterized by a slow gastric emptying time, is generally asymptomatic. The etiology is unknown, but it is speculated that the disorder may be due to a vagal neuropathy, since the atonic stomachs, when viewed radiologically, resemble those of patients who have undergone surgical vagotomy. The condition is most often found in Type I diabetics with other manifestations of neuropathy.

Delayed gastric emptying time may cause problems in the control of blood sugar levels, since the exogenous insulin may begin acting before the meal reaches the intestinal tract. The occasional patient who has symptoms experiences periodic nausea and vomiting. Bouts of vomiting have been reported to last several weeks, with weight loss of 5 to 30 pounds. The weight is regained rapidly when the patient stops vomiting.

Treatment is generally directed to increasing the gastric emptying time. Drugs such as bethanecol chloride (Urecholine) and ambinonium chloride (Mytelase) have been tried with variable success. The episodes are often self-limited and need no therapy except reassurance.

## Diabetic Diarrhea

This form of diarrhea is a frequent complaint, usually in younger Type I patients, but it is also seen in those over age 50. The etiology of this disorder is not well understood, but it is probably neurogenic. Recent studies have found excessive bacterial flora in the small intestine in only a small percentage of patients examined. Diabetic diarrhea can be severe, with the passage of watery stools every 30 to 60 minutes, especially during the night, sometimes with fecal incontinence. However, patients do not lose much weight, and their appetites usually remain good.

Since the symptoms can be characteristic of many other gastrointestinal conditions, it is sometimes necessary for the physician to order a complete gastrointestinal work-up to rule out other disorders, such as the malabsorption syndrome.

Treatment of simple diabetic diarrhea is as follows: For symptomatic patients, excessive bowel motility should be suppressed with diphenoxylate hydrochloride and atropine (Lomotil), codeine, paregoric, or tincture of opium. Tetracyclines have been effective when bacterial overgrowth has been found. It is worth a trial in most cases. The condition is frequently self-limiting, with a duration of 1 to 6 months. One should ascertain that the patient's diabetic control is adequate.

## Neurogenic Bladder

The paralytic bladder is a serious disorder that requires prompt attention and treatment by a competent urologist. The primary care physician must be alert to the early signs and symptoms of this disorder because the patient does not complain until a urinary tract infection takes place.

The patient's medical history is the clue in diagnosis. When asked, the patient mentions longer and longer intervals between voiding, until urine is passed only every 12 hours or longer. In addition, there is evidence of accompanying peripheral neuropathy. Along with infrequent voiding, the patient admits to weakness of urine stream, dribbling, and a feeling of incomplete bladder emptying. The serious complication of this disorder is infection, with frequently ascending pyelonephritis. Unless it is promptly treated, the patient may develop urosepsis and azotemia.

Treatment is medical and/or surgical. Medical therapy includes the use of an indwelling catheter for several weeks, with proper antibiotic therapy for the infection and the indicated parasympathetic drugs. Following removal of the catheter, the patient is encouraged to void his bladder every 3 hours, with help by manual pressure. About 40% of patients with a neurogenic bladder respond to such treatment. Surgical bladder neck resection is indicated if residual urine persists. This operation is ordinarily successful.

### Impotence

Impotence in diabetic men is fully discussed in the following chapter.

### Cardiovascular Manifestations

Cardiovascular manifestations of autonomic neuropathy include postural or orthostatic hypotension, resting tachycardia, and occasionally, painless myocardial infarction.

**Resting Tachycardia.** It has been observed that in some diabetics with other evidence of visceral neuropathy, resting tachycardia is frequent and constant, with rates between 90 and 100/min.

**Assessment of Cardiovascular Involvement.** Five simple, noninvasive tests can be used by the primary physician in determining the presence of autonomic neuropathy involving cardiac reflexes. They are the Valsalva maneuver, the beat-to-beat heart rate variation, and the lying-to-standing heart rate response, which assesses cardiac parasympathetic function. Two others, the measurement of postural hypotension and the response to a sustained handgrip are more likely to be positive when marked peripheral sympathetic damage is present. A brief description of the techniques involved in performing these tests follows.

***Valsalva Maneuver.*** The patient should blow into a mouthpiece connected to a manometer held at 40 mmHg pressure for 15 seconds, while a continuous ECG is recorded. The "Valsalva ratio" can be calculated by noting the ratio of the longest R-R interval to the shortest R-R interval, which compares the bradycardia overshoot with the strain bradycardia. The ratio of 1.21 or greater is normal, 1.11 to 1.20 is borderline, and 1.10 or less is abnormal. One can also compare the resting heart rate to bradycardia after strain.

***Beat-to-Beat (R-R Interval) Heart Rate Variation.*** There are several techniques for measuring this, but the simplest is the deep-breathing test. The subject, lying down, breathes deeply at the rate of 6 breaths per minute, and a monitor records the difference between maximum and minimum heart rate. Fifteen or more beats per minute are normal, and 10 or fewer are abnormal.

***Heart Rate Response to Standing.*** On changing from a horizontal to a vertical position, the normal person shows a rapid increase in heart rate, maximal about the fifteenth beat after standing, with subsequent bradycardia, maximal at about the thirtieth beat. Diabetics with autonomic neuropathy show only a gradual increase in heart rate. This response is mediated by the vagus nerve. In studies reported, the response correlates well with the Valsalva maneuver and the beat-to-beat heart rate variation tests.

***Blood Pressure Response to Standing or Orthostatic Hypotension.*** Orthostatic hypotension is not unusual in diabetics, probably owing to a disturbance of venous and arteriolar constriction on change of posture as a result of autonomic neuropathy. Vertigo, faintness, and even syncope on assuming the upright posture should alert the physician to the problem. It has also been reported that diabetic patients have problems with reflex alterations in heart rate in response to tissue needs, and one may observe resting tachycardia.

***Response to Sustained Isometric Muscular Exercise (Handgrip Test).*** Sustained muscular effort normally results in a moderate rise in diastolic blood pressure. A simple test uses a handgrip dynamometer set to 30% of maximum voluntary contraction. Normally, diastolic pressures rise 16 mm or more; a rise of 10 mm or less is abnormal.

Recent studies of diabetic patients have noted that parasympathetic function is affected more often than sympathetic function. What, if any, are the prognostic lessons to be learned from testing these functions? Since few diabetics have been thoroughly studied in this regard, more investigations of sudden deaths and myocardial infarctions in diabetics are needed. Ewing and colleagues reported from Scotland on a 5-year follow-up study of 73 diabetics with possible neuropathy. Of the 26 patients who died in this period, 21 had abnormal cardiovascular reflexes at the first testing. Half these patients died of renal failure, but the others died of causes that could have been attributed to neuropathy. Six of them died suddenly, apparently not owing to myocardial infarction.

In conclusion, this discussion covers the most common manifestations of diabetic neuropathy with sufficient information for the primary care physician to recognize and to treat the average patient with neuropathy. He should also be able to identify those diabetics with severe neuropathic involvement who need to consult the proper specialists. For in-depth reading, many articles and books by Dr. Max Ellenberg are available, and for an excellent review of diabetic autonomic neuropathy, one should see the issue of the Annals of Internal Medicine (92, February, 1980) devoted entirely to this subject.

# 22

# Sexual Dysfunction

The physician is frequently confronted with problems of sexual dysfunction, especially impotence, particularly in the Type I diabetic man who has had diabetes for 10 or more years. It is estimated that almost 50% of all diabetic men lose their ability to have erections, but this figure needs adjustment for age. The main problem is impotence in the young to middle-aged men, and most of this chapter deals with the proper diagnosis and available treatment for such patients. However, the sexual problems of diabetic women should also be mentioned.

Recently, studies of diabetic women have reported that almost one-third report a loss of orgasmic ability. In 1978, researchers in Czechoslovakia reported clitoral neuropathy in diabetic women. This report was based on autopsied clitoral tissue that showed degenerative changes in the clitoral nerve fibers in 6 of 17 specimens examined. The other 11 specimens showed some thickening of nerve fibers. Again, diabetics of more than 10 years' duration had the more severe degeneration. Another study of 40 diabetic women, with an average age of 49, stated that 35% reported loss of libido, 45% reported a lack of sensibility during sexual intercourse, and 32% could not reach orgasm. Control studies were not reported, however. Dr. Max Ellenberg studied diabetic women and found no difference in orgasmic response between diabetic and nondiabetic women. The question needs more study.

Dr. Ellenberg also reported a random survey of 200 diabetic men, of whom 59% reported impotence; 82% of these patients were found to have neuropathy. In a more detailed study of 45 impotent diabetic men, aged 21 to 68, 88% had clinical evidence of autonomic neuropathy. Dr. Ellenberg has stated that, of diabetic patients with erectile failure, more than 80% are organically impotent.

The rare diabetic may be impotent because of inadequate circulation, a result of advanced atheromatous changes. The Leriche syndrome is one cause; another is vascular degenerative disease of the penile artery. Vascular surgical procedures are sometimes helpful.

## DIAGNOSIS IN THE MALE

### Symptoms

Rarely does a patient volunteer that he is having problems. The physician should question every diabetic man concerning his sexual performance. It has been reported that the loss of erections may be the first symptom of diabetes.

It is important to remember that diabetic men can have either psychogenic or neurogenic impotence. One must make a careful differential diagnosis, since both the treatment and the outcome are different. It is well to ask the following questions, to help the physician to make this important differential diagnosis.

1. Was the onset abrupt or gradual? The latter suggests a neurogenic origin.
2. Is the inability to have an erection intermittent or constant? Although there is not always a clear-cut difference, the neurogenic etiology is usually accompanied by a complete loss of erections.
3. Does the patient note erections at any time, such as with attempted masturbation or during the night? If yes, a psychogenic etiology is suggested.
4. Was the onset of impotence related to emotional stress or marital problems? Other important questions may arise as the history-taking progresses, frequently questions about extramarital sexual activity.
5. Is libido maintained even in the absence of erectile power? It most often is in the diabetic with neuropathic impotence, since the real disorder is peripheral.

### Signs

The simplest and easiest test is palpation of the testes for pain sensitivity. Since the sacral nerves that convey pain impulses are similar to the nerves involved in the process of erection, the loss of testicular pain sensitivity suggests a neurogenic etiology.

A cystometrogram should be done, with the help of a urologist. Many patients with neurogenic impotence have neurogenic bladders. Fundamentally, neuropathy of the nerves to the penile arteries breaks the reflex of erection, and since the arteries are unable to dilate and to fill with blood with enough pressure to compress the veins, an erection cannot be sustained. Again, some of the same nerves that control bladder function also control erection.

If sleep-testing laboratory facilities are handy, one could order an assessment of spontaneous nocturnal penile tumescence. However, it is usually expensive. Home observations by the patient's bedpartner could be helpful, and a home testing device is now commercially available.

The physician should check for other signs of peripheral neuropathy because almost 90% of patients with neurogenic impotence have peripheral neuropathy. The physician should ask about pain, check the deep reflexes, particularly the ankle jerks, and check for sensory and vibratory loss in the lower extremities.

With an adequate medical history and the finding of important signs, one can usually make the differential diagnosis readily. It is important to repeat that the physician must not arbitrarily decide that since the diabetic patient is impotent, the cause must be neurogenic. The decision should be made only after careful evaluation of the patient's medical history, his physical findings, and the results of indicated studies.

## TREATMENT OF NEUROGENIC IMPOTENCE

### Education

The physician should inform the patient and his partner of the cause of the impotence. This in itself is of great importance and relief to both partners. In many marriages, neurogenic impotence, when not understood by both husband and wife, has caused many problems, even divorce. It is the same old story—the man formerly was potent and now is impotent and the wife likely believes he is unfaithful. An understanding of the organic basis of the impotence is most important.

### Surgical Implants

Surgical penile implants are a new and important addition to the therapeutic program. Before suggesting such an implant to the patient, the physician must make certain that the patient possesses a strong sexual drive or libido and has lost only the ability to attain and maintain an erection. If both libido and erectile potential are lost, implants are generally not indicated. In some cases, the implant may serve a primary purpose of satisfying the patient's partner sexually if the patient is no longer able to enjoy orgasmic sensation. This idea, too, should be discussed with both partners.

Two types of implants are currently available, various types of silicone rods and the inflatable prosthesis originally designed by Dr. F. Brantley Scott, Professor of Urology at Baylor University. The inflatable device uses inflatable Silastic tubing placed inside each corpus cavernosum that is connected by more Silastic tubing to an inflation-deflation pumping mechanism implanted in the scrotal pouch. There it can be manipulated by the patient. Fluid for inflation is in a reservoir implanted behind the rectus muscle. The system is filled with a 25% Hypaque solution, which permits roentgenographic visualization after implantation. The pump mechanism allows the patient to select a state of turgidity of the penis that is satisfactory both to him and to his partner. According to most reports, acceptance by both patient and partner has been excellent. Orgasmic sensation is most often preserved, and if ejaculation is present before the onset of impotence, it is unaffected. A few mechanical problems remain to be solved by engineering modifications.

### Sexual Therapy

For the organically impotent diabetic man and his partner, sexual therapy may be indicated, with emphasis on sexual practices that do not involve penile/vaginal intercourse. It would be appropriate to refer such a couple to a sexual therapy center, if possible. Information concerning such centers is available from Sexual Medicine Today, 641 Lexington Ave., New York, N.Y. 10022.

### Testosterone

There is absolutely no indication for administering testosterone to the impotent diabetic man. Measurements of testosterone in diabetics both with and without impotence have yielded normal results.

For the reader who is interested in a detailed discussion of this subject, the journal Diabetes Care contains an excellent symposium on sex and diabetes (*2*:4, 1979).

# 23

# Diabetic Nephropathy

Chronic renal failure is the leading cause of death in juvenile-onset diabetes. It accounts for around 50% of all deaths in patients who developed diabetes under 20 years of age and who have had diabetes for 10 to 19 years. The first visible sign of renal failure is persistent proteinuria, which develops 14 to 18 years from the onset of diabetes. The average duration of life from that time is about 5 years. It appears that diabetic nephropathy is irreversible in human beings. Recovery or cure has never been reported. In its latter stages, the condition is most often accompanied by retinopathy, neuropathy, and cardiovascular complications.

Briefly, the pathologic process consists of changes in the glomerulus, the renal tubule, and the arterial tree. Drs. Kimmelstiel and Wilson described some of these changes in 1936. The Kimmelstiel-Wilson lesion is nodular glomerulosclerosis, and these nodules are positioned within the capillaries, not between them. Additionally, there is capillary basement membrane thickening of glomerular capillaries and epithelial basement membrane thickening of the renal tubules. A combination of arteriosclerosis and arteriolosclerosis completes the degenerative picture.

## SYMPTOMS AND SIGNS

The patient may have persistent proteinuria for many years before symptoms or signs appear. As the daily excretion of protein in the urine approaches 2 to 3 g/24 hr (normal excretion is 150 mg/24 hr), one sees the beginning of the patient's nephrosis. It may start with anorexia and intermittent nausea accompanied by hypoglycemic episodes that require a reduction in the total insulin dose. The patient gains weight because of fluid retention, and he has obvious edema shortly thereafter. Hypertension may appear early in the course of renal decompensation and should be treated as vigorously as possible. Serum creatinine levels progressively rise, and the patient begins to look and to smell uremic. Indeed, the patient may develop uremic coma or semicoma for several days and later recover enough to leave the hospital and to pursue normal activities. However, the course of the disorder is steadily downhill, and the prudent physician enlists the help of a nephrologist and a dialysis center before the patient's kidneys have ceased functioning altogether.

## DIAGNOSIS

The physician should do a routine urinalysis at every visit, including careful microscopic study of the sediment. Persistent proteinuria is the earliest clue. Birefringent lipid material (Maltese crosses under polarized light) help to confirm the diagnosis. Hematuria is rare in diabetic nephropathy.

The provocative test may also be done. Recently, Mogensen from Denmark reported that vigorous physical exercise, by inducing high glomerular filtration pressure, increases albumin excretion in patients with thickened glomerular basement membranes and thus unmasks early renal abnormalities.

Azotemia is another clue in the diagnosis of nephropathy. The physician should determine the patient's serum creatinine level at least yearly after the first 10 years of Type I diabetes. Rising creatinine levels spell trouble, and the mean duration of life after the patient's creatinine level reaches 8 mg/dl is approximately 7 months.

Hypertension develops frequently. Edema with hypoproteinemia and anemia are found.

One of the best clues is the decreasing amount of insulin necessary for diabetic control. This decrease, of course, is brought about because insulin ordinarily is degraded by the kidney, and failing kidneys mean less insulin degradation. Not all diabetologists agree with this explanation.

Rising serum cholesterol levels are frequently found. There may also be an increasing severity of diabetic retinopathy.

## PREVENTION

There is increasing evidence that meticulous control of blood sugar levels minimizes or prevents the development of glomerulosclerosis. Some years ago, Dr. Howard Root and co-workers at the Joslin Clinic reported that in 61 patients maintained under excellent control for 10 to 34 years, only 1 developed glomerulosclerosis. More recent reports substantiate this evidence.

Table 23–1. Progression of Diabetic Nephropathy.

| Pathologic Process | Duration of Diabetes years | Serum Creatine mg/dl |
|---|---|---|
| onset of proteinuria | 17 | 1.2 |
| early renal failure | 19 | 2.8 |
| late renal failure | 21 | 8.5 |
| death | 22 | 12.4 |

(After Goetz, F. C.)

Fortunately, not all juvenile-onset diabetic patients face an untimely death from renal failure. Many seem to be immune to nephropathy, and this may be related to their metabolic control over the years. A small percentage of adult-onset diabetics suffer from renal failure. A recent report by Goetz presented a prognostic chart, based on the progression of proteinuria and serum creatinine, that may be of value to the practicing physician. Proteinuria, hypertension, and azotemia are the important leads to follow. The average case of diabetic nephropathy progresses as illustrated in Table 23–1. The amount of protein in the urine in 24 hours has an effect on the speed of progress of renal failure. Fewer than 3 g/24 hr means a slower progression. Table 23–1 represents patients with more than 3 g/24 hr.

Medical measures to relieve symptoms arising from renal failure include vigorous treatment of hypertension, administration of diuretics, low-protein high-carbohydrate diets, and treatment of urinary tract infections.

Evidence suggests that pituitary ablation may play a part in preventing diabetic nephropathy. In addition, it was reported recently that patients who had received cyclotron treatment for diabetic retinopathy in a series done at the Lawrence Laboratory of the University of California, Berkeley, have not experienced the expected incidence of nephropathy. This treatment was directed to the anterior pituitary, in an effort to subdue or to stop the secretion of growth hormone.

## TREATMENT

At present, long-term renal dialysis or kidney transplantation seems to provide additional years of useful life. The results of recent reports are summarized in the following sections.

### Hemo- or Peritoneal Dialysis

Early results of hemodialysis were poor. There was a high mortality rate (75%), accelerated retinopathy, progressive neuropathy, muscle wasting, fluid retention, and disability. Recent results have not been much more encouraging.

It has recently been reported that long-term peritoneal dialysis has many advantages and less morbidity, although the first-year mortality rate is about equal to that of hemodialysis. There is less progression of retinopathy and neuropathy, and dialysis can easily be accomplished by the patient at home or at work on a predetermined schedule.

### Renal Transplantation

Renal transplantation, from either a live donor or a cadaver, is the treatment of choice and should be undertaken early, when the patient's creatinine level is no higher than 5 to 6 mg/dl. Dialysis takes place only while awaiting transplant. A recipient of a cadaver kidney has a 50% chance of living for 5 years, and a recipient of a relative-donated kidney has a 50% chance of living for 7½ years. Survival of recipients of cadaver kidneys has been increased remarkably by pretreatment of the living donor with IV cortisone. Deterioration of eyesight is only half as great in transplant patients as in dialysis patients.

Thanks must be extended to the staff of the Division of Nephrology of the University of Minnesota who pioneered renal advances for diabetics. Over 500 of the 1200 patients with diabetes who have received dialysis in the United States have been treated at the University of Minnesota, as have 300 of the 400 diabetic patients who have received kidney transplants.

Survival of patients in the University of Minnesota renal transplantation program varied from 82% at the end of the first year to 60% at the end of 5 years. Graft survival went from 72% at the end of the first year to 43% at the end of 5 years. Some kidney grafts show changes consistent with recurrent diabetic glomerulosclerosis. However, no apparent problems with the function of these kidneys have arisen. Over two-thirds of the patients were able to return to work, housework, or school. Their neuropathy improved so much that most were able to walk well, whereas before transplantation 25% were confined to bed or chair. The longest surviving patient in the program is now in his tenth year (1979). Post-transplantation complications have included cataracts and unrelenting progression of arterial disease, including coronary, cerebral, and peripheral disease. An unusual number of amputations was noted. One wonders about the quality of life.

The physician should refer patients who have evidence of progressive renal impairment to a dialysis center for evaluation and treatment. One should not wait for complete renal failure to occur—it is then too late.

## INTRAVENOUS PYELOGRAPHY (IVP)

Diabetic patients with chronic renal decompensation risk exacerbating their renal failure if they undergo IVP. The most serious results are in those diabetics whose serum creatinine levels are 5.0 mg/dl or more; progressively less serious results are seen in patients whose serum creatinine levels are lower.

The physician should monitor renal function in potentially susceptible patients before and after dye administration. He should also consider alternate procedures, such as ultrasound.

In a recent report, Drs. Vesely and Mintz stated, "Of 53 patients with diabetes mellitus with acute renal failure following IVPs reported in the literature, all but two had creatinine levels of 2 mg/dl or more before their IVP" (Arch. Intern. Med., *138*:1858, 1978).

## AIDS TO PATIENTS

Patients with irreversible kidney failure may benefit from both information and possible financial assistance from the American Kidney Fund. They may write to the American Kidney Fund, 7315 Wisconsin Ave., Bethesda, MD 20205. Another supportive group is the National Association of Patients on Hemodialysis and Transplantation, 505 Northern Blvd., Great Neck, NY 10021.

# 24

# Risk Factors in Cardiovascular Disease: Hyperlipidemia and Hypertension

## CARDIOVASCULAR DISEASE

It is generally agreed that chronic hyperglycemia is etiologically related to the microangiopathic complications of diabetes, but it probably has little effect on atheromatous changes in the larger arteries, mainly the coronary, cerebral, and peripheral vessels. Risk factors for cardiovascular disease (CVD), which in diabetics are no different from those of nondiabetics, consist of hyperlipidemia, hypertension, cigarette smoking, obesity, and a family history of CVD. Nevertheless, the overall incidence of CVD is higher in the diabetic population of all ages.

In 1967, Epstein reported that from ages 15 to 44, diabetic women had a risk of CVD mortality 6.4 times higher and diabetic men 4.6 times higher than nondiabetics of the same ages. At ages 45 to 74 years, the risk was 2.0 higher for men and 3.2 higher for women. A recent report on the Framingham study showed similar figures (Table 24–1).

Table 24–1. The Average Yearly Incidence of Cardiovascular Disease per 1,000 Persons at Risk According to Age, Sex, and Diabetic Status.

| Age at Examination years | Men | | Women | |
|---|---|---|---|---|
| | Diabetics | Nondiabetics | Diabetics | Nondiabetics |
| 45–54 | 31.7 | 12.3 | 24.8 | 4.3 |
| 55–64 | 48.1 | 25.1 | 37.9 | 12.6 |
| 65–74 | 57.5 | 28.4 | 40.4 | 22.4 |
| Total average incidence | 39.1 | 19.1 | 27.2 | 10.2 |

(Modified from the Heart Disease Epidemiological Study, Framingham, Massachusetts.)

No one knows why diabetics are at greater risk of developing CVD. However, some factors bear mention here. The Framingham study is probably the single most reliable study ever undertaken in evaluating risk factors. Since 1948, a cohort of over 5000 men and women, aged 30 to 62 years at the time of the initial exam, have been followed twice yearly to ascertain the reason that some develop CVD and others do not. A portion of the study has dealt entirely with diabetics, in the hope of determining the impact of diabetes on the incidence of CVD. The study has attempted to determine (1) the absolute rate at which CVD develops in diabetics as compared with nondiabetics, (2) the relative risk for diabetics as opposed to nondiabetics, and (3) the fraction of the risk attributable to diabetes.

It is generally agreed that there is a higher incidence of peripheral arterial, coronary, and cerebrovascular disease in diabetics than in nondiabetics. In addition, the high relative risk of congestive heart failure may be due to small vessel disease, i.e., arteriolar sclerosis and proliferative lesions in cardiac muscle that cause cardiac myopathy. Of the major risk factors, hypertension was the most pernicious clinical finding in either sex. Cigarette smoking was the most detrimental influence among men. Although the incidence of coronary disease is less in women than in men, diabetic women have a risk of coronary disease identical to that of diabetic men.

## HYPERLIPIDEMIA

There is no question that hyperlipidemia is a major factor in all atheromatous events, and diabetics have higher low-density lipoprotein (LDL) cholesterol and very low-density lipoprotein (VLDL) triglyceride levels, but lower high-density lipoprotein (HDL) cholesterol values. Although the exact prevalence of hyperlipidemia is questionable, it has been stated that about 12% of all diabetics have Type II hypercholesterolemia (LDL) and about 25 to 30% have Type IV hyperlipidemia (increased endogenous triglyceride). I believe that these figures are too low.

A recent report from the University of Miami School of Medicine may furnish further evidence of the increased incidence of coronary disease in diabetics. The study concerned the ability of serum to solubilize a given amount of added cholesterol, and the researchers designated this ability the serum cholesterol-binding reserve (SCBR). This reserve was lower in patients who had premature myocardial infarction. Ordinarily, values for SCBR increased with rising levels of cholesterol and triglycerides in the serum of control subjects, but not in those with myocardial infarction. It was shown that SCBR could be attributed to the cholesterol-solubilizing capacities of HDL and VLDL. It would seem logical, then, that because HDL may be the "scavenger" lipoprotein that cleans the walls of atheromatous deposits, a low SCBR would reflect a deficiency in this capability. The study showed significantly lower SCBR values in diabetic patients.

## HDL Cholesterol

Since all lipoproteins carry cholesterol, hypercholesteremia may occur with an elevated level of any of them. LDL accounts for over 50% of the body's cholesterol in a fasting state in a normal individual, whereas HDL accounts for around 25% or approximately 35 to 50 mg/dl of all cholesterol by weight. Studies in Hawaii were among the first to show that lower levels of HDL were associated with a higher incidence of coronary disease. Further studies substantiated the inverse relation of HDL cholesterol to coronary artery disease. Little is known about HDL, and there is still a question as to whether the lipid or the protein is related to coronary heart disease. We do not know exactly how HDL works. Theoretically, it could be the disposal system, picking up cholesterol from the tissues and blood cells and returning it to the liver. Some theories suggest that HDL acts as a scavenger in the plasma and moves the cholesterol to a safe depository.

Some investigators feel that HDL is almost predictive of coronary heart disease. Dr. Castelli stated that the risk for coronary disease increases 25% for every 5 mg/dl decline in HDL below 45 mg/dl in men and 55 mg/dl in women. The average ratio of total cholesterol to HDL cholesterol among men having coronary disease in the Framingham study was 5.4:1. A ratio with a good prognosis should be 4.4:1 or less. There is little doubt that HDL levels are inversely related to coronary artery disease.

The factors that lower HDL levels are obesity, uncontrolled diabetes, a high carbohydrate diet, hypertriglyceridemia, and cigarette smoking. On the other hand, the factors that raise HDL levels and improve the situation are the converse of the foregoing factors, exercise, and 1 or 2 drinks of an alcoholic beverage daily.

### Serum Cholesterol Levels

In a study by Dr. Castelli, no cases of coronary heart disease (CHD) developed in persons who had cholesterol levels under 150 mg/dl. Those with levels of 200 mg/dl or less were found to be relatively safe, but about one-fourth of the CHD in our society occurs in persons whose cholesterol level is under 200 mg/dl. In this study, 225 mg/dl was the mean level of cholesterol, and 219 mg/dl was the mean level of patients who were free of CHD in the first 16 years of the study. The mean level of cholesterol of those who developed CHD in the first 16 years was 244 mg/dl. A cholesterol level of 260 mg/dl about doubles the standard risk, and a cholesterol level of 300 mg/dl or higher puts a patient into an inordinately high-risk group. Seventy-five per cent of coronary heart attacks occur in persons who have cholesterol levels considered to be "within normal limits." Although many physicians have been taught not to be concerned about cholesterol levels up to 250 mg/dl, this is the level at which patients have heart attacks.

Familial hypercholesterolemia occurs in about 1 in 300 births, and many of these patients have coronary heart disease between the ages of 20 and 50 years. It seems that one of the problems in this disorder is that cell receptors are not present to bind and to remove the circulating lipoproteins, and so these lipoproteins concentrate in blood vessels and cause atheromatous changes.

### Serum Triglyceride Levels

Triglyceride elevations are a frequent result of hyperglycemia, particularly in the new Type I diabetic. It is advisable for the physician to control the patient's blood glucose level before worrying about an elevated triglyceride level. If, after 6 to 12 months of good diabetic control, there is still a significant elevation of triglyceride, then one should study and treat the condition, if possible. Elevated triglyceride levels in patients over ages 60 to 65 are less of a risk factor. Normal triglyceride serum levels should be under 150 mg/dl.

If elevated triglyceride levels persist, one should look for other causes, such as:

1. Hypothyroidism, renal disorders, estrogen or glucocorticoid treatment, or excessive alcohol intake.
2. Insulin overdosage, which may occur when insulin is given to a Type II diabetic who is not insulinopenic.
3. Familial hypertriglyceridemia, more common in Type II diabetes.
4. The rare Thannhauser-Aldersberg syndrome, with marked elevation of triglyceride unaffected by hyperglycemia. The serum is lipemic, and patients have lipemia retinalis, abdominal pain, and usually diffuse vascular involvement. There is often a low renal threshold. Treatment consists of a low-fat diet and administration of phenformin (by permission of the FDA) and a new drug, gemfibrozil, not yet commercially available.

## Measuring Lipids

All diabetic patients over age 16 should have a lipid profile at regular intervals. If the original test results are normal in a patient under 30, it is enough to repeat the test every 2 to 3 years. Annual profiles are in order after age 40 in all diabetics. Triglyceride, total cholesterol, and HDL levels obtained after a 12-hour fast provide all the needed information. The serum cholesterol level alone gives important information concerning coronary risks for patients under 50, and the HDL determination is particularly valuable for the patient over age 50. Triglyceride levels do not indicate the risk of cardiovascular disease, but rather are used to determine LDL levels according to the Frederickson formula. This formula states that the LDL cholesterol level equals the total cholesterol level minus the HDL cholesterol level minus the $\frac{\text{triglyceride level}}{5}$. LDL, the cholesterol-rich lipoprotein, may be the most atherogenic. Lipid values may change throughout a person's lifetime, and normal values at age 20 do not guarantee normal values at age 30 or 50. Elevated triglyceride values occasionally are found in teenagers.

What are normal levels? Triglyceride levels should not exceed 150 mg/dl. HDL levels in women should be above 55 mg/dl and in men, above 45 mg/dl. Total serum cholesterol levels should be below 200 mg/dl. The ratio of total cholesterol to HDL cholesterol should be 4:1 or less. LDL cholesterol levels should be 150 mg/dl or less.

## Treatment of Hypercholesterolemia

Does lowering serum LDL cholesterol levels and raising HDL cholesterol levels decrease the risk of cardiovascular disease, particularly coronary heart disease? The theory that lowering LDL cholesterol levels can prevent heart disease has not been proved. However, Dr. Robert I. Levy, director of the National Heart, Lung, and Blood Institute, and other investigators have demonstrated in animal and human experimentation that lower LDL cholesterol levels not only prevent atherosclerotic progression, but also apparently produce regression of the condition. Generally, cholesterol levels in the population are lower today than they were 10 years ago by between 4 and 8%, particularly in more educated persons. The practical steps in the management of cholesterol abnormalities, until the many questions are answered, are outlined in the following paragraphs.

**Prudent Diet.** One should avoid high-cholesterol foods such as egg yolks, meats, and dairy fats and should minimize saturated fat intake by limiting dairy fats and fat animal meats, as well as hot dogs, cold cuts, potato chips and commercial baked goods, for example. Not more than 30% of the daily calories should be furnished by fat, and of this, not more than 10% should be saturated fat; 20% should be polyunsaturated. If hyperlipidemia is severe, fat calories can be lowered even more. Cholesterol content of the diet should be no more than 300 mg daily.

One cannot deny that diet has an effect on cholesterol levels. For example, the Japanese inhabitants of Japan have an average cholesterol level 100 mg/dl below that of Americans in the United States of the same age, and the Japanese have one-tenth the coronary artery disease rate that Americans have.

Recent studies of high-fiber diets indicate that the fiber may be responsible for lowering cholesterol and triglyceride levels in diabetics. More study is required before substantial conclusions can be drawn. For further details on diet, see Chapter 3.

**Drug Therapy.** This is designed mainly to lower LDL concentrations rather than elevated triglycerides. In most cases, an LDL level of 165 mg/dl or over should be treated with some form of medication. The first choice is probably cholestyramine, commercially known as Questran. The dose is 9 g b.i.d. An alternate drug is colestipol, 5 g b.i.d. In a month's time, serum concentrations can begin to be measured. A third drug that is successful if tolerated is nicotinic acid. The eventual therapeutic dose is probably in the range of 1000 mg b.i.d.; one must start with 100 mg b.i.d. and increase slowly, not more often than every 3 to 5 days.

**Sucrose Polyester.** Recently, an artificial fat, sucrose polyester, has been used in experiments on human subjects and has been found to reduce elevated cholesterol levels in those who were on a zero-cholesterol diet as well as those with intermediate and high levels of cholesterol. The product was synthesized some time ago by Proctor and Gamble. The substance is taken orally with meals. The investigators were able to lower cholesterol levels 15 to 20% in all subjects. In addition, LDL levels decreased by around 20%, and HLD levels showed a slight increase.

Sucrose polyester works by preventing absorption of dietary cholesterol. It is produced by attaching fatty acids to ordinary sucrose by ester linkage at 8 sites. It does not undergo hydrolysis in the digestive tract, cannot be absorbed, and goes through the digestive tract in an oil phase. Cholesterol, which has great affinity for oil, readily binds with the globules of sucrose polyester and is excreted in the feces with them. This process includes the binding of dietary cholesterol as well as that which is recirculated in the intestine following excretion in the bile. Further studies are being done by Dr. Charles Glueck and Dr. Fred Mattson of the University of Cincinnati's Lipid Research Group. The product has great promise.

**Exercise.** The effect of exercise in preventing coronary disease is still not determined, and more research is needed. One study showed that after 3 years, there was no improvement in survival of patients who underwent daily supervised exercises.

## HYPERTENSION

Hypertension occurs twice as often in diabetics of all ages as in nondiabetics and contributes to an increased incidence of coronary disease, congestive heart failure, and peripheral vascular disease. Even the microangiopathic changes of nephropathy and retinopathy progress more rapidly in the presence of hypertension. Since hypertension is such a formidable catalyst in these life-threatening disorders, it is imperative that the physician pursue a vigorous and planned program of antihypertensive treatment.

Three distinct categories of hypertension may occur in diabetes: (1) Diabetic nephropathy results in the most severe and irreversible hypertension ("diabetic hypertension"), and this form of glomerulosclerosis is the leading cause of death in young diabetics. Obviously, satisfactory reduction of blood pressure in the advanced stage of nephropathy is almost impossible without resorting to dialysis. (2) Essential hypertension is identical to that seen in the nondiabetic population, but the increased incidence in diabetes may be partially due to chronic hyperglycemia, which results in increased blood volume. In addition, many diabetics show low plasma renin activity. (3) Systolic hypertension is most frequently seen in the older Type II patient, and the loss of large vessel elasticity probably contributes to this condition. Diastolic pressures are usually normal. Other causes of systolic hypertension may be as in the nondiabetic person.

### Treatment

In planning a treatment program, the physician must be aware of the various side effects of antihypertensive drugs in relation to diabetes. Drugs in the potassium-losing diuretic group, such as the thiazides, furosemide, and ethacrynic acid, can contribute to hypokalemia, elevation of cholesterol, and elevation of blood glucose in Type I diabetics. The potassium-sparing diuretics, spironolactone and triamterene, may cause hyperkalemia with accompanying cardiac arrhythmias. If diabetic nephropathy exists, one should not use spironolactone or triamterene, since severe hyperkalemia may result.

Hypokalemia in the Type II diabetic may suppress endogenous insulin release and may contribute to hyperglycemia. Administration of oral potassium or a switch to potassium-sparing diuretics usually avoids this problem.

The beta-adrenergic blockers, propranolol and metoprolol, may obscure the sympathoadrenal-induced symptoms of hypoglycemia. Although this is usually not a major concern, patients taking such drugs should be informed of this possibility. In addition, these drugs should be used with caution in patients with cardiac disease. Beta-adrenergic blocking drugs may cause hyperglycemia in non-insulin-dependent diabetics, because beta blockade leaves alpha stimulation unopposed, and the result may be a decrease in endogenous insulin secretion.

Diabetics who have orthostatic hypotension due to autonomic neuropathy may show a severe drop in blood pressure in the upright position if they are taking any of the sympathetic inhibitor drugs, such as methyldopa, clonidine, reserpine, or guanethidine. Similarly, the alpha-adrenergic blocking agent, prazosin, can exaggerate orthostatic hypotension. For such patients, one should always check blood pressure in the supine and standing positions, using the standing pressure as a guide to proper dosage. The sympathetic inhibitors may also cause impotence, and in a male diabetic who already has some neuropathic impotence, the drug therapy may make it considerably worse.

Therapy of hypertension in the diabetic without renal disease follows the accepted methods used in the general population, but with continued awareness of the possible deleterious side effects on the diabetic state. Sodium restriction, thiazides plus beta-adrenergic blocking drugs, or a sympathetic inhibitor plus hydralazine or prazosin all may be used in the proper combinations to attain the desired results. Almost all hypertension can be controlled with a well-planned program.

Systolic hypertension usually responds to diuretics alone or in combination with methyldopa, reserpine, or propranolol. The physician must be cautious and must not reduce the systolic pressure too much, since the accompanying diastolic reduction could result in compromised blood flow to the heart, brain, and kidneys.

The physician must remember that the diabetic with renal disease has a low-renin hypertension accompanied by an increased blood volume and increased peripheral resistance. One should start treatment with a thiazide diuretic if the patient is not azotemic, but with furosemide if azotemia is present. If this regimen is not effective, one should add prazosin or hydralazine to overcome peripheral resistance. If necessary, add a beta-adrenergic blocker, methyldopa, or clonidine. Finally, guanethidine may be added if indicated.

The physician should consult the Physicians' Desk Reference for complete prescribing information as well as details concerning drug complications. It is imperative to have a thorough understanding of the adverse effects of antihypertensive drugs in diabetic patients.

## PLATELET ABNORMALITIES IN DIABETES MELLITUS

Research in recent years has revealed that platelet abnormalities may affect the etiology of vascular disease in diabetics, both in atheromatous changes and in the final obliterative stage of microvascular disease. Adhesiveness of platelets has been found in diabetics of all ages and severity. Factor VIII, the von Willebrand factor of plasma, may be involved in this abnormal adhesiveness.

The second abnormality that has been investigated is platelet aggregation, with increased sensitivity to aggregating agents. Platelet aggregation influences the primary formation of atheromatous plaques, according to recent studies. Fortunately, a simple solution was discovered when it was noted that aspirin blocks this increased platelet aggregation by inhibiting the cyclo-oxygenase enzyme, which catalyzes the conversion of arachidonic acid to prostaglandin $E_2$ (PG $E_2$) within the platelet.

Ten Veterans Administration hospitals in the United States are engaged in a large-scale study to determine whether antiplatelet-aggregating agents are helpful against peripheral vascular disease. A similar study is being undertaken by the National Eye Institute, with regard to retinopathy.

Dr. George Mann of the Vanderbilt School of Medicine, an outspoken critic of some of the alleged effects of cholesterol, does not think that the level of dietary cholesterol has any effect on elevated serum cholesterol levels. He thinks that platelet factors may be the most important factor in coronary heart disease. Dr. Mann has also stated that hydrogenating vegetable oils creates abnormal trans-fatty acids, which the body has trouble using. Feeding of transfatty acids to healthy young male volunteers elevates their cholesterol levels.

Few reports have been published on the results of several in-depth studies being carried on through the World Health Organization. The results of these studies should provide insight into prevention and treatment of hyperlipidemia and the significance of elevated lipid levels in the development of CVD.

# 25

# Substitute Insulin Delivery Systems

Sufficient evidence has now accumulated through both human and animal research to relate the serious microvascular and neuropathic complications of diabetes to the levels of blood glucose as well as to the metabolic abnormalities involving lipids and amino acids. We also are aware that conventional insulin therapy rarely achieves the goal of restoring body-fuel metabolism to normal. Under special laboratory conditions that involve multiple feedings and accompanying injections of regular insulin, one can greatly improve diabetic control. However, almost complete restoration of a normal metabolic profile can be seen in patients who are connected to a so-called artificial pancreas, a closed system of continuous monitoring of blood sugar levels and delivery of calibrated amounts of insulin throughout the 24 hours. This apparatus, known in laboratories as the "Biostator," is hardly the kind one would take home, but it is excellent for research purposes.

Because of available research funds, the past few years have noted tremendous progress and research, the aim being to produce a device to deliver insulin to the body in a manner most closely resembling the response of the islet cells in the intact pancreas. It would be useless to go into a detailed explanation of various devices in this manual, since research and development are moving so rapidly that what is new today is old in 6 months. However, a brief sketch is in order.

## PANCREATIC TRANSPLANTS

Several research centers have been performing pancreatic transplants, both whole and segmental, over the past 10 years. In the majority of cases, this operation has been reserved for diabetics who had already received a kidney transplant or who were scheduled to receive transplants of a kidney and the pancreas simultaneously. These patients were in many cases already controlled by immunosuppressive drug therapy, so the additional rejection phenomenon did not take place. In the majority of transplant patients, the pancreas functioned for a short time before being rejected. An occasional patient had adequate pancreatic function for 2 to 4 years before the transplant was rejected or the patient died. A few centers continue to investigate the feasibility of such transplants, but it seems unlikely that we could expect to provide a new pancreas for the more than one million insulin-dependent diabetics, even if the major problems of transplantation were solved. Recent reports on segmental pancreatic transplants indicate better results.

## ISLET-CELL INJECTION

Other research centers have used only islet cells, in the main derived from fetal pancreatic tissue. The group at the University of Minnesota pioneered this approach and found that if the islet cells were injected into the portal system, so that they "nested" in the liver, they became functional. Most subjects who received islet cells had previously received a kidney transplant, so they were already in a continuing program of immunosuppressive therapy. Again, 2 problems are obvious: a supply of islet cells for the number of insulin-dependent diabetics who might want them, and the need for a continuous intake of immunosuppressive drugs. As a research tool, this procedure seems justifiable.

## MECHANICAL DEVICES

Current research focuses on 2 types of insulin delivery systems, the first to be worn externally and the second to be implanted in the body. The focus is mainly on the externally worn infusion devices at present. Several hundred Type I diabetics in England, Canada, and the United States are now wearing an external infusion pump, and mechanical engineering improvements are being made frequently.

Delivery sites have included subcutaneous, intravenous, and intraperitoneal sites. Most patients presently wearing a pump are delivering the insulin subcutaneously, either with a conventional 27-gauge needle or a fine nylon catheter, the latter having the advantage of lasting up to 60 days before requiring changing. The pumps used are either syringe-driven, peristaltic, or continuous-bellow-driven. Miniaturization has enabled the pump to be not much larger than a walnut.

Insulin delivery is continuous with most systems, and programming is such that approximately 0.6 to 1.0 U insulin are delivered each hour. Control of insulin delivery is accomplished through mechanical switching, magnetic switching, or electronic regulation (remote). The device may be automatically programmed or programmed by the patient. Insulin delivery in the most recent devices is continuous. A basal rate averages 0.6 to 1.0 U/hr, and the premeal bolus, given approximately 30 minutes prior to eating, is usually about 8 to 10 times the basal rate. The most satisfactory method of giving the premeal bolus at present seems to be patient-controlled. The best devices contain automatic controls following delivery of the premeal bolus, with return to the smaller basal rate. The device is easily filled with insulin as needed, and many investigators are using regular purified pork insulin.

A few diabetics have worn such devices for a sufficient time to tell something about the results, which in some cases are almost unbelievable. Blood glucose values, which have almost approximated nondiabetic levels, are rarely lower than 50 mg/dl and are rarely higher than 150 mg/dl. Other metabolites, including growth hormone, amino acid blood levels, pyruvate, lactate, lipids, and glucagon levels have returned to normal or are nearly normal. Reversal of early nephropathic changes and of retinopathy has been reported, as well as marked improvement in long-standing neuropathy.

Insulin requirements were reduced by 10 to 25% in many cases. Glucosuria was absent in almost all patients, and hypoglycemia was mild and occurred infrequently. Neither prolonged fasting nor exercise had an adverse effect. The need for strict timing of meals no longer applied since the premeal bolus was controlled by the patient.

Experience with the insulin infusion pump in the United States is meager because it has been commercially available for only a short time, since the fall of 1980. At the present time, the demand is so great that the manufacturers cannot supply the numbers requested. Practicing physicians will have many calls from their Type I patients inquiring about the pumps. The following criteria will serve as a guide in determining the advisability of a pump for a given patient:

1. It would seem that age, per se, is not half as important as is the state of maturity of the person. Some youngsters are mature at age 14 or 15, whereas others obviously are not suitable candidates for the use of the pump until a few years later. There is no established cut-off age, and some 11 or 12 year olds might well be suitable candidates.

2. The patient must demonstrate that prior to considering using a pump, every effort has been made to attain maximum control of the diabetes with a well-managed program. This regimen would include taking 2 doses of insulin per day, following the diet meticulously, having a regular exercise program, and, one hopes, having mental tranquillity.
3. The patient must have previously monitored his own blood sugar levels accurately, as often as the attending physician felt necessary. He must demonstrate that he has taken a keen interest in his diabetic state, and has made the necessary adjustments in the insulin as the result of home glucose monitoring.
4. The patient must realize that the insulin infusion pump is not a device to be used mainly for the purpose of allowing complete indifference concerning meal plans or time of meals, but is an attempt to give him the kind of insulin delivery that a normally functioning beta cell would.
5. The patient must be serious, well motivated, and fully cooperative, particularly from the standpoint of keeping in close touch with the attending physician and following instructions conscientiously.

Two pumps are now available and can be purchased when prescribed by the attending physician. The Mill-Hill pump, originally designed and manufactured in England, has now been licensed to the Harvard Apparatus Company for manufacture and distribution in the United States. More patients have used this pump than any other since the researchers in England began its use several years ago. The second available pump is the Auto-Syringe, manufactured by an American company of the same name. Experience with this pump has been limited, but to date the patients who have used it seem favorably impressed.

Both pumps work on the same principle, that is, continuous or every-few-minutes delivery of small doses of insulin around the clock, then a larger dose given 15 to 30 minutes before eating, under control of the patient. The device is to be worn 24 hours a day, except for short intervals allowing for bathing, swimming, and other athletic activities. At the present time, we feel that the insulin infusion pump should be reserved for those persons who have severe Type I diabetes, with difficulty in controlling it by the conventional means of treatment. Later, it may be useful in the Type II diabetic who takes insulin to control high blood sugar levels.

It is generally understood that, when the pump is prescribed by the doctor, around 80% of the cost is paid by most insurance companies. The present cost of the pump is close to $1,000. The cost of the test stick is around 55¢. We have not been informed to date whether the insurance companies will pay for the sticks.

Since it is obvious that patients planning to use an infusion pump will need some detailed education, the diabetes education center of which I am director has started instruction courses for such persons.

We have an added advantage because one of our nurse-instructors is wearing such a pump. It would be prudent for physicians to require their patients to attend similar instruction courses before beginning to use an infusion pump.

## IMPLANTABLE DEVICES

Implantable device designs include 2 kinds: those that deliver insulin and those that contain islet cells. Insulin may be delivered either into the subcutaneous space, intravenously, or ideally directly into the peritoneal cavity with subsequent vascular transport to the liver. The pump's exact anatomic location is still under study, but the insulin reservoir will be located subcutaneously for ease of refilling. As with the externally worn pump, the implanted pump will deliver a continuous basal dose of insulin with an appropriate increase at mealtimes. Both basal and mealtime doses of insulin will be determined by an external program-transmitter, controlled by the patient.

At the time of this writing, Drs. D. Schade and P. Eaton of the University of New Mexico had just reported an intra-abdominal pump implantation in a young male diabetic. The device had been functioning successfully for 5 months. Insulin was delivered directly into the peritoneal cavity.

Dr. J. S. Soeldner at the Joslin Research Laboratory is working on a long-range project to develop a complete artificial pancreas to be implanted and to function autonomously. Glucose levels will be continuously monitored by a glucose sensor, and insulin requirements will thus be determined by a miniature computer, which will then program the pump to deliver the proper dose of insulin.

An implantable device known as the "hybrid pancreas," under development by Dr. W. Chick and colleagues of the Joslin Research Center, may provide a permanent substitute for the missing beta cells in Type I diabetes. This device will contain islet cells, probably of porcine origin, and will be connected to an artery and a vein, so that circulating blood will perfuse the islet cells. An ingenious innovation, a microporous substance, protects the islet cells from contact with 2 substances in the blood that are mainly responsible for rejection: large lymphocytes and globulins. Perfection of this device may come in this decade.

# 26

# Home Blood Glucose Monitoring

## RATIONALE FOR HOME MONITORING

The recent surge in popularity of home blood glucose monitoring is based on reliable data proving that most diabetics are controlling their blood sugar levels more closely than was ever possible with home urine tests and infrequent blood sugar determinations done in the physician's office. It became obvious several years ago that home monitoring was helpful when clinics began asking their pregnant diabetics to do home monitoring in an effort to reduce the risks associated with pregnancy.

In May of 1979, the Diabetes and Endocrine Center of the Brooklyn-Cumberland Medical Center sponsored an international conference on the subject of home blood glucose monitoring. The proceedings of that conference were published in the journal, Diabetes Care (3:57, 1980). If reports continue to show marked improvement in control of blood sugar levels resulting from home monitoring, and with the advent of improved instruments and methods, within the next few years most Type I, motivated diabetics will probably follow this procedure.

Many patients report a lack of correlation between blood sugar levels and urine test results and a tenuous correlation between home blood sugar levels and those determined in the physician's laboratory at similar times of day. Most clinics that have studied groups of diabetics who monitor their blood sugar levels at home have found that a gradual, stepwise approach to the program is most satisfactory. For the first week, the patients are asked to check blood sugar levels before and an hour after each meal, as well as any time that they feel hypo- or hyperglycemic. There is no change of insulin dosage during this week of observation. This period gives patients the opportunity to assure themselves that they can accomplish the test without difficulty and to note the vagaries of glucose control, finding that they frequently cannot correlate symptoms with blood sugar levels. The second week of the program is usually when adjustments in insulin dosage are made. The ultimate goal is to keep blood sugar levels between 70 and 140 mg/dl, similar to nondiabetic glucose excursions. In this type of program, patients become proficient at modifying their own insulin doses, to avoid hypoglycemia as well as hyperglycemia. Most patients are controlled with 2 doses per day of mixed insulin and are thoroughly instructed in the time-actions of the components. It has been generally observed that the first important step is to control the fasting blood sugar level, since the daytime sugar levels are subsequently easier to keep in a normal range.

It is obvious that allowing patients to be partners in the management of their disorder is advantageous to everyone. For the most part, compliance of the patient is good, and most patients are able to avoid both hypoglycemia and hyperglycemia. Dietary restrictions were relaxed in some of the programs without a rise in blood sugar levels. There are distinct economic advantages to such a program; it will result in fewer hospital trips for hypoglycemia, threatened acidosis, or "for control." Several clinics in Great Britain instruct all new Type I diabetic patients in home monitoring from the start, since they believe that this method should be the routine for all such patients.

## COLORIMETER DEVICES IN USE

These devices usually use capillary or fingertip blood. Glucose values for capillary blood compare almost equally with glucose values for venous plasma.

**Ames Dextrometer.** This device costs $340 (battery pack $35 extra). This method uses a glucose oxidase-based strip, which when saturated with blood, undergoes a colorimetric reaction proportional to the glucose concentration. The meter allows accurate reading of the Dextrostix. Capillary blood samples are procured by pricking the finger with a sharp lancet. One drop of blood is placed on the Dextrostix and is allowed to remain for exactly 60 seconds. The Dextrostix is then washed off with a special wash bottle that uses water, is blotted dry, and is inserted into the meter for reading. Standard reference strips are provided for calibration before each use, and in addition, a calibration and control set using simulated blood is provided for periodic checking. One can thus see that in order to be accurate, careful attention must be paid to the directions. Dextrostix cost 60 cents each.

**StatTek Twin-Beam Electronic Photometer.** Marketed by Biodynamics of Indianapolis, a subsidiary of Boehringer-Mannheim, this device is similar to the Ames system. The price is $675 and test strips are 55 cents each.

**Glucocheck.** This is made in England by Medistron, Ltd., and sells for $150. This instrument is small, portable, and battery-powered (rechargeable). It uses Dextrostix and has a built-in timer that automatically switches off. Because the machine is factory-calibrated, it requires no further calibration during its lifetime. It would seem that these are distinct advantages. At present, it is not available in the United States.

Undoubtedly other devices will appear on the market, and ultimately all will be simple, accurate, and reasonably priced.

## COLOR-STRIP METHODS

**Chemstrip-bG.** This method of checking blood glucose levels has just appeared on the market. A patient of mine, who wears an infusion pump, compared Chemstrip-bG to both the Ames system and the Beckman glucose analyzer and stated that they correlate well. This system is so simple that, if proven accurate, it may eliminate the need for photometer methods. Recent reports of larger numbers of comparative tests using Chemstrip-bG show a favorable correlation with standard laboratory methods for glucose measurement, with a variance under 15% generally.

Chemstrip-bG uses fingertip blood that, after the proper waiting time, is simply wiped off the strip and is compared with double color scales printed on the vial containing the test strips. Double color comparison adds to the accuracy, it is believed. Values can be read from 20 mg/dl up to 800 mg/dl in increments of 20, 40, 80, 120, 180, 240, 400, and 800 mg/dl. Variations in color tones allow the patient to approximate values between the color zones. The advantages are mainly in cost and convenience, since no instrument is involved. This method may be preferred in future. Chemstrip-bG is marketed by Biodynamics of Indianapolis, a subsidiary of Boehringer-Mannheim. The strips cost about 65 cents each.

**Ames Dextrostix.** The color appearing on the Dextrostix can be compared with a standard color strip, instead of using the Dextrometer, but it is felt that the inaccuracy of color matching precludes its being a satisfactory method, and it has generally been discontinued.

The types of patient for whom one thinks of home monitoring to establish the best possible diabetic control include the following:

1. Pregnant diabetics. Some clinics routinely have pregnant Type I diabetic patients use the home monitoring techniques all through pregnancy and have found it to be valuable in maintaining patients' euglycemia.
2. Patients with altered renal thresholds that render urinary tests completely unreliable. Many postpubertal teenage girls are in this category.
3. Patients in whom adequate control is difficult to attain and to maintain, and in whom unusual fluctuations of blood sugar levels are frequent and are difficult to interpret.
4. Patients who have frequent episodes of unrecognized hypoglycemia, particularly if associated with seizure disorders.
5. Patients who think that they are hypoglycemic when other indicators do not confirm this belief.

The frequency of home blood glucose determinations is established by the attending physician and depends on the patient. In most instances, after the original indoctrination period, the patient does home glucose tests q.i.d., the same schedule as that for urine testing. Some clinics ask for a diurnal profile done once a week, consisting of 7 determinations—before each meal, 2 hours after each meal, and at bedtime. Patients who may have nocturnal hypoglycemia can do determinations during the night, when the episode occurs.

The advantages of home blood glucose monitoring are as follows:

1. Testing takes place in normal home conditions of work, rest, exercise, and usual daily stresses, instead of in the artificial and sometimes stressful atmosphere of the laboratory or physician's office.
2. By comparing the results of both urine and blood tests, the patient can establish a true renal threshold.
3. A record of blood sugar levels allows the patient to evaluate the appropriateness of the diet and insulin therapy.
4. Similarly, the record of blood sugar levels can readily show the patient what can happen if the program is not followed.
5. It shows the patient the effect on blood sugar levels of exercise, mild illnesses, menstrual periods, and other stresses.
6. Blood sugar levels positively identify hypoglycemic levels and could uncover an otherwise unrecognized Somogyi effect.
7. Psychologically, home monitoring apparently has a tremendous effect by bolstering the patient's confidence in his ability to alter the insulin dosage and/or diet as indicated by the record of blood sugar levels. The patient shortly becomes an important part of the team and learns to share the responsibility for good control with the attending physician.
8. It is of the utmost value to pregnant diabetics and is indicated for almost all of them.

9. It is of similar value in the unstable diabetes so often noted in postpubertal teenage girls, whose renal thresholds are frequently unreliable.

Few problems have arisen in home glucose monitoring, among them the following:

1. The patient may experience technical problems with the procedure and/or the apparatus.
2. Some patients are not sufficiently motivated and/or educated to perform the procedure accurately and dependably.
3. A few patients are reluctant to do the repeated finger-pricks necessary to obtain blood specimens. (Several spring-loaded devices are now available that do the finger-prick automatically on release of a trigger, and some patients report this procedure to be more acceptable than the manual method.)

# 27

# Substitute Sweeteners

## NON-NUTRITIVE SWEETENERS

This category includes cyclamate, saccharin, and others.

### Cyclamate

Cyclamate was discovered incidentally in 1937 by Michael Sveda, a chemist at the University of Illinois. While working in his laboratory, he put his cigarette down; when he later picked it up, it tasted sweet. Dr. Sveda proceeded to taste the contents of all the chemicals in the area of the cigarette, and this was the beginning of the sodium cyclamate story. In 1950, Abbott Laboratories put cyclamate on the market, where it remained until it was banned by the FDA in 1970.

Cyclamate was a better sweetener than saccharin, which had been used for the previous 60 or so years and left a bitter aftertaste with many persons. There followed many artificially sweetened products, including canned fruits, mouthwashes, toothpastes, chewing gum, and diet soft drinks. It was not long before cyclamates became a billion-dollar-a-year, diet-product business.

When Abbott Laboratories petitioned the FDA to market cyclamate, they turned them down on the basis that the experiments were not conducted properly. The FDA then embarked on their own 2-year experiment, after which they approved cyclamate with the mild restriction that it must be labeled "should be used only by persons who must restrict their intake of orinary sweets." In addition, a committee of the National Academy of Sciences warned that "at intakes of five grams or more per day, cyclamate has produced a mild laxative effect." One had to consume 100 Sucaryl tablets per day or drink 3 quarts of diet beverages to consume 5 grams. In 1958, after the Delaney Amendment was passed, cyclamate was placed on the "GRAS" list, i.e., "Generally Recognized As Safe." In 1965, the FDA repeated that there was no evidence that cyclamate was a hazard to health. Ther cyclamate industry then grew to an annual consumption rate of 18 million pounds by 1967.

At this time there were many claims and counterclaims about the superiority of sugar over cyclamates. Abbott Laboratories had claimed that cyclamate was not metabolized in the body and was simply excreted unchanged, but Japanese scientists found a metabolic product called cyclohexylamine in both humans and dogs following ingestion of cyclamates. There was some earlier evidence that cyclohexylamine was not entirely safe for human use. Research projects sponsored both by Abbott Laboratories and the sugar industry followed, with conflicting results. The FDA asked the National Academy of Sciences National Research Council to appoint a committee to study cyclamates. In November of 1968, the National Academy of Sciences reaffirmed their previous position, that up to 5 grams of cyclamate per day posed no hazard to an adult. In December of 1968, the FDA cautioned the public to restrict its daily use to 3.5 grams for an adult.

Further research projects uncovered alarming changes in test animals. In June of 1969, researchers at the University of Wisconsin found a significant incidence of bladder tumors in white Swiss mice. Another Abbott Laboratories-sponsored research project found bladder tumors in rats that had been fed a mixture of cyclamate and saccharin in a ratio of 10 to 1, the ratio found in many soft drinks. Fifty per cent of the tumors were cancerous. As a result, cyclamate was removed from the GRAS list in 1969, and in August of 1970, the FDA ordered all cyclamate-containing products banned as of September 11, 1970.

On November 15, 1973, Abbott Laboratories submitted a petition to the FDA to permit the use of cyclamate as a sweetening agent in foods for special dietary use. About 300 reports on toxicology were submitted, but the FDA asked for more information. It would seem that this request imposed a formidable task on Abbott Laboratories. However, in 1980 they again petitioned the FDA to permit the use of cyclamate and again were refused. Abbott then announced that they had "surrendered" in their battle with the government.

## Saccharin

Saccharin, first synthesized in 1879 at Johns Hopkins University, became popular as an artificial sweetener during World War I, when the production of sugar was limited. Around 5 million pounds were used as a food additive in some form in 1976, almost 75% in diet drinks. The rest was used in cosmetics, pharmaceuticals, animal feed, canned fruits, chewing gum, and fruit preserves, for example.

Everyone seemed happy with the use of saccharin; it did not appear to be metabolized in the body, it was considered to be safe, and the FDA had placed it on their GRAS list. On June 25, 1971, however, the FDA published a proposal to remove saccharin from the GRAS list and to establish a provisional regulation prescribing conditions of safe use. Studies of saccharin's relationship with cancer were done mainly with rats, both first- and second-generation studies. The single-generation feeding studies involved feeding rats a 5.0% diet of saccharin, i.e., 2.5 g/kg body weight/day, equivalent to 800 diet soft drinks per person per day. Two-generation studies were carried out in a similar fashion. Seven single-generation rat studies reported no relationship between cancer and saccharin ingestion up to levels of 7.5% and up to 24 months. Monkey studies reported no abnormalities after more than 6 years of ingestion of variable doses of saccharin.

Three investigations of 2-generation rat studies formed the basis for the proposed ban of saccharin by the FDA. In these studies, the rats were exposed to saccharin *in utero,* during suckling, and throughout their remaining life. Each study found a significant increase in bladder cancer, mostly in male rats at high-dosage (5% or over) feeding. The first 2 studies were done by the FDA and the Wisconsin Alumni Research Foundation, and the third study was done by Canadians. The findings, which have been subjected to detailed studies by many scientists, are not repeated here. An outstanding criticism of these studies concerned the fact that fetal concentration of saccharin may have been high because saccharin, in crossing the placental barrier, is cleared more slowly by the fetus than by the parent. In addition, if the newborns were exposed to high levels during weaning, theoretically the urine concentration of saccharin could be high, with deleterious effect on the bladder mucosa. Eleven out of twelve human studies on bladder cancer and use of saccharin failed to show any association. The study that did show a significant increase in bladder cancer has been faulted by several critics. There was a sex difference. Women using saccharin were found to have less bladder cancer than the control subjects, whereas men were found to have more. No nonhormonal carcinogen in man is known to affect a single sex, so this came as a distinct surprise.

In April of 1977, the FDA proposed a ban on saccharin as a food additive. There was immediate public response against this ban, and Congress passed an 18-month delay of the ban. In June of 1979, a 24-month moratorium was declared by Congress. In July of 1978, the

American Diabetes Association, in a policy statement on saccharin, concluded that "much more research of broader scope and greater detail is needed before the saccharin controversy can be resolved. An appraisal of the experimental data through May 1978 has been published elsewhere. Surveillance of new information by the Association will continue. However, based on evidence now available, there appears to be little justification for placing further governmental restriction on the use of saccharin by the American public at the present time" (Diabetes Care, 1:209,1978).

The action of the FDA is thought to be mainly a result of the Delaney Amendment, passed by Congress in 1958, which states that any food additive that causes cancer in experimental animals cannot be used for human consumption. However, 2 qualifications in the Delaney Amendment can make decision by the FDA discretionary and not necessarily mandatory. The amendment states that 2 conditions must be met before it can be invoked, the first being that appropriate tests show a substance to be carcinogenic. Many scientists doubt that the investigations of saccharin were appropriate. The second condition is that the substance must induce cancer. The FDA feels that the tests are appropriate and that the substance does cause cancer.

The Canadian investigators, who arrived at different conclusions concerning the dangers of cancer from both cyclamates and saccharin, do not believe that cyclamates cause cancer in humans. Cyclamates are sold in Canadian pharmacies without a prescription. A simple label states "this should be consumed with the advice of a physician." Although the Canadian scientists feel that saccharin is carcinogenic, it also is available in pharmacies as a food sweetener, but it cannot be used in soft drinks. Many diabetic patients in the northern United States purchase cyclamate sweeteners in Canada for personal use.

Meanwhile, important studies are being done to determine whether saccharin causes cancer in human beings and to investigate the possibility that impurities in saccharin rather than saccharin itself may cause cancer. A most important study was conducted nationwide by the National Cancer Institute and the FDA, to determine whether saccharin does cause human cancer. This study, begun in March of 1978 and completed in December of 1979, was based on personal interviews with around 3000 persons with newly diagnosed bladder cancer. The age limits were over 21 and under 85. In addition, this study gathered information on any association between human cancer and cyclamates.

The study was reported by Dr. Robert Hoover in March, 1980, and briefly, this was the conclusion: "The evidence is that little, if any, current bladder cancer is due to the consumption of artificial sweeteners at the doses and in the manner in which sweeteners were commonly consumed in the past" (N. Engl. J. Med. *302*:573, 1980). Additionally, the researchers reported no evidence that diabetics have more cancer of the bladder than nondiabetics. A study recently reported by Dr. L. S. Morrison of the Harvard Medical School Department of Epidemiology concluded, "As a group, users of artificial sweeteners have little or no excess risk of cancer of the lower urinary tract" (N. Engl. J. Med., *302*:537, 1980). Drs. Wynder and Stellman of the American Health Foundation's recent study stated that "no association was found between the use of artificial sweeteners or diet beverages and bladder cancer" (Science, *207*:1214, 1980).

Saccharin probably should not be used by pregnant women, since it crosses the placenta and an accumulation could take place in the fetus. No definitive studies have been done on this problem, however.

We have no scientific way to evaluate artificial sweeteners, either in diabetics or in the obese. Would most diabetics drink sugar-sweetened soft drinks if diet drinks were not available? Would the obese do the same? The use of saccharin in foods and beverages has made dietary life more pleasant for diabetics, particularly the younger ones who are avid soft drink consumers. These products are probably of similar value and comfort to obese persons trying to reduce their caloric intake. In terms of relative values, how many lives are extended and saved by the use of artificial sweeteners and how many would be lost as a result of their use?

### Other Artificial Sweeteners

Various products have been suggested for use as artificial sweeteners.

**Dihydrochalcones.** These substances are synthesized commercially from naringen, a bitter component of grapefruit skins. The United States Department of Agriculture has been working with them for over 20 years. Neohesperidine dihydrochalcone (Neo-DHC) is 1500 times sweeter than sucrose. Several companies have applied to the FDA for approval for use in chewing gum, but the FDA has turned them down, stating that insufficient data exist concerning the safety of the substance. However, these products seem to have the most optimistic future.

**Miracle Fruit.** A berry found on a bush that grows in West Africa, this taste-modifying substance causes sour foods to taste sweet. After tasting the berry juice, sour foods such as lemons and limes taste wonderfully sweet. The Miralin Corporation, which planned to use miracle fruit concentrate in diabetic foods, was started in 1968 and went into bankruptcy in January, 1975. The FDA denied their petition to classify Miralin as GRAS, in spite of the fact that Africans have eaten it for hundreds of years and it was approved as safe by the Food and Agriculture Organization. In addition, the Miralin Company submitted copious data.

**Serendipity Berries.** These berries, indigenous to tropical West Africa, are borne on climbing vines and grow in grape-like clusters. The Monell Senses Center and the Unilever Research Laboratorium have called the berry "Monellin."

**Others.** Dynapol Corporation is developing a sweetener that is said to be nonabsorbable, water-soluble, and polymer-bound. The Stanford Research Institute is researching a new aldoxime sweetener. The National Institute of Dental Research is funding work on a new, noncariogenic sweetener. Hoechst-Roussel A. G. of Frankfurt is working on a sweetener called acetosulfam. Japan's Toray Industries is investigating new sweeteners.

In time, there will be artificial sweeteners that meet all the criteria for safety, stability, solubility, and taste. To be ideal it should have the taste of sucrose and the pharmacology of pure spring water.

## NUTRITIVE SWEETENERS

Almost all human beings, including those with diabetes, have a desire for sweetness that cannot be ignored. The ban on the nonnutritive sweetener cyclamate and the threat of a ban on saccharin, in addition to lack of other FDA-licensed chemical or natural sweeteners, lead investigators to research further the use of the nutritive sweeteners. Some interesting discoveries have been made that generally favor their use.

### Fructose

Also known as fruit sugar or levulose, fructose is found in many fruits, vegetables, berries, and honey (40%). Fifty per cent of sucrose (table sugar) is fructose; the other 50% is glucose. The amount of fructose in fruits and berries varies from 2 to 6%. Fructose can be formed in the body from glucose or sorbitol, and only traces of it circulate in human blood. It is 1½ times sweeter than sucrose, but the sweetness is more noticeable when it is cool. Fructose is soluble in water and withstands high temperatures in preparing foods and canning. Commercially, it is made by extraction from sucrose. There is no bitter aftertaste. Fructose yields 3.75 kcal/g.

Fructose is slowly absorbed in the jejunum by facilitated diffusion, and the majority of it is absorbed unmetabolized, with a slight conversion (5 to 8%) to glucose or lactate during absorption. It is metabolized mainly by the liver, by the fructose-1-phosphate pathway. The first reaction is catalyzed by fructokinase, an enzyme that functions independently of insulin; moreover, the entry of fructose into the liver does not require insulin. The next product of metabolism is fructose-1-phosphate, and the next is the trioses. Only the final destiny of these trioses depends on insulin. With adequate amounts of insulin, trioses are oxidized to pyruvate and are finally metabolized through the Krebs cycle. The metabolism of fructose in man is rapid, its half-life being about 18 minutes.

The effect of fructose on the diabetic state has been studied, in particular the rise in blood glucose levels on ingestion of fructose. In general, it has been found that the rise in plasma glucose levels after the ingestion of fructose may be even lower than after ingestion of complex carbohydrates. Several excellent clinical studies have shown that the isocaloric replacement of glucose by fructose decreases hyperglycemia and glucosuria in Type I and Type II diabetics whose disorder is controlled. Experiments using fructose as a powder on desserts, as a sweetener in coffee and tea, or sprinkled on cereals and fruits showed that the average well-controlled diabetic can consume 75 g/day of fructose without exacerbating hyperglycemia. However, the caloric value must be calculated into the diet. Generally, most physicians feel that 30 to 35 g/day should be sufficient as an added sweetener. This amount does not alter plasma glucose levels.

It has been reported that the daily ingestion of high amounts of fructose (200 to 500 g/day) can increase triglyceride levels, whereas moderate amounts (60 to 70 g) have no significant effect. Similar results were seen in a chronic consumption study (24 months), with no changes in triglyceride or cholesterol levels. A 2-year study on dental caries showed that patients using fructose had an incidence of caries that was 25% less than that of the control group, which used sucrose.

Since fructose is sweeter than sucrose, a lesser amount can be used. For instance, if a recipe calls for ½ c sugar, one should use ⅜ c fructose; for 1 c sugar, one should substitute ¾ c fructose. Fructose in both granular and liquid form is now available in most grocery stores. A high-fructose corn syrup contains about 90% fructose and about 8% glucose. The low-fructose corn syrup, which contains 42% fructose and 50% glucose, is contraindicated in the diabetic diet. If patients are interested in recipes using fructose, they should request them from Batter-Lite Foods Inc., P.O. Box 341, Beloit, WI 53511.

In summary, it appears that fructose will be used more extensively by the diabetic patient in the future.

## Sorbitol

Sorbitol is a sugar alcohol present in many plants and produced commercially. It causes osmotic diarrhea in doses of more than 30 g, so this limits the amount that can be used daily. It is absorbed by passive diffusion and is immediately oxidized to fructose. Sorbitol does not require insulin until the conversion product, fructose, reaches the triose stage, nor does it raise plasma glucose levels. Sorbitol has little advantage over fructose. It produces 4 cal/g. Oral sorbitol does not follow the "sorbitol pathway" we have referred to in discussing neuropathy and other complications, so the diabetic need not be concerned about the presence of sorbitol in foods.

## Aspartame

Aspartame, which is a product of normal protein metabolism (a dipeptide made up of L-aspartic acid and the methyl ester of phenylalanine), is 200 times sweeter than sucrose, and yields 4 cal/g. It has no known effect on glucose tolerance. The FDA's Bureau of Foods has studied the data and has given a favorable preliminary report. Aspartame may be released for general use in the near future.

## Xylitol

Another sugar alcohol, xylitol, is present in many plants, especially strawberries, raspberries, and of all things, cauliflower. It is produced commercially from hardwood and birch residues. Like sorbitol, xylitol causes osmotic diarrhea in large doses. Its sweetness is equivalent to fructose, and it is spicy. After absorption, it is efficiently taken up by the liver; the oxidative degradation to the trioses in the glycolytic pathway occurs in the liver. Xylitol is probably the least cariogenic of all nutritive sweeteners, and thus is the preferred agent in chewing gum and other substances likely to stick to the teeth. Xylitol does not increase blood glucose or triglyceride levels. It produces 4 cal/g.

In summary, from reports on fructose, sorbitol, aspartame, and xylitol, it is obvious that these substances are safe when taken orally, they do not cause hyperglycemia as do sucrose and glucose, and less insulin is needed to keep blood sugar levels constant after ingestion. In addition, they are absorbed from the bowel and are taken up by the liver without the need for insulin until their final metabolic conversion to glucose. These substances decrease ketogenesis and do not increase serum triglyceride levels. It is reported that patients who use these substances follow their meal plans more faithfully. One undesirable side effect has been noted with sorbitol and xylitol, i.e., the tendency to osmotic diarrhea with higher doses. Long-term studies to evaluate the effects of these sweeteners on diabetic control, complications, nutritional values, and general safety will be carried out in the near future. Aspartame may be released for general use in the near future.

## SPECIAL "DIET" FOODS

Special foods usually sold in "health food" stores are not needed to achieve the dietary objectives prescribed by the physician. These dietary objectives can be achieved less expensively and by choosing from commonly available food items. Foods carrying labels such as "diet," or "dietetic," or "diabetic" are interpreted differently by consumers, and if the patients do use them, they usually have no regard for the caloric content. An FDA survey reported that 22% of persons questioned thought the word "dietetic" on a label meant that it was for use in a reducing diet; 28% said that it was for diabetic use only. The use of such foods complicates the problem of maintaining a constant daily caloric intake for diabetics or obese persons. Complete labeling of all such foods has recently been made a requirement by the FDA, so that there will be less guessing of contents and caloric value. Most diabetologists feel that 2 types of special foods are worthwhile for diabetics, "diet" soft drinks and water-packed fruits.

In the future we shall probably see more jams, jellies, and bakery products made with fructose, sorbitol, or xylitol—they are already popular among diabetics in Western European countries. I suggest that the American Dietetic Association take immediate steps to formulate recipes for some "goodies" made with these sweeteners. The relative cost of fructose, for instance, is reduced with increased production and consumption. Diabetics would have a greater freedom of choice in heretofore forbidden types of foods without changing their overall diabetic control. The desire for sweetness is universal in human beings. Of 500 diabetics questioned in a study by Mehnert, 84 said they could do without sweet-tasting foods, but all 416 others used either artificial or nutritive sweeteners.

## FURTHER READING

Symposium on sweeteners. Diabetes Care, 1:209, 1978.

# 28

# Glycohemoglobin

Some years ago, it was noted that many diabetics had a much higher percentage of glycohemoglobin (HbA-1c) than nondiabetics, and there followed a series of studies regarding the value of this factor in appraising diabetic control. What is HbA-1c? Early studies of hemoglobin indicated that only 2 components existed, "A," for adult, and "F," for fetal hemoglobin. Further studies demonstrated that there were several variant hemoglobins. When separated by a chromatographic column, hemoglobin shows several fast-moving minor components, labeled HbA-1a through HbA-1c, in addition to other components. In uncontrolled diabetes, all HbA-1 components are elevated, but HbA-1c is present in the greatest amounts and is the easiest to measure. Most laboratory methods measure only HbA-1c, but some measure and report all 3, i.e., HbA-1a through HbA-1c, in which case the normal values are higher.

Glycosylation of hemoglobin is a postsynthesis, nonenzymatic chemical reaction between glucose and phosphorylated sugar (glucose-6-phosphate) with the N-terminal valine of the B-chain of the hemoglobin molecule. Since hemoglobin is exposed to the ambient glucose concentration in the blood, a higher concentration will result in more glycohemoglobin formation. The result is that this hemoglobin becomes an important index of the long-term control of diabetes and may be a more reliable index than the degree of hyperglycemia or glucosuria. In a nondiabetic, HbA-1c is between 3 and 8% of all hemoglobin, whereas in patients with poorly controlled diabetes, it may be anywhere between 8 and 20%. The advantage of measuring glycohemoglobin as a parameter of diabetic control is that it indicates the level of control of the disorder for the previous 60 days, when the RBCs are about halfway through their 120-day cycle.

## LABILE FORM

Recently reported studies suggest that a small percentage (10 to 15%) of glycohemoglobin comprises a labile form that is responsive to sudden changes in plasma glucose, whereas the major portion is stable, once formed. The labile portion can change after 12 hours of euglycemia; after 48 hours of euglycemia, only the stable glycohemoglobin remains, according to a report from the Joslin Clinic. In performing the test for glycohemoglobin, the laboratory can remove the labile form by incubating the RBCs in normal saline solution at 37°C for 5 hours.

## INTERPRETATION OF TEST RESULTS AND ADVANTAGES

These results vary with the method used. An indication of normal diabetic control is HbA-1c of 3 to 8.5%. Transitional diabetic control is signified by 8.5 to 12%, and 12 to 20% HbA-1c indicates uncontrolled diabetes.

The distinct advantages of using glycohemoglobin as a measure of diabetic control are as follows:

1. It measures control of diabetes over a period of the past 60 to 70 days.
2. Diabetics who "go into training" by skimping on food and/or taking extra insulin in the 24 hours before a blood glucose test find that such manipulations have only a slight effect, if any, on the outcome of a glycohemoglobin determination.
3. Blood can be drawn any time of the day, unrelated to food intake, exercise, or emotional upsets provided the laboratory method is used that eliminates the labile form.
4. It may establish a better standard for measuring the degree of control than blood or urine glucose measurements.
5. It is useful in patients with abnormalities of renal thresholds in whom testing for glucosuria is of little value.
6. It is also useful for unstable diabetics whose blood sugar levels vary from day to day or even from hour to hour.
7. It might indicate to the physician the time to prescribe insulin for a patient taking oral agents.
8. It is certainly not a test to be done frequently, but rather twice or 3 times a year, or more often if indicated.

Pediatricians are generally impressed with the value of this test in younger patients, especially those under age 10, in whom blood glucose determinations are affected by so many emotional factors and are not reliable. Many pediatricians use glycohemoglobin values and the results of 24-hour quantitative urine glucose measurements for guidance in establishing good diabetic control. They order these tests as often as indicated by the patient's control, usually about every 3 months.

## UNANSWERED QUESTIONS

There is undoubtedly excellent correlation between the levels of blood glucose and HbA-1c. However, some pertinent questions remain unanswered. We need to know whether the mean daily blood glucose level is the main factor affecting HbA-1c levels and whether short periods of high blood glucose levels can produce the same effect as smaller elevations over a longer period of time.

## NONDIABETIC FACTORS

A physician should keep in mind that RBC disorders and hemoglobinopathies alter the laboratory findings, so one should order RBC, hemoglobin, and hematocrit tests for each patient. The following changes may occur:

1. Anemia from bleeding or hemolysis lowers HbA-1c.
2. Hemoglobinopathy renders the findings unreliable.
3. Patients who have undergone splenectomy may have elevated HbA-1c levels because of the lengthened RBC survival time.

At present, the most important benefit derived from this determination is the evaluation of the degree of long-term diabetic control. In the past, evaluation of a patient's state of diabetic control by other means (hyperglycemia, glucosuria) has been subject to various interpretations. There were no standardized criteria. Glycohemoglobin determinations may provide the standard measurement.

An important aspect of glycosylation of proteins other than hemoglobin has been introduced by the studies done with HbA-1c. If, as some investigators believe, glycosylation of structural proteins, such as those in basement membranes, is involved in microvascular complications of diabetes, then the measurement of HbA-1c may give important but indirect information regarding the degree of glycosylation taking place in other organs.

## 2-3 DIPHOSPHOGLYCERATE

Early work showed that the dissociation of oxygen from HbA-1c was slower than from other hemoglobins, but because of its limited amount this is not of practical importance in terms of tissue anoxia.

In contrast, Dr. Ditzel, in his extensive studies, has shown that there is a decrease in the compound 2-3 diphosphoglycerate (2-3 DPG) in the RBCs of many diabetics. This compound ordinarily enhances the release of oxygen from hemoglobin. He also believes that a phosphate-rich diet with additional calcium diphosphate might help, since he has shown in his own patients that he can increase 2-3 DPG in nondiabetics. Further studies are needed before any positive conclusions can be drawn.

# 29

# Diabetes Secondary to Other Disease States and Rare Types of Diabetes

## PANCREATITIS

Diabetes may occur secondary to both acute and chronic forms of pancreatitis.

### Acute

Almost all patients with acute pancreatitis have impaired glucose tolerance, and frank hyperglycemia occurs in about one-third of all cases. The carbohydrate intolerance returns to normal in almost all patients following recovery from pancreatitis; only about 2% develop permanent diabetes. Treatment of the diabetes during the acute stage depends on the degree of hyperglycemia, and small doses of insulin may be required for a short time in some cases.

### Chronic

Diabetes is commonly associated with chronic pancreatitis. It occurs in about 15% of patients with pancreatitis who do not have calcinosis, but in about 50% of patients with calcific deposits. The diabetes is usually mild and easily controlled, but an occasional case is severe. About two-thirds of these diabetic patients require insulin for control. Retinopathy and nephropathy have been observed in patients with diabetes resulting from chronic pancreatitis.

## PANCREATECTOMY

Ninety per cent of the pancreas must be removed before clinical diabetes results. In patients undergoing subtotal pancreatectomy, the resulting diabetes is usually mild, stable, and controlled without insulin. After total pancreatectomy, the diabetes is frequently severe and difficult to control, with wide fluctuations of blood sugar levels; these patients are often prone to ketoacidosis. Their insulin requirements average around 25 U/day.

## TRAUMA TO PANCREAS

Occasionally, one hears of a lawsuit in which the onset of diabetes is claimed to result from a crushing abdominal injury, presumably with pancreatic injury. There is no substance to such a claim, since an injury sufficient to destroy 90% of the pancreas would certainly result in the patient's death. The trauma of an accident, with an increased concentration of stress hormones, could conceivably uncover a latent diabetic state.

## EXOGENOUS CORTISONE AND DIABETES

Even long-term treatment with exogenous cortisone for various disorders produces glucose intolerance of variable degrees in only 1 to 2% of patients, and most of these have a family history of diabetes. In most instances, the glucose tolerance returns to normal after cessation of therapy. If a diabetic requires corticosteroid therapy when no other therapy will help, there is no contraindication to giving such treatment. The physician has to realize that hyperglycemia increases and that insulin may be required if the patient has previously controlled his diabetes without it. In patients who already take insulin, the requirements increase, sometimes by almost 100%. When the dose of cortisone is reduced, the physician must cautiously avoid severe hypoglycemia, since the adrenal glands are relatively inactive at first and resume full activity slowly.

Steroid-induced diabetes occurs frequently (10%) after renal transplantation in adults, usually within 3 months of transplantation. Some patients require insulin for diabetic control, but the degree of hyperglycemia and the requirement for insulin decrease with time. The hyperglycemia has disappeared on discontinuance of the steroid treatment in all cases reported.

## CUSHING'S SYNDROME

About 80% of patients with Cushing's syndrome have either frank diabetes or impaired glucose tolerance, mainly owing to the excess of glucocorticoids. The diabetes is usually stable, mild, and easily controlled. Many of these patients have hypernormal amounts of serum insulin and may have cell receptor decreases, as in the obese Type II diabetic. Occasionally, an obese patient with hyperglycemia may be in the early stages of Cushing's syndrome, and the alert physician must take the necessary diagnostic steps. One should look for central obesity, cutaneous striae, osteoporosis, weakness, hypertension, plethora, and hirsutism. The physician should draw blood for a serum cortisol test. For details of diagnosis, the reader is referred to endocrinology textbooks. When Cushing's syndrome is cured, the diabetes disappears.

## ACROMEGALY

Diabetes occurs in 30 to 35% of all acromegalics, and another 30% show impaired glucose tolerance. The diabetes may be of variable severity, from mild to severe, and may require large doses of insulin for adequate control. With treatment of the acromegaly, carbohydrate intolerance frequently improves, but some acromegalics continue to require insulin for diabetic control. Studies in progress relate concentrations of growth hormone to carbohydrate intolerance in treated acromegalics.

## PHEOCHROMOCYTOMA

An occasional patient with a pheochromocytoma develops mild diabetes, which promptly disappears after removal of the tumor.

## HEMOCHROMATOSIS

"Bronze diabetes" is a label given to the diabetes resulting from the deposit of hemosiderin crystals in the beta cells in the course of the disorder called hemochromatosis. The skin pigmentation, occurring in some cases, results from deposits of both melanin and hemosiderin and has a bronze cast; hence the name. Hemochromatosis results from an excess accumulation of iron in the body, starting with excessive iron absorption from the gut that elevates serum iron concentration and increases saturation of the iron-binding proteins. Iron deposits in the liver cause cirrhosis of variable severity. This disorder is far more common in men than in women, and about 65% of all patients with hemochromatosis develop diabetes. The diabetes follows a pattern similar to that of primary diabetes, and all the complications have been observed in some patients.

The average primary physician may see one such case in a lifetime. The clues to diagnosis include the patient's age (commonly 40 to 60 years), skin pigmentation as described, hepatomegaly with some hepatic dysfunction, occasional evidence of hypogonadism; not infrequently cardiac failure, and diabetes. Laboratory confirmation shows increased serum iron and iron-binding saturation.

Treatment consists of the usual diabetic diet and necessary insulin—sometimes large doses are required—and repeated phlebotomies, done frequently enough to reduce excess iron stores. In most cases reported, the diabetes has been permanent, although insulin reqirements may reduce after several years of treatment. The prognosis is guarded.

## HYPERTHYROIDISM

Occasionally, hyperthyroidism is accompanied by the onset of diabetes mellitus. One should be alert to this possibility. In addition, the incidence of hyperthyroidism is higher in persons with diabetes than in the general population. If a diabetic develops tachycardia or atrial fibrillation, weight loss, and perhaps heat intolerance, the physician should suspect hyperthyroidism and should order the appropriate tests.

## RARE FORMS OF DIABETES MELLITUS

Many rare forms of diabetes are seldom seen by the primary care physician. I mention them here only in brief; further discussion is found in more detailed books on the subject.

**Lipoatrophic Diabetes.** This is also known as the Lawrence type of diabetes and is characterized by partial or total absence of adipose tissue and by severe hyperlipidemia, insulin resistance, lack of ketoacidosis in spite of poor diabetic control, and hepatomegaly. Two subtypes have been described under this heading, congenital generalized lipodystrophy and acquired lipodystrophy.

Congenital generalized lipodystrophy (Bernardinelli-Seip syndrome) is recessively inherited. Patients have no fat in adipocytes; adipose tissue is absent in the entire body, including the cheeks and perianal area. Their growth rate is increased in the first few years, and then follows a period of normal growth; skeletal maturation is increased. Female patients have clitoral hypertrophy. Diabetes is usually seen between 7 and 12 years of age. Patients have elevated plasma insulin levels and apparent insulin-resistance, since large amounts of exogenous insulin are required for control of the disorder. There is severe hyperlipidemia, hepatomegaly, and acanthosis nigricans.

The several types of acquired lipodystrophy have manifestations similar to those of congenital lipodystrophy.

**Congenital Temporary Diabetes.** This rare syndrome develops in the first 6 weeks of life and disappears completely within 4 months.

**Tropical Diabetes.** Several types of diabetes occur in tropical countries, usually associated with marked malnutrition and/or pancreatitis. Some are associated with a copious intake of tapioca.

**Glucose Intolerance.** There are around 30 disorders associated with variable degrees of glucose intolerance, including inborn errors of metabolism, inherited neuromuscular disorders, progeroid syndromes, and some cytogenetic disorders.

**"Vacor" Rodenticide and Diabetes.** For several years, the chemicals alloxan and streptozotocin have been used experimentally to produce diabetes in laboratory animals. Several cases of diabetes mellitus have occurred in humans after the accidental or intentional ingestion of a rodenticide, marketed as "Vacor," that is structurally related to alloxan and streptozotocin. Vacor is N-3 phridyl-methyl-N′4 nitrophenyl urea. Five deaths have occurred in this country among 18 reported cases. Most survivors develop a brittle type of diabetes and marked postural hypotension. In most reported cases, there has been a period of several days between ingestion of the toxin and development of diabetes, with several patients developing ketoacidosis. Immediate treatment is lavage of stomach contents and administration of large doses of nicotinamide, which apparently protects against the cytotoxic effects on the beta cells if received within 2 hours of ingestion of the Vacor. The recommended dose is up to 3 g IV in divided doses over a 24-hour period. No one has determined how long such a patient should receive nicotinamide, but it has been suggested that a 7-day course may be sufficient.

# 30

# Lactic Acidosis

Lactic acidosis (LA) is a state of clinical acidosis in which the accumulated acid is almost entirely lactate. Normal persons experience a benign increase in lactate in response to physical exercise or hyperventilation. The difference between this condition and the state of clinical lactic acidosis is the relation of pyruvate to lactate. Any condition that elevates lactate normally is accompanied by a corresponding increase in pyruvate, and the ratio of these 2 substances remains the same. A normal adult produces about 1500 mmol of lactic acid every day, mainly from muscle, skin, brain, and red blood cells. Under normal circumstances, lactate is oxidized back to pyruvate in the liver and enters the Krebs or Cori cycles. As long as lactate use equals lactate production, no problem exists.

Tissue hypoxia seems to be the prerequisite for excess lactate production. Hypoxia may be due to problems in the delivery of oxygen at the cardiorespiratory level or to the metabolic use of oxygen. Lactic acid accumulation is frequently seen in hospital patients as a result of circulatory collapse and/or shock. The weapons to combat such conditions include oxygen, blood transfusion, vasodilators, and usually an immediate infusion of sodium bicarbonate. When the circulatory collapse or shock is reversed, the lacticemia recedes.

## LACTATE-PYRUVATE RATIO

The normal lactate-pyruvate ratio is 10:1, meaning that if the normal lactate level is 1.0 mEq/L or 9 mg/dl, then the normal pyruvate level is 0.1 mEq/L or 0.88 mg/dl. One should remember the glucose-6-phosphate pathway:

$$\text{G-6-P} \rightarrow \text{pyruvate} \rightarrow \text{oxidized to acetyl CoA} \rightarrow CO_2 \text{ and } H_2O$$

Anoxia, from any cause, stops the chain at pyruvate and accelerates the pyruvate-lactate conversion, and thus lactate accumulates.

## ETIOLOGY

1. Shock, from any cause that produces tissue hypoxia.
2. Diabetes mellitus, especially prior to 1978, if the patient had taken phenformin (DBI, Meltrol), which is known to promote lactic acid production. In the majority of patients taking phenformin who developed LA, a pathologic process produced tissue anoxia, such as renal or cardiac decompensation.
3. Glycogen storage disease.
4. Alcohol excess, especially in the person with diabetes.
5. Idiopathic—universally fatal.
6. In patient with leukemia.
7. Simultaneous occurrence with diabetic ketoacidosis (DKA).

## SYMPTOMS

The symptoms of lactic acidosis are as follows:

1. Sudden onset.
2. Marked hyperventilation.
3. Dehydration.
4. Possible coma, with shock-like features.
5. Low blood pressure and frequent bradycardia.
6. Similarity of symptoms to DKA and, as stated, the 2 conditions may occur together.
7. Possible intoxication.

## LABORATORY FINDINGS

1. Normal blood lactate levels, measured by usual laboratory methods, are 0.55 to 1.5 mEq/L or 5 to 15 mg/dl. Significant elevations begin at 2.0 mEq/L or 20 mg/dl. One can approximate the lactate level with the following formula:

$$(Na + K) - (CO_2 + CL) = L-13$$

   If the L factor is over 20, the condition is definitely lactic acidosis.
2. There is a marked increase in the amount of undetermined anions—usually the anion gap is greater than 25 mEq/L.
3. Blood glucose levels are frequently increased in diabetics, whereas in others, they are normal or even low.
4. The patient's serum bicarbonate level is usually below 15 mEq.
5. There is little or no acetonuria, unless the condition is accompanied by DKA. In the occasional case of accompanying DKA, the majority of ketone bodies may be in the form of $\beta$-hydroxybutyrate,

which does not appear on the Acetest or Ketostix tests. In such a case, one must ask for serum determination of $\beta$-hydroxybutyrate.

6. The patient's pH is lowered.
7. The serum osmolality is normal, unless the condition occurs in conjunction with DKA. One can approximate the serum osmolality with the following formula:

$$\text{Osmolality} = 2 \times \text{Na (in mEq/L)} + \frac{\text{glucose mg/dl}}{18} + \frac{\text{B.U.N.}}{2.8}$$

The normal serum osmolality is 280 to 300 mOsm/kg $H_2O$.

## DIFFERENTIAL DIAGNOSIS

The physician must distinguish between LA and the following conditions:

1. DKA—can sometimes occur in conjunction.
2. Hyperosmolar coma (HOC).
3. Methyl alcohol poisoning.
4. Ethylene glycol poisoning.
5. Paraldehyde intoxication.
6. Salicylate poisoning—also can show increased lactate.
7. Azotemic renal failure.

Table 30–1 outlines some important points in the differential diagnosis between DKA, LA, HOC. The patient with LA is briefly described as being comatose, with mild to moderate elevation of blood sugar levels, a decreased serum bicarbonate level and pH, and no increase in plasma ketones, but a marked increase in lactic acid. The key is the absence of ketones in the presence of much lactic acid, assuming that there is no accompanying DKA.

## TREATMENT

**Shock.** The physician should maintain adequate cardiac output and normal blood pressure. Lactic acidosis decreases the patient's ventricular contraction force, produces bradycardia, and decreases response to catecholamines when pH is below 7.10.

**Insulin.** One should give insulin as indicated.

**Sodium Bicarbonate.** No one is sure how much to give because there is a divergence of opinion about the amounts needed to neutralize the acidosis. It has been pointed out that when a patient's bicarbonate level is low (under 5 mEq/L), the amount required is more than expected, since the apparent space of distribution is closer to 100% of body weight and not the usual accepted figure of 50% of body weight. For example, a patient with a bicarbonate level

Table 30–1. Differential Diagnosis of Metabolic Comas.

| | Diabetic Ketoacidosis | Lactic Acidosis | Hyperosmolar Coma |
|---|---|---|---|
| AGE | any age | usually elderly; rarely occurs in young diabetics | usually 60 years or over; can occur in younger age groups |
| ETIOLOGY | infection or trauma; omission or decrease of insulin dosage; and onset of diabetes | commonly accompanied by debilitating chronic disease; precipitation by alcohol; intercurrent infections; renal impairment | intercurrent illness resulting in hyperglycemia, causing osmotic diuresis that brings about hyperosmolality |
| SYMPTOMS | acute illness with nausea, vomiting, dehydration, hyperventilation, lethargy, stupor, and finally coma; strong acetone breath; symptoms usually lasting 12–36 hours | gradual or rapid onset of coma, with shock-like syndrome; low blood pressure, bradycardia; symptoms lasting 1–6 days | polyuria, polydypsia, weight loss, followed by rapid onset of coma; MARKED DEHYDRATION; symptoms frequently lasting 10–12 days |
| DIABETES PRESENT | always | maybe | in 50%, usually mild |

| | | | |
|---|---|---|---|
| LABORATORY DETERMINATIONS | | | |
| blood glucose | high (400–1200 mg/dl) | increased, usually moderately | high (500–2000 mg/dl) |
| $CO_2$ | below 15 mEq/L | low, usually below 15 mEq/L | no change or low |
| acetonuria | 4+ | none to slight | none to slight |
| serum acetone | Marked elevation | none | none to slight elevation |
| pH | lowered, usually below 7.2 | lowered, usually below 7.37 | no change or lowered |
| lactic acid | normal | elevated, above 2 mEq/L | normal |
| serum osmolality (normal–290 mOsm/kg $H_2O$) | slight to marked elevation | normal | hypernormal, up to 450 mOsm/kg $H_2O$ |
| DIFFERENTIAL DIAGNOSIS | Acute illness, sometimes comatose patient; strong acetone odor; usually $h_x$ of diabetes; marked hyperglycemia, ketonuria, and lowered pH | comatose patient who may or may not have moderate elevation of blood sugar; decreased $CO_2$; no increase in urinary ketones or plasma ketones; marked increase in lactic acid (over 2 mEq/L) | disoriented or comatose patient with marked elevation of blood sugar; normal or slightly lowered $CO_2$; usually no increase in plasma acetone; marked evidence of dehydration with elevated Na, BUN; marked increase in serum osmolality (Normal–290 mOsm/kg $H_2O$) |
| MORTALITY RATE | less than 5% | over 50% | 40 to 50% |

of 2.4 mEq/L was given 360 mmol sodium bicarbonate, which raised the plasma bicarbonate level to 10.8. Then an additional 198 mmol bicarbonate was required to raise the plasma bicarbonate level to 25.2.

Actually, no specific guideline can be given for the exact amount of sodium bicarbonate, since there is so much individual variation. It is suggested that frequent monitoring of the acid-base indices as well as observation of the clinical response are the best guides. However, one must remember that complete and immediate correction of the acidosis is not the aim of treatment, since it could result in volume overload and in possible hypokalemia, hypocalcemia, and the development of spinal fluid acidosis.

One investigator has suggested that a reasonable program is to raise plasma bicarbonate levels by 4 to 5 mEq/L initially, with a goal of raising it to 14 to 16 mEq/L in 24 hours. In such a case, the amount given can be based on the original assumption that the volume of distribution is 50% of the patient's body weight unless the plasma bicarbonate level is under 4 mEq/L. For a 70-kg man, this means 140 mEq of sodium bicarbonate, to raise the plasma bicarbonate level 4 mEq/L.

If, on the second determination several hours later, the bicarbonate level of the 70-kg patient is still between 5 and 10 mEq/L, one should give 50 to 100 mEq.

**Dichloroacetate.** This new drug, now being investigated for treatment of LA, apparently acts by increasing the physiologic use of pyruvate. It activates PDH, the enzyme responsible for initiating the oxidation of pyruvate to acetyl CoA. The drug may also aid in peripheral glucose oxidation. Dichloroacetate is being investigated in clinical diabetes, and it is reported that it can reduce plasma glucose, plasma lactate, alanine, cholesterol and triglyceride levels, and ketones. Peripheral neuropathy has been reported in some patients using this drug.

**Hemodialysis.** This procedure is of questionable value. A recent study reported a 48% mortality rate in patients undergoing dialysis and a 42% mortality rate in patients not undergoing dialysis.

One must always think of lactic acidosis as a possible cause of acidotic coma.

## FURTHER READING

Kreisberg, R.A.: Lactic acidosis. Ann. Intern. Med., 92:227, 1980.

# 31

# Hyperosmolar-Hyperglycemic Coma

For this life-threatening complication of diabetes, prompt recognition and treatment are essential. The mortality rate is high—45%, and the pathogenesis is unknown.

## MEDICAL HISTORY

The average age of patients who develop hyperosmolar-hyperglycemic coma is 62. Half these patients are not known diabetics at the time of onset of this condition. When diabetes is present, it is usually mild. Victims of hyperosmolar-hyperglycemic coma are frequently nursing home patients. The condition occurs in patients subjected to stress factors that cause hyperglycemia, such as infections and illnesses, as well as the administration of concentrated carbohydrates, e.g., hyperalimentation, peritoneal dialysis solution, or sugar-containing soft drinks.

Certain drugs, for example, thiazide diuretics, steroids, and phenytoin (diphenylhydantoin) are also stress factors. The symptoms are often present for 10 to 12 days. Many patients (80%) have chronic renal or cardiovascular disease. This type of coma has been reported in children and in insulin-dependent diabetics, although infrequently. Some patients have developed hyperosmolar coma while in a hospital.

## CLINICAL FINDINGS

Patients may have a long prodromal period of polyuria and polydipsia, or they may have some acute or chronic illness. Weakness is an outstanding feature of this condition. Patients usually show signs of extreme dehydration and volume depletion, including dry mouth and skin, decreased jugular vein pressure, tachycardia, orthostatic hypotension, and perhaps shock. This condition causes a disordered mental state, ranging from lethargy to coma, and patients may have focal seizures. About one-third are comatose at the time of hospital admission. Frequently, an erroneous diagnosis of cerebrovascular accident has been made.

The physician should consider the diagnosis in all dehydrated elderly patients who show even subtle changes in their mentation. See Table 30–1 for the differential diagnosis of metabolic comas.

## LABORATORY FINDINGS

If adequate laboratory facilities are available, the physician should order tests for blood glucose, osmolality, electrolytes, venous pH, serum ketones, and creatinine. If no laboratory facilities are available, the diagnosis can be made with 2 simple bedside tests, blood sugar and ketones. The former test indicates the patient's high glucose level, and the latter reveals the absence of ketosis.

1. Hyperglycemia—average is close to 1000 mg/dl.
2. Hyperosmolality—average is 380 mOsm/kg $H_2O$.

$$\text{osmolality} = 2 \times \text{Na in mEq/L} + \frac{\text{glucose mg/dl}}{18} + \frac{\text{B.U.N.}}{2.8}$$

3. Absence of ketosis. Ketostix on urine and serum is negative.
4. Serum K—usually normal at first, but a severe depletion of body K becomes apparent with treatment.
5. Acidosis—if any is present, it is mild.
6. Marked glucosuria.
7. Electrolyte values—Na, 145 mEq/L; Cl, 103 mEq/L; K, 5 mEq/L; and $HCO_3$, 18 mEq/L. These values are average and may vary widely among individual patients.

## TREATMENT

Prompt treatment is crucial, and one should be able to recognize the condition easily in elderly patients who have severe hyperglycemia without ketosis and with physical evidence of marked fluid volume depletion.

**Flow Sheet.** Starting a flow sheet for the patient is the first step in treatment.

**Correction of Volume Depletion and Hyperosmolality.** Volume depletion is usually 30% or greater. If the patient is hypotensive, one should start with normal saline or plasma volume expanders, 0.9%

saline solution at 500 to 1000 ml/hr. If he is not hypotensive, one should administer 0.45% saline solution.

When the patient's blood pressure becomes normal, the infusion should be changed to hypotonic saline solution, 0.45% saline solution at 500 ml/hr. As serum osmolality decreases, fluids can be given at a slower rate. Urine output should be at least 30 ml/hr.

Most patients who have survived have received at least 5 L in 12 hours. One research series reported an average of 8.2 L per patient. The physician must check the patient's serum osmolality frequently.

**Correction of Hyperglycemia.** Insulin may be administered in any of several methods. Low-dose infusion of regular insulin has proved satisfactory. However, a few cases of extreme insulin resistance have been reported, so larger doses may be indicated.

One should start with 10 U IV and continue with 50 U in 500 ml saline solution infused at the rate of 1 ml/min (6 U/hr). The infusion rate should be controlled with a pediatric minidrip and an electronic drip-counter apparatus. When the patient's plasma glucose level is 300 mg/dl or lower, one should decrease the insulin infusion to 0.5 ml/min (3 U/hr) and administer 5% glucose at the rate of 150 ml/hr. The physician should maintain the patient's plasma glucose level between 100 and 300 mg/dl by adjusting the infusion rate of the glucose solution, starting with about 150 to 200 ml/hr.

Insulin and glucose infusions are usually required for about 12 to 24 hours. Patients should eat something as soon as nausea subsides.

**Correction of K Depletion.** Physicians must use caution in the presence of severe renal failure or low urinary output. If the patient's original serum K is normal, he should be given 10 to 15 mEq/hr in the IV fluid (usually KCl). If hypokalemia is severe (under 2.0 mEq/L), one can give up to 60 mEq/L. The physician should check the patient's serum K and/or his ECG for progress. The patient's serum K should be checked every 2 to 3 hours until stable.

**Other Considerations.** If nausea and vomiting are present, the patient may need a nasogastric tube. He should be catheterized if absolutely necessay, and then for a short time only. These patients acquire urinary infections easily.

The diabetic state is probably permanent in those who are not known diabetics at the onset of the episode. Therefore, one must outline a program adequate to control their blood sugar levels through diet and insulin or tablets, as indicated.

## PATHOPHYSIOLOGY OF NONKETOTIC HYPEROSMOLAR COMA

The marked hyperglycemia is responsible for the elevation in plasma osmolality, since each 180 mg glucose has an osmotic pressure of 1 mOsm. The increased osmolality then causes fluids to shift from intracellular sites to the extracellular compartments; this shift leads to cellular dehydration. This extracellular hypertonicity and relative cellular dehydration are responsible for the stupor and coma. Sustained hyperosmolality can eventually rupture cerebral veins and cause intracranial hemorrhage, which leads to death.

Glucose tubular reabsorption falls behind, glucose loads increase, and this excreted glucose causes osmotic diuresis that results in a marked loss of water and sodium. As dehydration progresses, the renal blood flow and the glomerular filtration rate are reduced; oliguria and azotemia follow.

## PREVENTION OF RECURRENCES

Repeated episodes were reported in as many as 6 out of 8 patients in one research series. Therefore, education of the patient is most important, as it is for all diabetics who have never experienced hyperosmolar coma. Nursing home personnel should be particularly alert to early warning signs and symptoms of an impending coma.

Physicians must use caution when prescribing agents that may aggravate carbohydrate intolerance. This group includes such commonly prescribed drugs as thiazides, phenytoin (diphenylhydantoin), and steroids.

Patients and families should be taught that any acute illness should be brought to the attention of the family doctor at once. A decrease in the high mortality rate will only be brought about by early recognition, treatment, and prevention of its occurrence. A complete treatise on hyperosmolar coma is found in one of the "Current Concepts" manuals published by the Upjohn Company in 1974. It is free for the asking.

# 32

# Etiology and Genetics of Diabetes Mellitus

The fundamental cause of diabetes mellitus is still unknown, but distinctions can be made between what we choose to call Type I or insulin-dependent diabetes mellitus (IDDM) and Type II or non-insulin-dependent diabetes mellitus (NIDDM).

Type I diabetes is probably inherited. There probably is a genetic predisposition to a defect in the immune system that can result in clinical disease in association with viral infections or other unknown environmental factors. In this chapter, I discuss the genetic research that suggests that there may be a biochemical marker, such as the HLA antigens. Further identification of Type I DM may be possible by finding islet-cell antibodies.

Type II diabetes is a different syndrome and is unassociated with the genetic markers described. Because over 60% of Type II diabetics are obese at the time of the onset of their disorder, some investigators state that obesity is the main cause of Type II diabetes; reversal of the obesity usually results in normal glucose tolerance. However, this theory does not tell us why some and not all obese adults develop diabetes. Studies of blood insulin concentrations in adult-onset diabetics tell us what is happening, but not why it is happening. The obese nondiabetic has marked elevations of serum insulin, whereas the obese diabetic has adequate levels of insulin when compared with lean diabetics, but not nearly as much insulin as obese nondiabetics. Obesity itself increases the demand for insulin. It appears that the obese diabetic has a decreased number of cell receptors for insulin. There may exist a decreased "affinity" between insulin and the cell receptors. One theory proposes that insulin itself may affect the "down-regulation" of receptors. Weight reduction usually reverses receptor anomalies.

## ISLET CELL ANTIBODIES AND AUTOIMMUNITY IN TYPE I DIABETES

On rare occasions, Type I diabetes has been associated with other disorders that have an autoimmune pathogenesis, such as lymphocytic thyroiditis and Addison's disease. "Islitis" or inflammation of the pancreatic islets has been found at autopsy in patients who developed Type I diabetes shortly before death.

In 1974, Bottazzo and colleagues in London reported the finding of islet-cell antibodies (ICA) in many Type I diabetics studied shortly after the onset of diabetes, even though the presence of ICAs was not associated with other autoimmune disorders. ICAs have been found in 75% of Type I diabetics studied soon after the onset of their diabetes. A further observation is that a high percentage of Type II diabetics found to have ICAs later become Type I diabetics. In addition, the study showed that Type I diabetics with HLA B8 antigens had higher titers of ICA longer than did diabetics with other B antigens. No ICAs were found in those patients with B15 antigens. The question remains as to whether ICA presence indicates a primary immunologic reaction to pancreatic islet cells or a secondary response to islet cell injury, such as injury by a virus.

## VIRUS THEORY IN TYPE I DIABETES

There is increasing evidence that the insulin-deficient Type I diabetes in children may well result from an inflammatory process in the islet tissue (islitis) that leads to complete or partial destruction of beta cells. Three etiologic factors are involved: genetics, viral infection, and autoimmunity. It is postulated that certain HLA antigens confer additional susceptibility to infection by an invading virus. Coxsackie B-4, mumps, congenital rubella, cytomegalovirus, infectious mononucleosis, and varicella viruses have all been studied. Coxsackie B-4, mumps, and rubella viruses are prominent among these. In 1979, Coxsackie B-4 virus was isolated from the pancreas of a 10-year-old boy who died from ketoacidosis. The virus was transferred to mice, beta cell destruction took place, and diabetes ensued. There may be a great variation in the temporal relationship, and diabetes may appear weeks after coxsackie viral infection, months to several years after mumps, and up to 15 to 20 years after congenital rubella.

Obviously, all children who contract such viral infections do not develop diabetes, and many children who develop diabetes do not have a history of such diseases. Additionally, many school-age children have been immunized against mumps. About half the population of the United States has antibodies to coxsackie viral infection, whereas juvenile diabetes develops in only about 0.1% of the population. Congenital rubella usually causes multiple defects in the fetus, including damage to eyes, ears, central nervous system, and heart. Forty-five Australian children born with rubella-induced damage have been studied since 1967 by Dr. Margaret Menser and colleagues. Twenty per cent of this cohort developed diabetes sometime in their 20s, although each of them had had other defects since birth.

A vaccine against coxsackie virus is in the making, but this does not mean that it will afford universal protection from diabetes to children receiving the vaccine. Many other viruses may be implicated in beta cell destruction. Such destruction may be effected through direct cellular invasion or, perhaps more likely, through an autoimmune mechanism, as is seen in many other chronic diseases. British studies reported evidence that the primary autoimmune type of diabetes is a distinct clinical entity, showing islet-cell antibodies and an abnormally high incidence of HLA B8 antigens.

It has been suggested that anti-inflammatory or immunosuppressive therapy at the time of diagnosis of Type I diabetes could be useful in altering the course of the disorder, by preventing complete destruction of beta cells. Diabetes has been produced experimentally in mice with variants of 2 human viruses, reovirus type III and coxsackie B-4.

In juvenile-onset diabetes, the peak incidences occur at ages 5 and 11 in both sexes, but especially at age 11. More boys than girls develop the disease between birth and age 4; the disease is more common in girls aged 5 to 9 years, and then again in boys aged 10 to 15 years. Overall, more boys than girls develop diabetes. It is difficult to reconcile these facts with the viral theory. If, as many scientists believe, juvenile-onset, Type I diabetes is an autoimmune response to a virus, it would appear that differences at the HLA D locus are most crucial in determining such a response.

If one takes a practical look at the idea of a vaccine to prevent diabetes in children, there are many barriers. If one assumes that 10% of all Type I diabetes is virally induced, and 1 in 1000 such individuals develops diabetes each year, we would have to immunize 10,000 persons to prevent diabetes in 1 person.

## HLA ANTIGENS IN TYPE I DIABETES

The genetic nature of diabetes is undisputed, but there remains disagreement about the specific mode of inheritance. Most investigators feel that there is much genetic heterogeneity, in light of recent findings concerning HLA antigens in juvenile-onset or Type I diabetes. It seems worthwhile to discuss briefly these findings, since they will have application in the future management of diabetes.

To begin with, I shall review a few definitions that may be new to some. *HLA* means H (human) L (leukocyte) A (antigen), the major histocompatibility complex of man. It is a gene complex located on the short arm of chromosome 6. Four HLA loci have been defined—A, B, C, and D. The *gene*, the biologic unit of heredity, is located on a chromosome at a definite position (locus). *Alleles* are alternate forms of a gene that occur at the same locus on a chromosome. A haplotype is a neologism defined as the haploid genetic composition of a chromosomal region. Thus, an individual inherits 1 HLA haplotype from each parent; together, the 2 haplotypes form the HLA genotype of the individual. HLA antigens are cell-membrane-associated glycoproteins of 45,000 molecular weight expressed by all nucleated human cells.

The exact function of HLA antigens is unknown at this time. Their antigenicity may not be related to their function. HLA antigens are determined by genes located on the sixth pair of autosomal chromosomes, and they thus could well provide markers for a special type of diabetes.

It has now been clearly demonstrated that some patients with juvenile-onset or Type I diabetes have an increased frequency of HLA antigens. Three distinct types have been identified in Type I diabetes. The first type is associated with HLA B8 and Dw3, the second type with B15 and Dw4, and the third or combined type is associated with all four: B8, Dw3, B15, and Dw4.

Studies done on identical twins showed no difference in HLA types between maturity-onset Type II diabetic twins and control nondiabetic twins, whereas Type I twins, some with and some without diabetes, showed an increase of HLA B15. HLA B8 was increased only when both twins had Type I diabetes. This finding also suggests a genetic predisposition to the disease. There are Type I diabetics who do not have any of the foregoing HLA antigens. These persons must represent a different subtype of diabetes. It is now thought that the presence of HLA Dw2 renders protection against Type I diabetes, since the antigen has never been found in a Type I diabetic to date.

A distinct connection between HLA types and many diseases has been shown in the past few years, although the mechanism by which HLA factors confer disease susceptibility still remains unclear. HLA B8 and Dw3 are not only increased in Type I diabetes, but also in other conditions with autoimmune etiology, such as Graves' disease, idiopathic Addison's disease, and celiac disease. The type associated with HLA B8 and Dw3 is the autoimmune form. It involves an increased prevalence of pancreatic islet cell antibodies, a lack of antibody response to exogenous insulin, and perhaps an increased susceptibility to microangiopathy. The other type, associated with HLA B15 and Dw4, is not associated with autoimmune factors or islet cell antibodies and involves an increased antibody response to exogenous insulin. The third, or combined type, infers a much higher risk for diabetes and appears more frequently in concordant twins and in families with multiple cases of diabetes.

Dr. Nerup of Steno Memorial Hospital in Copenhagen recently stated that HLA B8 and/or B15 was demonstrated in 65% of their Type I patients, as compared with 39% of the general population. He further stated that individuals with HLA B8 or B15 have a 2.5 times greater risk of developing Type I diabetes; those with HLA Dw3 have a 4.2 greater risk; those with HLA Dw4 a 8.9 greater risk; and if both HLA Dw3 and Dw4 are present, there is a 20 times greater risk.

For the reader who is interested in pursuing this subject, a concise and comprehensive article by Drs. Jerome Rotter and David L. Rimoin entitled "Diabetes mellitus: the search for genetic markers" appears in Diabetes Care (2:215, 1979).

## INHERITANCE IN TYPE II DIABETES

Type II maturity-onset diabetes is apparently not HLA-related. From studies done in the last few years, it is clear that the genetic factor seems to be more important in Type II than in Type I diabetics. Evidence indicates that Type II diabetes is probably inherited as an autosomal dominant trait, because about 85% of such diabetics have a diabetic parent, and about half the siblings in such a family have diabetes. In one study, 46% of families showed a direct vertical transmission of diabetes through 3 generations. In the same study, only 11% of juvenile-onset diabetics had a diabetic parent, and a 3-generation vertical inheritance was found in only 6 of the families. Further, only 8 of the 74 tested had siblings with diabetes mellitus. If a parent has Type II diabetes, the risk to the offspring of becoming diabetic at some time is about 25%, whereas if both parents have Type II diabetes, the risk doubles. On the other hand, if a child is born of a Type I diabetic mother, the risk of that child's becoming diabetic at any time is between 5 and 10%. Another important contribution to our knowledge was made by Dr. Pyke and colleagues with identical twins. When the index twin developed diabetes before age 40, only 50% were concordant (i.e., both developed diabetes before age 40), whereas when the index twin developed diabetes after age 50, 100% were concordant. Of the 125 pairs studied, 85 pairs were concordant and 40 were discordant.

Fajans and Tattersall at the University of Michigan first described an unusual type of diabetes they called maturity-onset diabetes of the young (MODY). These patients are young at the onset of the disorder, have few if any symptoms and no ketonuria, and can control their diabetes without insulin. These persons have not become more severely diabetic in over 20 years of study. This disorder is apparently a separate entity, neither Type I nor Type II. Of those studied, 85% had a diabetic parent, 53% of siblings tested had diabetes, and 46% of the families showed 3 generations of direct vertical transmission of the trait, suggesting autosomal dominant inheritance. These diabetics add more evidence to the heterogeneity of diabetes.

In time, the genetic puzzle will be solved, and a positive marker may be found that will truly predict diabetes. Meanwhile, the family physician can reassure diabetic parents about the chances of their offspring's developing diabetes with our present knowledge. Certainly, the diabetic mother should be assured that her children have no more than a 10% chance of becoming diabetic.

# 33

# Multiple Hormones Involved in Diabetes

In 1921, 51 years after Langerhans in Germany had described the islets of cells in the pancreas that bear his name, Banting and Best discovered the secretion of the beta cells of these islets and called the substance *insulin.* A few years later, it was discovered that the alpha cells of these same islets secrete a substance called glucagon. In 1973, we learned that the delta cells of the islets are the source of another hormone, somatostatin, and now there is growing evidence that a fourth type of cell may secrete another polypeptide.

Glucagon raises the blood sugar level and somatostatin partially controls the ultimate serum concentration of glucagon. It appears that, in some diabetics, there is an abnormality in this somatostatin-glucagon relationship, particularly when there is a shortage of insulin. Evidence suggests that the interactions of insulin, glucagon, and somatostatin that provide an appropriate physiologic mixture require a high degree of coordination between the alpha, beta, and delta cells of the islets. Dr. Unger and his colleagues have demonstrated the presence of intercellular junctions of 2 types, "tight" and "gap" junctions, which likely serve as means of communication among the 3 types of cells. It is now possible by immunoassay to measure accurately serum levels of insulin, glucagon, and somatostatin. The circulating half-life of these hormones is approximately 5 minutes.

## INSULIN

### Structure

In 1960, Dr. Sanger in England analyzed insulin and found that it contained 2 polypeptide chains with a disulfide linkage (S-S) at

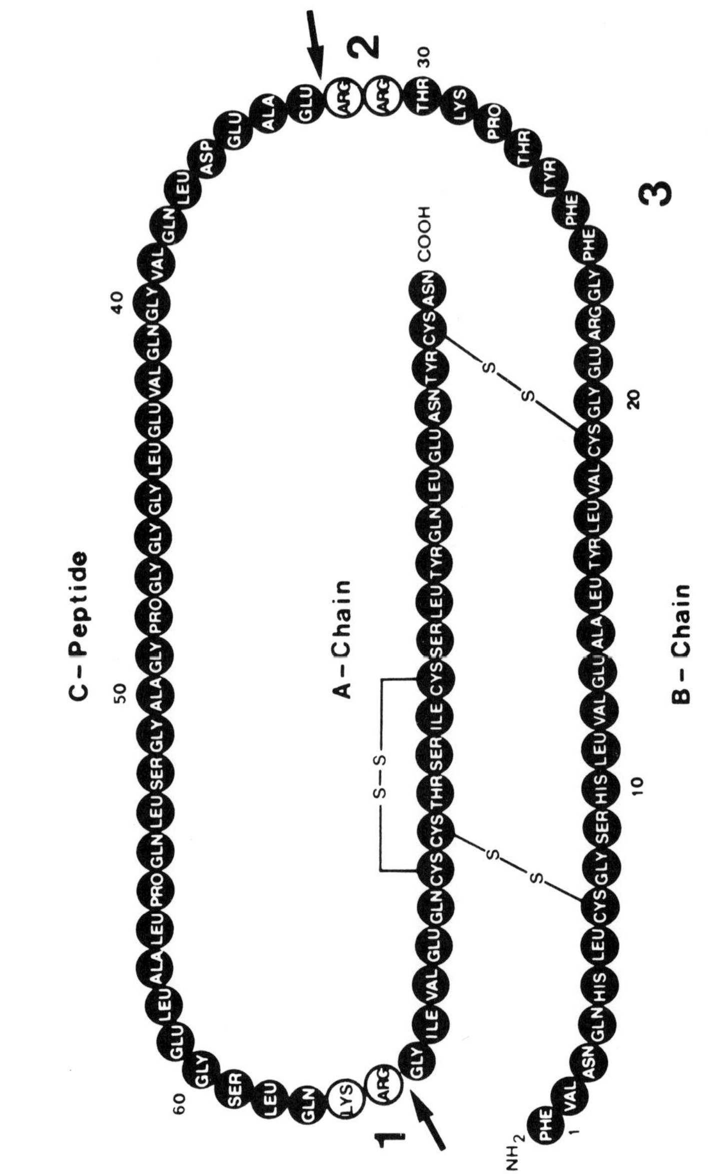


**Fig. 33–1.** Human proinsulin. (From Gabbay, K.H.: Insulinopathies (editorial). N. Engl. J. Med., *302*:165, 1980.)

positions A-7, B-7, A-20, B-19, and 1 in A-20, between cysteine 6 and 11. The A-chain has 21 amino acids and the B-chain has 30 (see Fig. 33–1). Amino-acid sequences vary among animal species, and this variation has stimulated interesting research. The rat makes 2 different varieties of insulin.

The structure of insulins of various animal species studied all differ from one another and from human insulin in the sequence and position of the amino acids. Pork insulin is most like human insulin, differing by only 1 amino acid at position 30 on the B-chain; in the pig, it is alanine and in the human being, threonine. It is now possible to desalinate pork insulin. This insulin has been used in cases of severe insulin resistance and in investigative studies. Pork insulin has proven over the years to be the least antigenic, and it is indicated in cases in which antigenicity becomes a problem (see Chap. 13). Recently, Lilly has marketed a new purified pork insulin that should be even less antigenic than the original pork product.

Once in a while, a defect occurs in the structure of human insulin. A recent report described a 51-year-old diabetic man who had both hyperglycemia and hyperinsulinism. A study of his insulin showed a structural abnormality, since it contained a leucine instead of a phenylalanine at position 24 or 25 of the B-chain. These positions are areas of active receptor-binding. The patient also secreted normal insulin, but the abnormal insulin apparently antagonized the action of the normal insulin.

### Secretion

The average adult pancreas contains 500,000 to 1 million islets. Of the 3 well-identified types of cells within each islet, 65% are beta cells secreting insulin, 25% are alpha cells secreting glucagon, and 15% are delta cells secreting somatostatin. When Type I diabetes has been present for a variable period of time, some diabetics suffer a complete loss of beta cells, so that the relative percentages of pancreatic islet cells could show 0% beta cells, 75% alpha cells, a threefold increase, and 25% delta cells, a slight increase. In Type II diabetics, several different changes may take place in the islets, but there is usually some slight reduction in beta cells, although earlier investigators proposed that there was hypertrophy of beta cells. As Type II diabetes continues, there may be a further decrease in the number of beta cells, so that insulin production falls below that required and the patients become insulin-dependent.

The secretion of insulin by the beta cells is a result of the relative glucose concentration of the blood. Insulin is first evolved as the proinsulin molecule, consisting of the 21 amino-acid A-chain and the 30 amino-acid B-chain connected to the 35 amino-acid C-peptide chain. Proteolytic conversion of proinsulin with cleavage sites, as shown in Figure 33–1, results in equimolar concentrations of C-peptide and insulin that are stored within the beta cell granules and are liberated together during exocytosis. During cleavage, 3 arginine and 1 lysine amino-acid molecules are expelled, so that the C-peptide chain now contains 31 amino acids. Cleavage occurs at the position of the arrows in Figure 33–1.

## Physiology

What are the main physiologic functions of insulin? A brief review is in order because knowledge of these functions helps one to understand the metabolic abnormalities that occur in diabetes. Insulin is anabolic in all its actions—it is the energy storage hormone.

1. First, insulin, through its receptors attached to the cell wall of muscle cells, fat cells, and connective tissue cells, allows translocation of glucose into the cell. Many cells of the body do not require insulin for glucose entry, notably brain and nerve tissue, renal tissue, gastrointestinal mucosa, and RBCs.
2. Insulin acts on the liver to accomplish 2 things: to promote glucose uptake by the liver, where it is stored as glycogen, and to inhibit gluconeogenesis by the liver. Finally, insulin inhibits the release of glycogen by the liver.
3. Insulin suppresses the synthesis of fatty acids by the liver and stimulates the deposit of fat in the adipocytes.
4. Insulin blocks the output of amino acids from muscle cells.

The reader is referred to textbooks on metabolism for detailed information.

## Cell Receptors for Insulin

Recent studies have indicated that practically all hormones have cell receptors specific for each hormone, to carry out their physiologic functions. This receptor-hormone alliance may be on the surface or within the cell. Insulin attaches to a specific insulin receptor on body cells, mainly on those cells that require insulin for glucose metabolism such as fat, muscle, and liver cells, but to a lesser extent on cells such as monocytes and erythrocytes. In Type I diabetics, there is either an absolute absence of insulin or a diminished supply, and there are excess numbers of cell receptors for insulin. On the other hand, in Type II diabetics, especially in the obese, there is a diminished supply of insulin receptors. Cell receptors are studied *in vitro*, using monocytes or erythrocytes and incubating them with radioactive-labeled insulin.

In the presence of diabetic ketoacidosis, it has been noted that receptor affinity for insulin is greatly diminished. In cases of prolonged, untreated DKA, there may be a diminished number of receptors. This receptor deficiency is restored with adequate hydration and electrolyte replacement.

Some recent studies have shown that exercise has a beneficial effect on diabetics by increasing the number of insulin receptors. High-fiber diets may also increase the number of insulin receptors. Reduction of caloric intake by the obese diabetic increases the number of receptors, as does the administration of oral antidiabetes tablets (sulfonylureas).

There is a rare type of diabetes occurring in thin adults who have greatly elevated levels of insulin and a normal number of receptors. These receptors, however, are "inactivated" theoretically by autoantibodies. When the antibodies disappear, either spontaneously or following immunosuppressive therapy, both insulin and glucose levels return to normal and the receptors become normally active.

Autoantibodies that block insulin activity by virtue of their attachment to receptors have been found to mimic insulin activity in some target cells. If this receptor-antibody combination is able to mimic insulin activity, it seems that the information for activation of the cells rests with the receptors rather than with insulin. In theory, substances might be found that could be taken orally and would be capable of binding to receptors and producing "insulin-like" activity. The future may hold such a substance.

## Insulin Production

A few years after Dr. Sanger analyzed insulin, Dr. Katsoyannis at the University of Pittsburgh was first able to synthesize insulin. This breakthrough raised hopes that eventually all diabetics would use synthetic human insulin and would thus avoid the antigenicity of animal insulin. Unfortunately, this has not proved to be true, since the cost of synthetic insulin is prohibitive and no production facilities can economically produce large amounts.

All commercially available insulin today is extracted from the pancreases of healthy slaughterhouse animals, now entirely beef and pork. The magnitude of such production can be better realized from these facts: It requires 8000 lb animal pancreases to yield 1 lb pure zinc insulin crystals, enough insulin for approximately 750 diabetics with average requirements for 1 year. Pancreases from 8500 cattle and 15,000 hogs amount to 8000 pounds.

## Recombinant DNA Technique to Produce Human Insulin

In October of 1978, the City of Hope National Medical Center in Duarte, California, announced that they had produced human insulin from *E. coli*. Researchers at Harvard University had produced rat insulin by the same process only a few months earlier.

All living cells are directed by the DNA that they contain. The beta cell contains the gene for assembling the amino acids into their proper sequence to produce insulin. Therefore, it was obvious that if the researchers could introduce beta cell DNA into bacteria, insulin would be produced. The information in the DNA must be transcribed into molecules of messenger RNA (mRNA), which can then be transported within the cells to direct the assembly of insulin. The scientists reversed the process of transcription by synthesizing a DNA copy called cDNA, to be inserted into the bacteria. The process was made easier because *E. coli* and other bacteria have 2 sources of DNA, their main chromosome and small rings of DNA called plasmids. Therefore, cDNA was incubated with plasmids in such a way that it was introduced into a specific region of the plasmid that directs the production of a bacterial protein, penicillinase, normally excreted by *E. coli*. In this way, the insulin produced was also excreted by *E. coli* instead of being digested. The next step was the incubation of the modified plasmids with *E. coli*, so they were taken up by the bacteria. Then the bacteria were grown on nutrient plates and were transferred to vats. At the present time the *E. coli* are programmed to make either the insulin A- or B-chain; the chains are then combined in the laboratory.

We shall look for commercial amounts of human insulin within a few years. We can anticipate freedom from antibody formation, and thus the average human insulin requirement may be considerably less. We can assume that there will be a plentiful supply and that eventually, this will mean a less costly product. We can also assume that there will be relative freedom from immunologic reactions to insulin. We cannot anticipate what any new problems might be, however.

## Circulating Serum Insulin Determinations

Circulating insulin levels in healthy subjects and in diabetics not taking exogenous insulin can be readily measured by means of radioimmunoassay techniques. However, this method is not satisfactory for diabetics who take exogenous animal insulin because of the development of antibodies and the similarity of animal insulins to human insulin. Obese Type II diabetics usually have large amounts of circulating endogenous insulin.

Occasionally, in a 25- to 40-year-old obese diabetic, it is clinically helpful to know whether this patient is an obese Type II or a possible Type I diabetic. Serum insulin levels are helpful. Single serum insulin determinations are not as satisfactory as multiple determinations. Generally, the blood samples are taken while the patient is fasting. Then 100 g glucose are given, and the blood samples are taken 30, 60, and 120 minutes after the glucose ingestion. Detailed instruction should be procured from the laboratory involved.

### C-peptide Immunoassay

When one needs to know the amount of endogenous insulin being secreted by diabetics who take exogenous insulin, a C-peptide determination can be ordered. This test reflects beta cell secretory capacity, and neither insulin antibodies nor insulin interferes with C-peptide determinations.

Another unusual but important indication for the determination of C-peptide level is the suspicion that a person is taking insulin surreptitiously to produce hypoglycemia. The malingerer is frequently a nurse who has some understanding of insulin action and who can readily produce hypoglycemia with the proper amounts of exogenous insulin. This person's medical history and symptoms suggest the presence of an insulinoma. C-peptide evaluations clarify the diagnosis. The usual finding with surreptitious insulin injection is a low C-peptide level in relation to the serum insulin level, since exogenous insulin suppresses the secretion of endogenous insulin.

C-peptide measurement is valuable in determining other causes of spontaneous hypoglycemia, such as mesenchymal tumors or hepatic or renal failure. It is also useful in evaluating the postsurgical patient who has had a "total" pancreatectomy for nesidioblastosis or carcinoma, to be certain no residual pancreatic tissue remains.

## SOMATOSTATIN

Somatostatin unfortunately inhibits not only glucagon synthesis, but also growth hormone, insulin, thyrotropin, and others, including some gastrointestinal hormones. Somatostatin was originally isolated from the hypothalamus, but subsequently it has been found in the cerebral cortex, sympathetic neurons, thyroid, stomach, small intestine, and islets of Langerhans. It is now believed that somatostatin acts as a neurohormone, to regulate some pituitary hormone secretions, with other roles in other tissues.

There is experimental evidence that this hormone is able to decrease both fasting and postprandial hyperglycemia, to help to forestall the onset of ketoacidosis, and possibly, to improve diabetic control in Type I patients. Since the half-life of somatostatin is about 30 minutes, it must be given by intravenous drip for a sustained effect. Consequently, a search is under way to synthesize analogs of somatostatin with longer action and a more limited spectrum of activity. Some encouraging progress is being made.

It seems obvious that improvement in diabetic control must be brought about through somatostatin's ability to inhibit both glucagon and growth hormone secretion. In a recent report, Dr. John E. Gerrich of the Mayo Clinic stated that an encouraging analog of somatostatin that has been synthesized can decrease growth hormone and glucagon levels by 60% without affecting insulin levels. The analog does not affect carbohydrate absorption and is active for up to 4 hours when given subcutaneously to rats. Eventually, a derivative such as this will be suitable for clinical use in the treatment of diabetes.

## GLUCAGON

Glucagon is a 29-amino-acid polypeptide secreted primarily by the alpha cells of the islets, but also by similar cells in the walls of the stomach and duodenum. Glucagon is partially responsible for maintaining glucose production at a rate sufficient to meet the needs of the cells, especially those of the central nervous system. A declining insulin-to-glucagon ratio stimulates hepatic glycogenolysis. When the liver glycogen is depleted, glucagon then stimulates gluconeogenesis and ketogenesis by the liver. Normally, ketones are used as an alternate fuel by the central nervous system. Thus, glucagon is crucial in preventing serious hypoglycemia in the physiologically normal person.

Since 1969, it has been known that excessive levels of glucagon are found in both Types I and II diabetes in relation to levels of glucose. High fasting glucagon levels are not suppressed by high glucose levels, and even hypoglycemia in Type I patients does not elicit an adequate glucagon response. Restoration of adequate insulin levels frequently restores glucagon response to almost normal. Amino acids and gastrointestinal hormones can stimulate the alpha cells to produce more glucagon. Low levels of blood glucose stimulate glucagon production, whereas high levels inhibit glucagon production.

## GASTROINTESTINAL HORMONE

A fourth hormone involved intimately in diabetes control is the gastric-inhibitory polypeptide, primarily a gastrointestinal hormone, which inhibits gastrin-stimulated gastric secretion and stimulates insulin response to glucose in nondiabetics. However, in diabetes, it stimulates glucagon release and causes an excess of glucagon, according to recent studies.

## COUNTER-REGULATORY HORMONES

Many hormones besides insulin, glucagon, and somatostatin have important roles in diabetes through their participation in carbohydrate metabolism. Not many are helpful to diabetes, and by understanding their effects, one may envision the changes in hormonal secretion that impair the diabetic state. Counter-regulatory hormones exert their influences in carbohydrate metabolism in both nondiabetics and diabetics. However, the lack of endogenous insulin in the Type I diabetic to overcome the antagonistic actions of these hormones, and the loss of coordinated action between insulin, glucagon, and somatostatin in the islet cells, creates a further state of impaired carbohydrate metabolism.

Dr. Peter Forsham, an outstanding diabetologist at the University of California Medical Center in San Francisco, has categorized the counter-regulatory hormones into 2 divisions: insulin antagonists and hyperglycemic hormones.

### Insulin Antagonists

1. Catecholamines (epinephrine and norepinephrine), which inhibit release of insulin by beta cells.
2. Growth hormone (GH), which stops the effectiveness of insulin at the cell surface by direct antagonism.
3. Progesterone, which antagonizes the action of insulin at the cell surface (important to keep in mind for diabetics taking oral contraceptive pills).
4. Other inhibitors of insulin secretion, which are somatostatin and prostaglandin E. Prostaglandin E is probably synthesized in plasma membrane of certain islet cells. Recent studies have reported that prostaglandin E inhibits glucose-induced insulin secretions in humans, and this effect can be neutralized by administering sodium salicylate. It is postulated that the effect of salicylates may be to decrease synthesis of prostaglandin E.

### Hyperglycemic Hormones

1. Glucocorticoids, which act by mobilizing amino acids that are then deaminated in the liver and raise liver glycogen and blood glucose levels (clinical example, Cushing's syndrome with diabetes).
2. Thyroid hormones, which liberate glucogen from the liver and may increase the rate of absorption of glucose from the intestine.

3. Glucagon, which has been discussed previously.
4. Catecholamines, which (a) stimulate endogenous glucagon secretion and thus raise glucose levels, (b) stimulate glycogenolysis, (c) stimulate ketone production by liver, and (d) possess lipolytic activity (clinical example, pheochromocytoma with impaired glucose tolerance).

The "stress hormones" frequently discussed in relation to diabetes are principally glucagon, the catecholamines, the glucocorticoids, and growth hormone.

## GROWTH HORMONE AND DIABETES

Growth hormone (GH) plays a primary role in the development of diabetes mellitus as well as in the stimulation of vascular complications, according to many investigators. There is much evidence to support this implication, but there is also some evidence to dampen it. A brief review is in order.

In 1930, Houssay and Biasotti demonstrated the importance of the pituitary gland in diabetes when they performed hypophysectomies in experimental animals who had been made diabetic by previous pancreatectomy. The researchers noted that the severity of the diabetes decreased remarkably. Then, by injecting an extract of the pars distalis of the pituitary gland, they were able to increase the severity of the diabetes to its former state. Thus, the researchers could turn diabetes on and off with pituitary extract.

Later investigations showed that GH was the active substance in pituitary extracts that induced diabetes in animals. It was also shown that when human GH (hGH) was given to nondiabetic persons who had undergone hypophysectomy, a mild diabetic state could be produced. Additionally, it was shown that hGH given to diabetics caused deterioration of the diabetic state, particularly when hGH was given to juvenile diabetics who had undergone hypophysectomy.

Other investigations showed impaired IV glucose tolerance in normal subjects after 4 days of hGH administration. However, in acromegaly, fewer than 50% of the patients show overt diabetes.

The relationship of GH to vascular disease is not fully understood. However, there is evidence relating GH to diabetic retinopathy. Some years ago, a young diabetic woman with advanced retinopathy was the victim of Sheehan's syndrome following delivery of a child. In a few months' time, it became obvious that she was regaining vision and was showing anatomic improvement in the retinopathy. There followed a rash of pituitary operations throughout the world in an effort to halt progressive and blinding retinopathy. The operative mortality rate was high until a simple method of pituitary destruction evolved by the transsphenoidal approach. The object of the operation was to remove the source of GH. In some patients, the results were successful, and progression of the retinopathy was halted. A pleasant fringe benefit was a decreased insulin requirement, with many patients requiring 50% or less of their former dose. Some patients even developed a severe insulin sensitivity, with frequent hypoglycemic episodes.

Another group of patients with progessive retinopathy was treated with the cyclotron (proton beam). Improvement in retinopathy was not so noticeable. However, recently it has been reported that few of these treated persons have any evidence of nephropathy, the incidence being much less than would normally be expected. Could this phenomenon be related to GH?

There is not much evidence that an increase of GH stimulates the production of vascular disease. Some investigations have shown that there is not an abnormal increase in GH in the well-controlled Type I diabetic. If hGH is a primary factor in vascular disease, there should be evidence of this in acromegalics who have a long-standing elevation of GH. This is not generally the case. However, it is well known that diabetics who are pituitary dwarfs do not develop retinopathy despite many years of insulin dependence.

Recently, another hormone has been isolated from human pituitary glands that is different from GH and has diabetogenic properties. Thus, GH has diabetogenic properties, but one can have diabetes even without GH. One of these days, the pieces will fit together.

# 34

# Pathways of Glucose Metabolism and Glucose Homeostasis

## GLUCOSE METABOLISM

In untreated diabetes, glucose in physiologic concentrations is unable to penetrate certain types of cells. Primarily, 3 types of cells are involved: fat cells, muscle cells, and connective tissue cells. Most brain and central nervous system cells allow glucose to penetrate the cell barrier without insulin, as do renal cells, RBCs, gastrointestinal mucosal cells, and perhaps liver cells. Insulin makes cells permeable to glucose. In the absence of insulin, some glucose (10%) enters cells at high glucose concentrations, but at physiologic or normal glucose levels, insulin is needed for normal metabolism.

Figure 34–1 illustrates a simplified scheme of glucose metabolism. Diabetes affects the metabolism of all foodstuffs, not only carbohydrates. This is important to remember, since an understanding of the basics of glucose metabolism enables one to understand the more serious complications of diabetes. Foodstuffs are of little value if they remain in the bloodstream—they must penetrate the cell barrier to be metabolized. The first obstacle to the penetration of the cell by glucose is the cell membrane, and this is where insulin exerts a prime influence. Once in the cell, glucose can proceed in several directions, some physiologic and some pathologic, as shown in Figure 34–1.

**Conversion to Glycogen.** Glucose-6-phosphate can be converted to glycogen and can be stored as such. Insulin also affects the activa-

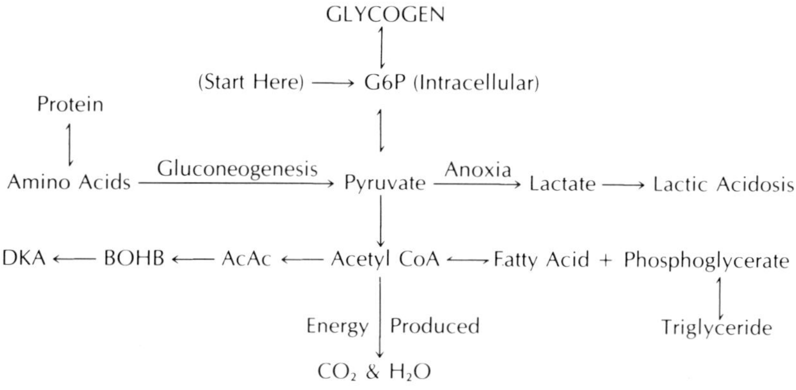


**Fig. 34–1.** Pathways of glucose metabolism.

tion of this pathway. Insulin seems to favor build-up or anabolism for further storage of materials, never their breakdown.

**Oxidation.** The second pathway of glucose metabolism is to oxidation, through pyruvate, which is then oxidized to acetyl coenzyme A (CoA) to $CO_2$ and water, with a liberation of energy. Pyruvate is decarboxylated ($CO_2$ removed) with the aid of CoA to form acetyl CoA, and this with nicotinamide adenine dinucleotide (NAD) acts as a transfer vehicle for the acetyl group.

**Anoxia.** If for any reason a condition of anoxia ensues and causes glucose metabolism to stop at pyruvate, then pyruvate is reduced to lactate, and the scene is set for the development of lactic acidosis.

**Fat Metabolism.** A typical fatty acid (FA) consists of 16 carbon atoms and is built from 8 molecules of acetyl CoA. FAs cannot be stored in the body without disrupting the cells, so the body hangs them on a compound that is a by-product of carbohydrate metabolism, phosphoglycerate. This has 3 OH groups for the attachment of 3 fatty acids. This forms a triglyceride or neutral fat, which is a blob of oil and can be easily stored in a fat cell. It thus becomes evident that every carbon, oxygen, and hydrogen atom composing the triglyceride came from glucose originally. The triglycerides of animal fats that we eat are mainly made from glucose. Thus, fat is a storage form of carbohydrate, and when it is needed for energy, which is almost all the time, it is broken down to fatty acid, and the fatty acid is broken down to acetyl CoA.

**Ketoacidosis Pathway.** Insulin favors fat synthesis and inhibits fat breakdown. If a severe deficiency of insulin occurs for any reason, there is a breakdown of glycogen and fat. Lipolysis then causes an enormous increase of acetyl CoA in the liver, which in turn is not able to transform all of it to $CO_2$ and water. The acetyl CoA combines with itself to form acetoacetate and $\beta$-hydroxybutyrate, and ketosis ensues. The pathway in Figure 34–1 between fatty acid and acetyl CoA refers to a reversible reaction of fatty acids that produces acetyl CoA. Acetoacetate, a useful molecule that is produced continuously in normal physiology, is burned in muscle cells for the production of energy. It is, however, a strong organic acid that lowers the $CO_2$ combining power. When the level of bicarbonate decreases, so does the pH, and ketoacidosis occurs. Insulin given in ketoacidosis stops the liberation of fatty acids and allows the acetoacetate to be excreted and oxidized.

**Relation of Insulin to Protein.** This relationship is less well understood. Amino acids are deaminated in the liver, and the remaining portion is converted to sugar, first by being transformed to pyruvate, a process called gluconeogenesis. Insulin inhibits this process and favors anabolism, just as it does with carbohydrate and fat. Insulin thus favors resynthesis of protein from amino acids. All other hormones are not primarily anabolic in their actions.

Thus, having seen where insulin exerts its effects and how the metabolic paths of the 3 foodstuffs intertwine, what could one expect to see when there is little or no insulin available? One sees a low glycogen level, a low amount of fat, increases in lipolysis and ketosis, a negative nitrogen balance with a loss of amino acids and urea, and difficulty in penetration of the cell by glucose, with resultant hyperglycemia.

## GLUCOSE HOMEOSTASIS

In normal, nondiabetic persons, blood glucose levels rarely rise above 140 mg/dl after meals or fall below 70 mg/dl between meals or after the overnight fast. The ability of the body to maintain such glucose levels is the result of the action of hormones and enzymes on exogenous foods for utilization or storage. The body then uses these stored foods for the production of heat and energy in times of relative fast.

Glucose use is around 2 mg/kg/min, and the brain uses about 80% of that amount, or about 6 g/hr. A normally active, 70-kg person uses about 8 to 10 g glucose/hr. Liver glycogen is the only significant reservoir for the maintenance of blood glucose concentration. This store represents about 6% of the weight of the liver, and for the average, 70-kg adult this is probably around 108 g glucose (for an 1800-g liver). Between meals, the glycogen is constantly converted to glucose; the supply is restored with each meal from the absorbed glucose, fructose, and galactose. In addition, proteins are a good source of glucose through gluconeogenesis, and this conversion process is carried on by both the liver and the kidneys. Approximately 58% of ingested protein is converted to glucose. Some carbohydrate can be formed from the glycerol fraction of the body lipids. The stored glycogen of the liver is readily convertible to glucose, which can enter the bloodstream in an effort to maintain normal blood glucose levels. This ease of conversion is due to a special phosphatase enzyme present only in the liver.

The glycogen stored in muscles, about 350 g for the average, 70-kg adult, is there mainly to furnish energy for muscle metabolism. Muscle glycogen cannot act directly as a source of blood glucose because no special phosphatase enzyme is present. The conversion of glucose to glucose-6-phosphate in muscle is a one-way street involving the enzymes hexokinase, the phosphate donor adenosine triphosphate (ATP), and potassium and magnesium ions. When muscle glycogen breaks down to glucose-1-phosphate, the latter is carried through the series of reactions to pyruvic acid or lactic acid, but it does not form glucose. However, muscle glycogen can contribute to blood glucose levels by the following means: When mild exercise is undertaken and plenty of oxygen is present, glucose is used through the pyruvic acid pathway, and the end point is carbon dioxide and water. With sustained exercise, during anaerobic activity, muscle contraction releases variable amounts of lactic acid into the bloodstream and the liver, where it is converted into glycogen. Glycogen can again be converted to glucose, which can diffuse into the bloodstream and thus raise the blood sugar level. So, in sustained exercise, the diabetic probably is helping to replenish the stores of his liver glycogen through the lactic acid cycle.

The time required to build up glycogen in the liver is probably directly proportional to the availability of blood glucose for this purpose. During a meal, with ingestion of high amounts of carbohydrates, glycogen storage in the liver probably begins to build up within a few minutes of absorption of glucose, roughly 15 to 30 minutes after one starts eating. Ordinarily, a full storage of glycogen in the liver is enough to last the average person 6 to 8 hours with sedentary activity. Studies done under periods of experimental starvation in nondiabetics have proved that blood glucose levels drop only to about 50 to 70 mg/dl and stay there for many days. This is brought about because the body is accelerating gluconeogenesis and is making glucose from proteins and glycerol. Actually, soldiers in starvation camps during World War II died from acidosis rather than hypoglycemia. It apparently takes the added stimulus of an overdose of insulin, or exercise and an inadequate supply of glucose, to produce the severe hypoglycemic reactions seen in diabetics.

Investigation of glucagon levels in diabetics with hypoglycemia have shown that insulin depresses alpha-cell function (glucagon), and therefore, an excess of insulin contributes to the severity of hypoglycemia. Unger and colleagues in Texas and others have measured serum glucagon levels in hypoglycemic diabetics and have reported an inadequate glucagon response.

# 35

# University Group Diabetes Program (UGDP) Study

For 15 years following the introduction of the sulfonylurea drugs (1955 to 1970) for the treatment of Type II diabetes, there was almost complete satisfaction with the use of these agents, since clinical results were satisfactory and acceptance of them by patients was excellent. In 1970, however, the first report of the University Group Diabetes Program study, in progress since 1961, was published. The UGDP study was designed to see whether control of blood glucose levels helps to prevent or to delay vascular disease in diabetics who do not require insulin for the prevention of ketoacidosis.

## OBJECTIVES AND METHODS OF THE STUDY

The UGDP had 3 major objectives:

1. Evaluation of the efficacy of hypoglycemic treatments in the prevention of vascular complications in a long-term, prospective, and cooperative clinical trial.
2. Study of the natural history of vascular disease in maturity onset, non-insulin-dependent diabetes.
3. Development of methods applicable to cooperative clinical trials.

Twelve diabetes clinics throughout the United States were invited to participate in the study; the first 5 joined in 1960 and the rest between 1961 and 1963. Recruitment of patients began in 1961 and was completed in 1966; 1027 patients were enrolled. Patients admitted to the study were limited to those whose diabetes had been present for not more than 1 year prior to enrollment and who had a minimum life expectancy of at least 5 years.

Data from the 12 clinics were sent to a coordinating center at the University of Maryland Medical School, where the analysis was supervised by a biostatistician. Patients were randomly assigned to 1 of 5 treatment groups receiving the following:

1. Placebo
2. Fixed dose of tolbutamide (1 g before breakfast and 0.5 g before evening meal, total 1.5 g)
3. Fixed daily dose of insulin (either 10, 12, 14, or 16 U/day, depending on body size)
4. Variable dose of insulin (sufficient to maintain "normal" blood sugar level)
5. Fixed dose of phenformin (50-mg time-disintegrating capsule twice daily, total 100 mg)

At the end of the enrollment there were more than 200 patients in each of the 5 study groups. By 1979, approximately 15 million dollars had been granted by the National Institutes of Health (NIH) for this study.

## REPORT ON TOLBUTAMIDE

The first UGDP report stated that not only was tolbutamide not effective in lowering blood sugar levels, but the use of this drug was associated with a significantly increased risk of cardiovascular death. Shortly thereafter, UGDP spokesmen stated that the findings in this study pertained only to tolbutamide and extrapolation to other oral antidiabetes agents would not be proper. However, the American Medical Association (AMA) Council on Drugs stated that because sulfonylurea drugs are structurally similar, they should be considered to be similar to tolbutamide until proved otherwise. The UGDP group discontinued the use of tolbutamide in their study in 1969.

## RESPONSE TO THE UGDP REPORT

A news leak provided the Wall St. Journal with the tolbutamide story on May 20, 1970, several weeks before the report was scheduled to be delivered at the annual meeting of the American Diabetes Association (ADA) in St. Louis. This put many physicians who had prescribed tolbutamide for patients on the defensive, since most physicians had not then heard of the UGDP study. Two days after the Wall St. Journal report, the FDA endorsed the study, even though they had not seen the UGDP data and their advisory committee advised against endorsement. Three days later, the FDA announced that it was going to require warning labels for all oral antidiabetic drugs, in spite of the fact that the UGDP studies had still not been presented to the scientific audience.

Shortly thereafter, a group of prominent diabetologists, who not only disagreed with the UGDP findings, but also opposed the intent of the FDA to change the labeling of the oral agents, was organized by Dr. Robert Bradley of the Joslin Diabetes Clinic in Boston and Dr. Peter Forsham, chief of the Metabolic Unit of the University of California Medical Center in San Francisco. The original group, composed of 182 well-known, practicing diabetologists, was named the Committee for the Care of the Diabetic (CCD). Nonetheless, the FDA stated: "The FDA is required to determine the conditions of use under which the drug has been proved safe and effective by substantial evidence. This requires the FDA to act as independent arbiter on medical issues, and means that inevitably its decisions will not meet with unanimous scientific agreement. If an attempt is made to present both sides of a scientific controversy in the package insert, it would overwhelm and hopelessly confuse the practicing physician. . . ." (J. Med. Assoc. Georgia, 65:411, 1976). Then the CCD hired a lawyer, and on the second try for a restraining order that included testimony of a consumer, the motion was granted. Since that time, the issue has been in and out of court.

Following the oral presentation of the first UGDP report at the ADA meeting in St. Louis, the ADA endorsed the study's conclusions. Six months later, when the results were published, they were endorsed by the Council on Drugs of the AMA.

## CRITICISM OF THE UGDP STUDY

Many scientists questioned the validity of the report, the methods of reporting, the statistical analysis, and the selection of patients for the study. Numerous reports began to appear in the medical press, written by both the proponents and opponents of the UGDP conclusions. There was apparent discontent among some original investigators about the conduct of the study, and in November of 1970, 2 of them resigned, Dr. Angela Bowen and Dr. Robert Reeves of the Virginia Mason Clinic in Seattle.

In 1971, phenformin was also withdrawn from the study.

In an article in the Journal of Clinical Pharmacology and Therapy (19:78, 1976), Dr. Alvin Feinstein reported the following:

"1. The UGDP study omitted, distorted, or falsified vital clinical data in order to satisfy statistical methodology.

2. The study has become a clinical and statistical "debacle," an object lesson in unacceptably poor medical care offered to some 822 subjects for nearly 10 years.
3. About 50% of all the patients were on a fixed dosage of hypoglycemic drugs with no regard for adequate blood sugar control.
4. Glucose tolerance tests were done incorrectly in 4 clinics and thus kept 69 patients in this study who apparently did not have diabetes.
5. Patients with poor blood sugar control had twice the cardiovascular mortality of those who were well controlled."

The CCD wished to obtain the raw data (patients' records) from the UGDP study. On August 7, 1975, the assistant secretary of the United States Department of Health, Education, and Welfare (HEW), Theodore Cooper, wrote a letter to the attorney representing the CCD, stating, "I have made further extensive inquiries of both the National Institutes of Health and the Food and Drug Administration. Neither agency has ever had the raw data in its possession." Cooper further said the raw data was stored on microfilm. Apparently Mr. Christian Klimt, biostatistician for the study, controlled the raw data. In 1978, some of the records were turned over to the FDA at their request, and shortly thereafter, the CCD was able to obtain some of them.

The release of the raw data permitted members of the CCD to review carefully the patient records, and some important information surfaced. There were contradictions noted in the allocation of patients to different treatment groups and the assignment of baseline risks by the FDA and by the UGDP group. Many areas were open to criticism and reinterpretation, such as the causes of death in some patients, the inclusion in a particular treatment group of patients who either did not take the medication prescribed or took it for only brief periods of time, the inclusion of patients in the placebo group who at times took large doses of insulin or oral antidiabetes agents, the questionable diagnosis of diabetes in some patients, the questionable type of therapy given to some patients, and the different weight given to risk factors by the FDA and the UGDP.

Dr. Charles Kilo and Dr. Joseph Williamson, original UGDP investigators and both members of the faculty of the Washington University School of Medicine in St. Louis, spent hundreds of hours reviewing the data. The following is from a letter that they sent to various colleagues on December 20, 1978:

"We have reviewed the data on approximately 1,000 diabetics recently released by the UGDP coordinating center and our findings refute the basic conclusions of the UGDP investigators. Most importantly, in respect to the present communication, we found that virtually all of the excess cardiovascular mortality reported by UGDP investigators in tolbutamide-treated patients occurred in diabetics who were poorly controlled (with FBS values in excess of 200 mg%) and inappropriately treated. Since it is generally agreed that the response to tolbutamide is inadequate if FBS values cannot be maintained below 170-180 mg%, it is clear that one-half of the tolbutamide subjects who died of cardiovascular causes should not have been on the tolbutamide treatment regimen utilized in the UGDP study. Virtually any pharmacologic agent can have toxic effects if misused, therefore, we believe it is inappropriate to condemn tolbutamide under the circumstances under which it was used in the UGDP study. Independent of these considerations, we have provided strong evidence indicating that the difference in cardiovascular death rate in tolbutamide-treated and placebo-treated subjects was due to a spurious, low cardiovascular death rate in the placebo group, rather than to an absolute increase in the death rate in the tolbutamide-treated subjects. Lastly, we have shown that UGDP investigators were in error in concluding that insulin treatment was of no value in preventing cardiovascular complications in diabetics.

"These findings are discussed in more detail in the enclosed copies of material we have submitted to the FDA. Since labeling changes on oral agents proposed by the FDA would have potentially important medical-legal implications regarding the use of oral agents, we believe that any proposed labeling changes should be based on sound evidence. In view of our findings in the UGDP data, together with the numerous problems raised by many other investigators, it is our considered opinion that there is no evidence documenting cardiovascular toxicity, when tolbutamide is used properly in accordance with conventional guidelines. This opinion is shared by members of the Committee for the Care of the Diabetic, as well as by many diabetologists and statisticians who have critically reviewed the UGDP study." (Reproduced by permission of the American Diabetes Association, Inc.)

The last publication from the UGDP in 1978 reported on the study of patients receiving insulin therapy. The UGDP concluded that the cardiovascular death rate in insulin-treated, mild, maturity-onset diabetics with well-controlled blood sugar levels was no different from that in patients taking placebos. The UGDP concluded that insulin treatment to normalize blood sugar levels in these patients had no long-term protective value.

Kilo and Williamson made a detailed study of these data and reported the following: Kilo and Williamson first eliminated patients who had died or had dropped out the first year of the trial, those who were not available for follow-up for a year or more, and/or those who had changed their medications for a year. That left only 58% of that group available for fair analysis. Then they eliminated patients with increased cardiovascular risks at entry—subjects over age 70 and hypertensive patients with diastolic pressures above 110. Fifty percent of the insulin variable group, but only 34% of the placebo group, were thus at increased risk.

Thus, with inappropriate patients dropped from the study, Kilo and Williamson reported that "cardiovascular deaths in the placebo group were 4 times as frequent as those in the insulin-variable group." Also, they said, "insulin-standard patients had a threefold increased death rate, compared with those in the insulin-variable group." Kilo and Williamson concluded that "these preliminary findings alone call for a retraction of the UGDP conclusion that insulin (properly used) is ineffective in the prevention of diabetic vascular complications" (J. A. M. A., *243*:450, 1980).

## Position of the American Diabetes Association

On January 22, 1979, at the annual winter meeting of the ADA, the Board of Directors issued a new position statement on the UGDP study. The following information is quoted from the statement of the scientific advisory panel of the Executive Committee of the ADA published in Diabetes Care (*2*:1, 1979):

"Because of the continuing controversy over the UGDP study; because of the voiced concerns about the UGDP conclusions by many experienced diabetologists; because of the newer therapeutic attitudes toward maturity-onset diabetes; and especially because of the personal concerns of the affected diabetic people themselves, it is appropriate that the American Diabetes Association reassess its position concerning the UGDP reports. The timing of this reassessment has been made appropriate by the recent publication of the FDA audit analysis and the reopening of the comment period.

"The following statements reflect the current viewpoints of the ADA toward the UGDP study and the controversy surrounding it.

(1) The scientific literature does not reflect a clear consensus on the interpretation of the UGDP findings.

(2) The recent audit by the FDA has reassured the ADA only so far as its analyses were carried. Data on only 159 participants out of 1,027 of the UGDP study were addressed. No review of the primary clinical data or follow-up analysis on morbidity and mortality of the remaining 868 patients has been undertaken as yet. Clinical data from the twelve centers were not systematically examined.

(3) Significant differences do exist between the therapeutic designs of the UGDP protocol initiated in 1961 and the medical strategies commonly applied in 1979 by physicians with respect to the management of maturity-onset diabetes. Thus, the UGDP protocol used only one sulfonylurea drug, tolbutamide, at a single, fixed dosage. Neither tolbutamide nor other sulfonylureas were used in variable doses as is common practice. Of course, daily insulin dosage was varied in only one of the two study groups using insulin. More aggressive attempts at achieving weight control in the obese patient are pursued today and attention to biochemical control of blood glucose levels is the rule irrespective of whether an oral hypoglycemic agent or insulin is used in addition to diet. These actions often require more frequent patient-physician encounters than were part of the standard UGDP protocol.

(4) It is proper that resolution of the controversies about the UGDP findings and their clinical significance be pursued within the medical community from data published in refereed scientific journals. It is distressing to read hyperbole in publications, comments which generally polarize rather than clarify the issues.
(5) The patient-physician interaction should continue to be the primary arena of decision-making regarding the appropriate therapy for the individual diabetic patient whether that therapy is diet alone, diet plus insulin, or diet plus an oral sulfonylurea.
(6) The unique nature and size of the UGDP study, its multicentered base, the time now elapsed from the inception of the study, and the previously proposed governmental decisions concerning the nature of professional advice that physicians should give their diabetic patients suggested that access to and review of data from the twelve centers of the UGDP should be carried out by ad-hoc review groups which would include clinical diabetologists. However, the magnitude of the task in time, money and manpower lessens the feasibility of this approach and the likelihood of a successful outcome and, therefore, renders it impractical at this time.
(7) Sufficient uncertainty now prevails regarding the UGDP data on sulfonylureas to warrant reconsideration of any restrictive governmental actions based on the initial findings of the UGDP study. At this time, we oppose any formal governmental restrictions on use of the sulfonylurea agents which are based on the initial interpretations of the UGDP findings until newer analyses, some of which are already available (19), can be evaluated.

"From these foregoing viewpoints, the American Diabetes Association recommends that:
(1) Only data presented in refereed scientific publications concerning the UGDP be given professional credence.
(2) Physician judgment on management of the maturity-onset diabetic patient should be based on an assessment of all therapeutic information available including
    (a) data on known cardiovascular risk factors;
    (b) data on the positive influence of metabolic control of the diabetic state on vascular disease;
    (c) data pointing to the clear importance of dietotherapy in the obese diabetic patient;
    (d) data emphasizing the importance of regular physical activity;
    (e) data on objective reports in the scientific literature which pertain to the UGDP study;
    (f) data on objective reports in the scientific literature which relate to the long-term use of the sulfonylureas.
(3) Physicians continue to emphasize dietotherapy as the prime form of treatment for maturity-onset diabetes with appropriate use of an oral sulfonylurea or insulin only after diet therapy alone has clearly failed to achieve desired therapeutic goals. The choice of a sulfonylurea or insulin will be left to the judgment of the physician after discussion with the patient.

(4) Until a review of all newer data which relate to the UGDP findings has been completed, any formal recommendations on the use of tolbutamide in maturity-onset diabetes which are based on the initial findings of the UGDP study should be held in abeyance.

(5) A package insert be developed by the ADA and the FDA for the professional and consumer community which will recognize the state of the art regarding therapy of maturity-onset diabetes current to 1979. This insert should offer physicians data and references from various studies which impinge on the modern management of maturity-onset diabetes including the use of diet, insulin, and the oral sulfonylurea drugs in achieving acceptable goals of diabetes control. Emphasis on avoiding cardiovascular risk factors should also be included.

"Furthermore, the ADA comments with reference to prospective multicentered clinical studies that:

(1) Despite the controversies surrounding the UGDP study, well-planned and executed multicentered clinical trials should continue to be supported by appropriate governmental agencies because this is the only mechanism by which certain clinical problems in diabetes can be properly studied.

(2) When such multicentered clinical trials occur in the future, provision should be made at the inception of the study for monitoring of the study by an independent referee(s) who is not a collaborating participant(s).

(3) The activities of the independent referees would enhance the perception by the medical community on the significance of the findings by the study group."

## REVIEW OF THE UGDP STUDY

In March of 1979, the Americal Medical Association notified HEW, NIH, and the top medical organizations in the United States that its Council on Scientific Affairs had been directed to review the UGDP study and related reports, in order to reassess its position on the use of the oral antidiabetes drugs. AMA Executive Vice President Dr. James H. Sammons sent telegrams to these agencies that stated: "Several recent publications and a statement by the American Diabetes Association have raised questions concerning the validity of the UGDP study on oral antidiabetes drugs. As a result, the AMA has asked its Council on Scientific Affairs to review the study and related reports, in order that the association may reassess its position on the use of these drugs."

In April of 1979, Dr. Rolf Luft, professor of endocrinology at Karolinska Institute, Stockholm, and president of the International Diabetes Federation, said that he agrees with the American Diabetes Association in calling for a halt to any governmental actions based on the controversial findings of the UGDP. Dr. Luft, a long-time investigator of the sulfonylureas, made this statement to the FDA: "It is my considered opinion that the UGDP should not be used as an argument against the proper use of sulfonylureas in diabetic patients. My main reason for this view is that, so far, the original material has not been made available for evaluation by an unbiased group of experienced scientists and statisticians."

Concerning the findings of the UGDP of an excess cardiovascular death rate, Dr. Luft said: "In my own clinical work with thousands of diabetic patients in Sweden, I have *never* encountered any one case where a cardiac condition or coronary infarct could possibly be attributed to the use of sulfonylureas. In addition, studies performed in Sweden, which have been most carefully planned and controlled, have suggested that sulfonylureas may even be beneficial and may be used to decrease the risk of cardiac attacks in diabetics." Dr. Luft continued: "Both as a physician responsible for the care of thousands of diabetic patients and as president of the International Diabetes Federation (in which capacity I am not involved with any pharmaceutical companies manufacturing these drugs), I would deplore any curtailment of the proper use of sulfonylureas, which would adversely affect vast numbers of patients throughout the world, without reliable unbiased proof of their alleged harmful effects."

The Canadian government has not taken action regarding labeling changes or other regulations of oral antidiabetes drugs. Similarly, Great Britain's drug agency, the Scowen Committee on the Safety of Drugs, and the British Diabetic Association both declared that they saw no need to take action on the basis of the UGDP study.

One can conclude from all that has transpired since 1970 that both respect for the validity of the UGDP study and faith in its conclusions have declined, as demonstrated by the position statements of the American Diabetes Association, the Committee for the Care of the Diabetic, the International Diabetes Federation, and the American Medical Association.

Many of today's younger practicing physicians were in medical school or residencies when the reports of the UGDP study first were published, and they may have been taught not to use the oral antidiabetes drugs because of these reports. At the same time, they may not have been aware of the numerous studies whose conclusions were exactly opposite those of the UGDP. Dr. Harry Keen's study from England, Dr. Paasakivi's study from Finland, Dr. Goodkin's study in the United States, as well as Dr. Marble's report from the Joslin Clinic, all showed results contrasting with the UGDP conclusions concerning tolbutamide. It is difficult for some of these physicians to change their beliefs concerning the benefits of the oral agents. Fortunately, physicians are still allowed their choice in selecting a treatment program for patients, and one hopes that they always will be.

# Appendix

## Reading List for Diabetic Patients

### BOOKS ON FOOD

American Diabetes Association: A Guide for Professionals: The Effective Application of Exchange Lists for Meal Planning. American Diabetes Association (2 Park Ave., New York, NY 10016), 1977. Gratis

Cinnamon, P., and Swanson, M.A.: Everything You Always Wanted to Know about Exchange Values. University Cities Diabetes Education Program (733 Taylor Ave., Moscow ID 83843), 1976. $2.25

Deaconess Hospital Diabetes Education Center: Diabetic Diet Instructions. Diabetes Education Center (Deaconess Hospital, W. 800 Fifth Ave., Spokane, WA 99210), 1978. $3.00

Jones, J.: Cake Mix Magic with Batter-Lite. Batter-Lite Foods, Inc. (P.O. Box 341, Beloit, WI 53511), 1976. $1.00

Jones, J.: Cookie Mix Magic with Batter-Lite. Batter-Lite Foods, Inc. (P.O. Box 341, Beloit, WI 53511), 1976. $1.00

Jones, J.: Diet Delight Cookbook. California Canners and Growers (Cookbook Dept., 3100 Ferry Bldg., San Francisco, CA 94106), 1975. Gratis

Jones, J.: The Calculating Cook. 101 Productions (834 Mission St., San Francisco, CA 94110), 1977. $6.95 (hardback), $4.95 (paperback)

MacRae, N.: How to Have Your Cake and Eat It Too! Alaska N.W. Publishing Co. (130 Second Ave. South, Edmonds, WA 98020), 1975. $6.95

Middleton, K., and Hess, M.A.: The Art of Cooking for the Diabetic. Contemporary Books, Inc. (180 N. Michigan Ave., Chicago, IL 60601), 1978. $12.95 (hardback), $6.95 (paperback)

University of Kentucky Diabetes Research and Education Fund: High Carbohydrate and Fiber (HCF) Diets: A Dietician's Manual also Suitable for the Diabetic Patient. University of Kentucky Diabetes Research and Education Fund (c/o Dr. James Anderson, 1872 Blairmore Road, Lexington, KY 40502), 1978. $3.00 (tax-deductible)

University of Kentucky Diabetes Research and Education Fund: HCF Diets: A Professional Guide for Dieticians and Doctors. University of Kentucky Diabetes Research and Education Fund (c/o Dr. James Anderson, 1872 Blairmore Road, Lexington, KY 40502), 1979. $5.00 (tax-deductible; discounts on orders of more than 5 copies)

University of Kentucky Diabetes Research and Education Fund: HCF Diets: A User's Guide for High Carbohydrate, High Fiber Diets. University of Kentucky Diabetes Research and Education Fund (c/o Dr. James Anderson, 1872 Blairmore Road, Lexington, KY 40502), 1979. $4.00 (tax-deductible)

Wedman, B.: Canning and Freezing with Low Salt and No Added Sugar. B. Wedman (40 S. Clay St., Hinsdale, IL 60521), 1979. $1.00

Wedman, B.: Jams, Jellies, Marmalades. B. Wedman (40 S. Clay St., Hinsdale, IL 60521), 1978. $1.00

## GENERAL BOOKS

Biermann, J., and Toohey, B.: The Diabetic Sports and Exercise Book. J. B. Lippincott Co. (East Washington Square, Philadelphia, PA 19105), 1976, $5.95

Biermann, J., and Toohey, B.: The Diabetic's Total Health Book. J. P. Tarcher, Inc. (Los Angeles, CA), 1980. $10.95

Duncan, T.: The Good Life with Diabetes. Hampton Graphics (Southampton, PA 18966), 1973. $6.85

Krall, L.: Joslin Diabetes Manual, 11th Ed. Lea & Febiger (600 Washington Square, Philadelphia, PA 19106), 1978. $8.50

Musky, S.: Vacationing with Diabetes Not from Diabetes. E. R. Squibb and Sons, Inc. (Professional Services Dept., 5 Georges Road, New Brunswick, NJ 08903), 1973. Gratis

Olson, O.C.: Instruction Book for Diabetic Patients, 11th Ed. Diabetes Education Center (Deaconess Hospital, W. 800 Fifth Ave., Spokane, WA 99210), 1981. $3.00

E. R. Squibb and Sons, Inc.: Don't be Afraid of Diabetes. E. R. Squibb & Sons, Inc. (Professional Services Dept., 5 Georges Road, New Brunswick, NJ 08903), 1971. Gratis

Travis, L.B.: An Instructional Aid on Juvenile Diabetes Mellitus, 5th Ed. South Texas Diabetes Association, Inc. (ADA South Texas Affiliate, Inc., P.O. Box 12946, Austin, TX 78711), 1978. $3.75

## FREE BOOKS FOR CHILDREN

Ames Company: Care of the Child with Diabetes. Ames Company (Division of Miles Laboratories, Elkhart, IN 46514), 1977.

Ames Company: Straight Talk about Diabetes. Ames Company (Division of Miles Laboratories, Elkhart, IN 46514), 1977.

Wenger, D.M.: Mr. Hypo Is My Friend. Ames Company (Division of Miles Laboratories, Elkhart, IN 46514)

## PERIODICALS

ADA Forecast (Bimonthly). American Diabetes Association (2 Park Ave., New York, NY 10016). $6.00/yr.

Diabetes in the News (Quarterly). Diabetes in the News (233 East Erie Street, Chicago, IL 60611). Gratis

## Instruction Sheet for Nonprofessional Emergency Treatment of a Diabetic With Low Blood Sugar (Insulin Reaction or Hypoglycemia)

All personnel working with or around persons with diabetes should know that this person has diabetes, and further, should understand what to do in case of a reaction resulting from a blood sugar level that is too low. This situation can occur at any time of the day (mainly in diabetics who take insulin), but most frequently occurs during or following exercise or just prior to the next meal. The body sends out warning signs, and in most instances, the diabetic persons recognizes these and knows that he must take some form of sugar. If the early warning signs are not recognized, and sugar is not taken, the patient may become disoriented. In a few minutes, he becomes unconscious and may have convulsions.

### WARNING SIGNS AND SYMPTOMS OF IMPENDING LOW BLOOD SUGAR LEVEL

1. Usually excessive hunger
2. Sweating in almost all patients; skin feels cool and clammy
3. Shakiness
4. In children: sudden change in behavior; frequently a "glassy stare;" irritability, crying or confusion without adequate cause
5. Headache and drowsiness
6. Incoordination, including staggering, slurring of speech, double vision
7. Semiconsciousness, rapidly moving into complete unconsciousness with convulsions

## TREATMENT

The patient must have sugar immediately, preferably in one of the following forms:

1. Table sugar—2 tsp taken in a little water
2. Life Savers—4 to 5, chewed and swallowed, or other similar hard candy
3. Fruit juices of any kind—⅓ to ½ cup
4. Soft drinks—sugar-containing, *NOT* diet drink—6 oz or more
5. Syrup, honey, jelly, jam, or any other substance furnishing large amounts of sugar—1 tablespoon
6. If no other sugar-containing food is available, a candy bar may be given.

## IF PATIENT IS UNCONSCIOUS AND UNABLE TO SWALLOW

If the patient rapidly becomes unconscious, one should not attempt to give anything by mouth, since the swallowing reflex may be absent. It is then necessary to take the diabetic patient to the nearest medical facility for rapid treatment.

## RECOVERY

Recovery should occur within 15 to 25 minutes of ingestion of sugar-containing foods or fluids. The patient should then eat some substantial food such as a sandwich and a glass of milk. If it is just before mealtime, the patient should proceed with the meal at once.

# Index

Page numbers in *italics* indicate figures; "t" indicates tabular matter.


Abdomen, as injection site, 47
Acetoacetate, 264
Acetohexamide, 50t
Acidosis, bicarbonate in, 107–108, 110
  during pregnancy, 152
  lactic. See *Lactic acidosis*
Acromegaly, 232
Adolescents, diabetic control in, 7, 75
Adult-onset diabetic(s), 76
  nonobese, 76
  Type I, diabetes education for, 78
    diagnosis of, 77
    diet for, 77
    exercise by, 89
    follow-up visits by, 78–79
    hospitalization of, 82
    insulin for, 77, 78–79
    management of, 77–79
  Type II, control in, 83
    diet for, 79
    exercise and, 89
    follow-up of, 80–81
    general advice for, 81
    hospitalization of, 82
    insulin use by, 80
    newly diagnosed elderly, 84
    obese, 80
    office management of, 79–82
    special procedures for, 81
    typical, 79
    urinalysis in, 80
Age distribution, 4, 4t
Alcohol intake, 98
Aldose reductase, 168, 179
American Diabetes Association, recommendations for oral glucose tolerance test, 11–13
  University Group Diabetes Program study and, 272–274
Ames Dextrometer, 213–214
Ames Dextrostix, 214
Amniocentesis, 158–159
Amputation(s), infection as cause of, 143
  lower extremity, 137
  prevention of, 140
Amyotrophy, 180–181
Angiography, 173
Anoxia, 263
Antibodies, in Type I diabetes, 246
Antidiabetes agent(s), oral, 49–58
    acceptance of, 49–51
    clinical experience with, 49
    contraindications to, 51–52
    diet therapy and, 19
    for obese diabetics, 123
      Type II, 80
    hypoglycemia when taking, 98–99
    in pregnancy, 157
    indications for use of, 51
    mode of action of, 51
    postoperative resumption of, 129–130
    second-generation, 57–58
    surgical procedures and, 126
    University Group Diabetes Program study of. See *University Group Diabetes Program (UGDP) study*
Antigens, HLA, 247–249
Antihypertensive drugs, 204
Antiplatelet-aggregating agents, 205
Antiseptics, diabetic feet and, 142
Appetite, insulin doses and, 112
Artificial pancreas, 7–8, 207, 211
Aspartame, 224

Aspirin, in diabetic retinopathy, 176
in increased platelet aggregation, 205
Athlete's foot, 141
Athletics, hypoglycemia and, 100
Attitude of patient, 7
Autoimmunity, 246
Azotemia, 193

Bacteremia, 132
Bacteria, laboratory reporting of, 135
urinary tract infection and, 134
Basement membrane, capillary, diabetic control and, 170
hyperglycemia and, 167
Beef insulin, 31, 114
Beef-pork insulins, 34
Benedict's test, 64
Bernardinelli-Seip syndrome, 233–234
Beta-adrenergic blockers, 204
Bicarbonate, for acidosis, 107–108, 110
plasma, 237–240
"Biostator," 207
Bladder, cancer of, 219, 220–221
neurogenic, complications of, 185
diagnosis of, 185
in neurogenic impotence, 189–190
treatment of, 185–186
Blood pressure, in neuropathy, 187
Blood sample, in oral glucose tolerance test, preservation of, 12–13
processing of, 12
timing of, 12
Blood sugar. See *Glucose, blood*
Blood vessels, disease of. See *Vascular disease, peripheral*
Body, insulin injection sites on, 47–48
Books, dietary instruction, 24, 26
for diabetic patients, 277–279
Brain, hypoglycemia and, 93–94
Brittle diabetics, 73–74
"Bronze diabetes," 232–233
Bullae, on extremities, 136
Burger's exercises, 139–140

Calorie(s), expenditure of, 91
requirements of, for adults, 20
for children, 20
Cancer, saccharin and, 219, 220–221
Candy, diabetic, 24
Carbohydrate(s), in ideal diabetic diet, 23
in pregnancy, 153
meals loaded with, 10
tolerance to, age and, 8
Carbutamide (B–Z 55), 49
Cardiovascular disease, Framingham study of, 197–198, 198t
risk factors in, 197–206
Cardiovascular system, in neuropathy, 186–187
Cataract(s), juvenile-onset, 178
metabolic, 178
"senile," 178
sorbitol in, 168
Catecholamines, 259, 260
Catheterization, 102
Cellulitis, 132–133
Cerebral edema, 110
Cesarean section, 161
Chemstrip-bG, 214
Children, diabetes occurrence in, 5
dietary guidelines for, 20–21
free books for, 278–279
injection sites in, 48
insulin requirements of, over 25 units daily as, 35–37
under 25 units daily as, 34–35
oral glucose tolerance test in, 11
Chlorpropamide, 50t
hypoglycemia and, 98–99
side effects of, 54
Cholecystitis, 132
Cholesterol, abnormalities of, 202–203
high-density lipoprotein, 199
in coronary heart disease, 199–200, 201–202
level(s) of, coronary heart disease and, 200
exercise and, 87
high-fiber diets and, 24–25
serum, determination of, 201
normal, 201
low-density lipoprotein, 198, 199
in coronary heart disease, 201–202
Cholesterol-binding reserve, 199
Cholestyramine, 202
Circulation, constriction of, 142
Classification, of diabetes mellitus, 2–3
former, 1
requirements of, 2
Clinitest, 59–61
2-drop, 61
Colestipol, 202
Colorimeter glucose monitoring devices, 213–214
Color-strip glucose monitoring devices, 214
Coma, hyperosmolar. See *Hyperosmolar coma*
in diabetes, differential diagnosis of, 97–98, 238–239t
Compliance, dietary, 26, 27
Complications, diabetic, diet and, 21t
triopathy of, 165, 171
See also *Degenerative complications* and specific complications
Congenital malformations, 148, 163
Congenital temporary diabetes, 234
Consultations, for physician, 82
Contraception, 163–164

Contraceptives, oral, 163
Contraction stress test (CST), 160
Control, diabetic. See *Diabetic control*
Corns, treatment of, 141
Coronary heart disease, cholesterol levels and, 200
  high-density lipoprotein, 199–200, 201–202
  low-density lipoprotein, 201–202
 familial hypercholesterolemia and, 200
 platelet factors in, 205–206
Corticosteroid therapy, 231
Cortisone, 231
Counseling, for diabetics, elderly, 124
  juvenile, 68
  Type II, 79
Coxsackie B-4 virus, 246
C-peptide immunoassay, 257
Cushing's syndrome, 232
Cyclamate(s), discovery of, 217
 FDA and, 217–218
 sale of, 220
 studies of, 218
Cyclohexylamine, 218
Cyclotron therapy, in nephropathy, 194
 in retinopathy, 261

Degenerative complications, diabetic control and, 165–169
  studies on, 169–171
 risk of, 165–166
Delaney Amendment, 220
Dextrose solution, 96
Diabetes mellitus, rare forms of, 233–234
 secondary to other disease states, 230–233. See also *Adult-onset diabetic(s); Juvenile diabetes; Juvenile diabetic(s); Type I diabetes; Type II diabetes*
Diabetic control, degenerative complications and, 165–169
  studies in, 169–171
 evaluation of, 35
 importance of, 165–167, 177
 retinopathy and, 170, 171, 175–176
Diabetic ketoacidosis (DKA), abnormalities in, 106
 bicarbonate in, 107–108
 cerebral edema following, 110
 differential diagnosis of, 102, 238–239t
 during pregnancy, 152
 etiology of, 101
 exercise and, 87
 follow-up care in, 109–110
 glucose metabolism and, 263–264
 insulin administration in, 108–109
 insulin receptors in, 255
 laboratory findings in, 104–105
 potassium replacement in, 107
 prevention of, 110
 prognostic signs in, 111
 signs of, 102
 stress hormones and, 110–111
 symptoms of, 101–102
 treatment of, 106–110
  emergency, 102–104
  flow sheet in, 102, *103*
  orders subsequent to, 109
 volume depletion and hyperosmolality in, 106
Diabetic nephropathy, 192–196
 diabetic control and, 171
 diagnosis of, 193
 information to patients with, 196
 intravenous pyelography in, 196
 medical measures in, 194
 prevention of, 193–194
 progression of, 194, 194t
 symptoms and signs of, 192–193
 treatment of, 194–196
Diabetic neuropathy, 179–187
 differential diagnosis of, 182
 hyperglycemia and, 165, 166
 manifestations of, 179
 pathogenesis of, 179–180
 peripheral, 180–184
  treatment of, 182–183
  upper extremity involvement in, 181–182
 visceral, 184–187
  articles on, 187
  cardiovascular manifestations of, 186–187
  organ systems affected by, 184
Diabetic retinopathy, background, 173
 diabetic control and, 170, 171, 175–176
 florid, 174
 hypertension and, 176
 incidence of, 172
 ophthalmoscopic findings in, 172–174
 pathogenesis of, 174–175
 pituitary ablation in, 260–261
 prevention of, 175–176
 progress of, 173
 progressive, 261
 proliferative, 174
 treatment of, 176–177
Diabinese, 50t
Diagnosis, of diabetes mellitus, 9–17
  allowance for age in, 10
  announcement of, 17
  criteria for, 9–10
  procedures in, 16–17
Dialysis, hemo-, in lactic acidosis, 240
  in nephropathy, 195. See also *Hemodialysis; Peritoneal dialysis*
Diarrhea, diabetic, 185
 osmotic, 224–225
Diary, diabetic, 65, *66*
  for new juvenile diabetic, 71
  for Type II diabetic, 80

Diastix, 61
Dichloroacetate, 240
Diet(s), cholesterol abnormalities and, 202
  compliance of patient with, 26, 27
  composition of, ideal, 23, 27
  diabetic complications and, 21t
  education in, 18–19
  foods in, special, 24, 225
  for diabetics, elderly, 124
    gestational, 148
    new juvenile, 71
    obese, 122–123
    pregnant, 152–153
    Type I, 20–22
      adult-onset, 77
    Type II, 22–23, 26–27, 79
      elderly, 84
  high carbohydrate/high plant fiber (HCF), foods in, 25
    studies in, 25
  high-fiber, 24–26
  in preparation for glucose tolerance test, 11
  indiscretions in, 37–38
  instruction books on, 24, 26
Dietary management, 18–27. See also *Diet(s)*
Dietitian, instruction of patient by, 21–22
Dihydrochalcones, 221
2-3 Diphosphoglycerate, 228–229
Diuretics, 204, 205
Driving, by diabetics, 99–100
Drug(s), antihypertensive, 204
  as stress factors, 241
  beta-adrenergic blocking, 204
  cholesterol abnormalities and, 202
  diabetic feet and, 142
  interactions of, 55
  sulfonylurea. See *Antidiabetes agent(s), oral; Sulfonylurea(s), oral*
  sympathetic inhibitor, 204
  urine tests and, 60t, 65
Dymelor, 50t

Education, diabetes, for new juvenile diabetic, 68, 71
    for nurse, 78
  for Type II diabetic, 80
  in impotence, 190
  in prevention of diabetic ketoacidosis, 110
  in recognition of preacidosis, 111–112
Elderly diabetics, newly diagnosed, 84
  nursing home care for, 84–85
Emergency treatment, for diabetics, 280–281
Emphysematous cholecystitis, 132
Energy, expenditure of, 20
  sources of, 86–87
    requirements of during exercise, 87
Equipment, for insulin injection, 44
*Escherichia coli*, 256
Estriol excretion, 159
Etiology, of diabetes, 245–250
Exchange lists, 23
Exchange system, 24t
Exercise(s), 86–92
  effects on diabetics of, 87–90
  for new juvenile diabetic, 71
  hypoglycemia and, 88–89
  in peripheral vascular disease, 139–140
  in prevention of coronary disease, 203
  insulin injection sites and, 89
  kinds of, 90
  obesity and, 91
  precautions in, 90–91
  prescription of, 89–90
  sustained isometric muscular, 187
  walking as, 90, 91
Exercise test(s), 193
Extremity (extremities), amputations in, 137
  impaired, 137–145
  peripheral neuropathy and, 181–182
  recurrent bullae on, 136
Eye(s), disorders of, 172–178
  of Type II diabetics, 81
  transitory refractive changes in, 177–178

Fasting, for glucose tolerance test, 12
Fatty acid(s), free, 87
  glucose metabolism and, 263
Fetus, assessment of health of, 158–160
  survival of, 151–152
    rate for, 148
Fiber, dietary, 24–26
Flow sheet, for diabetic ketoacidosis treatment, 102, *103*
Fluid depletion, in diabetic ketoacidosis, 106
Food(s), books on, 277–278
  "diet," 225
  following hypoglycemic episode, 97
  for exercising diabetics, 88–89
  metabolism of, 262
  portions of, 23
  special diet, 24
Food and Drug Administration, cyclamates and, 217–218
  saccharin and, 219–220
Foot (feet), diabetic, burning or freezing of, 142
    care of, 140–142
    cleanliness of, 141
    cuts and irritations of, 141
    drugs and antiseptics on, 142
    dry, 138
    infection(s) of, 144–145

microangiopathy of, 138
neuropathic, 137–138
of Type II diabetics, 81
pressure on, 143–145
saving of, 143–145
self-observation of, 138
surgical management of, 145
ulcers of, 138
Framingham study, 197–198, 198t
Frederickson formula, 201
Fructose, 24
absorption and metabolism of, 222–223
effect on diabetes of, 223
properties of, 222
use of, 223
Fruit, miracle, 221–222
Fruit sugar. See *Fructose*
Fundoscopic examinations, 173, 177
Fungal infections, 133, 134

Gangrene, amputations in, 137
gas, 133
Gastrointestinal hormone, 258–259
Gastroparesis diabeticorum, 184
Genetics of diabetes, 245–250
Gestational diabetes, 10–11
definition of, 148
dietary regulation in, 148
fetal survival rate in, 148
management of, 156–157
oral contraceptives and, 163
pathogenesis of, 148–149
predisposition to, 149
screening for, 149–150
Glaucoma, 175
Glibenclamide, 49
Glibornuride, 49
Glipizide, 49
Globin insulin, 28, 29t. See also *Insulin(s)*
Glomerulosclerosis, nodular, 192
prevention of, 193
Glucagon, discovery of, 251
functions of, 258
hypoglycemia and, 96, 266
production of, 258
somatostatin and, 251
Glucocheck, 214
Glucocorticoids, 259
Gluconeogenesis, 264, 265
Glucose, blood, age and, 8
control of, complications and, 6
education of patient in, 6
importance of 193
meticulous, 6–7
mortality and, 169
retinopathy and, 175
determination of, in hypoglycemia, 96
pre- and postoperative, 127
exercise and, 87
fasting, urine testing of, 62
home monitoring of, 212–216
advantages of, 213, 215–216
approach to, 212–213
colorimeter devices for, 213–214
color-strip methods for, 214
during pregnancy, 156
frequency of, 215
need for, 67
patients for, 214–215
problems with, 216
rationale for, 212
in diabetic ketoacidosis, 104
in elderly Type II diabetic, 84
in pregnancy, 164
perinatal mortality and, 151
low, emergency treatment of, 280–281
signs of, 280
normal levels of, 264
reduction of, 166, 177
for glucose tolerance test, 12
high-fiber diets and, 24–25
in treatment of hypoglycemia, 96, 98
IV infusions of, 128
metabolism of, 262, *263*, 264
monitoring of, home. See *Glucose, blood, home monitoring of*
plasma, normal level of, 10
stores and sources of, 86, 87
uptake of during exercise, 87
urine, measurement of, 62–64
Glucose homeostasis, 264–266
Glucose intolerance, 234
Glucose test(s), plasma, fasting, 16–17
postprandial, for gestational diabetes, 149
1-hour and 2-hour, 150. See also *Glucose tolerance test(s)*
Glucose tolerance, associated with disorders, 3
impaired, classification of, 15–16
diagnosis of, 10
monitoring in, 16
"impaired gestational," 11
potential abnormality of (Pot. AGT), 3
previous abnormality of (Prev. AGT), 3
Glucose tolerance test (GTT), criteria for, 11
oral (OGTT), abnormal, 13
age and, 10
contraindications to, 13
criteria for children, 11
disagreement regarding, 13–14
gestational diabetes and, 149, 150
impaired glucose tolerance and, 16
in diagnosis, 9
interpretation of, 10
positive, 151
postponement of, 12

Glucose tolerance test (GTT), *cont.*
preparatory phase of, 11–12
procedures for, 11–13
in pregnancy, 150
processing of blood sample in, 12–13
testing phase of, 12
Glucose-6-phosphate pathway, 235
Glucosuria, diabetic ketoacidosis and, 104
insulin administration in, 35
Glucosyltransferase, 167
Glycogen, conversion to glucose of, 264–265
liver, 264–265
muscle, 86, 265
sources of, 86
Glycohemoglobin, as index of control, 226
advantages of, 227
determinations of, interpreting results of, 227–228
nondiabetic factors influencing, 228
labile form of, 227
unanswered questions concerning, 228
Glycosylation, 167–168
Group therapy, for obese diabetic, 122
Growth, hyperglycemia and, 171
Growth hormone, as insulin antagonist, 259
diabetes and, 260, 261
vascular disease and, 260–261
Guar gum, 25

Handgrip test, 187
Heart disease, coronary. See *Coronary heart disease*
Heart rate, in neuropathy, 186–187
Hemochromatosis, diabetes in, 232–233
treatment of, 233
Hemodialysis, in diabetic nephropathy, 195
in lactic acidosis, 240
Hemoglobin, 226
HLA antigens, 247–249
"Honeymoon period," 72
Hormone(s), counter-regulatory, 259–260
gastrointestinal, 258–259
growth. See *Growth hormone*
hyperglycemic, 259
in diabetes, 251–261
stress. See *Stress hormones*
Hospitalization, of diabetic(s), at present, 30
in past, 29
new juvenile, 69–71
older, 82–84
indications for, 82
prior to delivery, 160, 161
Type II, for major elective surgical procedures, 126
Hostility, in diabetic child, 74
Human leukocyte antigens, 247–249
Hydration, in preacidosis, 112
Hypercholesterolemia, familial, 200
treatment of, 201–203
Hyperglycemia, atheromatous changes and, 171
capillary basement membrane thickening and, 167
glucose metabolism and, 264
growth and, 171
in hyperosmolar coma, 243
insulin administration in, 35
maternal, fetal damage from, 151
fetal hyperinsulinism in, 162
platelet function and, 169
sorbitol pathway during, 168
sulfonylureas in, 54
systemic complications and, 165, 166
temporary, 14
triglyceride elevations in, 200
Hyperglycemic hormones, 259–260
Hyperinsulinism, fetal, detrimental features of, 151
neonatal problems from, 162
reactive, 100
Hyperlipidemia, 198–199
Hyperosmolality, in diabetic ketoacidosis, 104
in hyperosmolar coma, 242–243
Hyperosmolar coma, clinical findings in, 241–242
differential diagnosis of, 238–239t
etiology of, 241
laboratory findings in, 242
medical history in, 241
nonketotic, 243–244
recurrence of, 244
treatment of, 242–243
Hyperosmolar-hyperglycemic coma. See *Hyperosmolar coma*
Hypertension, categories of, 203
"diabetic," 203
disorders secondary to, 203
essential, 203
retinopathy and, 176
systolic, 203
treatment of, 205
treatment of, 204–205
Hyperthyroidism, 233
Hypoglycemia, 93–100
adrenal stage of, 94–95
blood glucose determination in, 96
causes of, 55, 94
cerebral stage of, 95
dangers of, 93–94, 95
death from, 98
drug interactions causing, 55
during surgery, 125–126
effect on brain of, 93–94

exercise and, 88–89
glucagon in, 96, 266
in children, 95–96
control of, 70
in elderly diabetic, 85
in neonate, 162
instructions to patients on, 99–100
nocturnal, 95
nonprofessional emergency treatment of, 280–281
oral antidiabetes tablets and, 98–99
prevention of, 55, 99
reactive, 100
signs and symptoms of, 95–96
"stroke pattern" during, 55
treatment of, 96–97
nonresponders to, 97–98
emergency, 180–181
Hypotension, orthostatic, 187

Identification, for patients, 40
Illness, acute, 12
diabetic control during, 55–56
Immunofluorescence test, 134
Impotence, causes of, 188–189
differential diagnosis of, 189–190
sympathetic inhibitors and, 204
treatment of, 190–191
Incidence of diabetes, 5
Infection(s), 131–135
foot, 144–145
amputation and, 143
fungal, 133, 134
incidence of, 131
renal parenchymal, 134
skin and soft-tissue, 132
streptococcal, 133
urinary tract. See *Urinary tract infection(s)*
vaginal, 133
Injection(s), insulin. See *Insulin injection(s)*
Insulin(s), autoantibodies blocking activity of, 255
beef, 31, 114
beef-pork, 34
cell receptors for, 254–255
change to sulfonylureas from, 53–54
circulating, 256–257
commercial production of, 255
C-peptide immunoassay in measurement of, 257
currently available in U.S., 30, 32–33t
decreased requirements of, 41–42
diabetic ketoacidosis and, 108–109
discovery of, 251
dosage of. See *Insulin dosage*
during illness or surgical procedures, 55–56
in IV infusions, 126–127, 128
excess production of, 121
exercise and, 87, 88
for diabetic(s), elderly, 85
for Type II, 80
obese, 123
pregnant, 154–155
globin, 28
hazardous situations when taking, 99–100
human, 256
implantable delivery device(s) for, 211
types of, 211
in long-distance travel, 40–41
in nephropathy, 193
infusion pump(s) for, 210
cost of, 210
instruction in use of, 210–211
principle of, 208–209, 210
results of experience with, 209
selection of patients for, 209–210
injection of. See *Insulin injection(s)*
Lente, 28
measurement of, 43
mixing of, 45–46
noninsulin ingredients in, 114, 115
NPH, 28
physiologic functions of, 254
pork, 31–34. See also *Pork insulin*
postoperative, 128–129
predelivery administration of, 160
proinsulin content of, 115
protamine zinc (PZI), 28
protein and, 264
purification of, 30–31
purified, 115
purified pork, 31–34
reaction(s) to, cutaneous, 115–116
emergency treatment of, 280–281
immunologic, 114–119
systemic allergic, 116–117
See also *Hypoglycemia*
recombinant DNA, 256
regular, 28
administration of, 83–84
neutral, 115
requirements of, of fewer than 25 units daily, 34
in children, 34–35
of more than 25 units daily, 35–37
of new juvenile patients, 69–70, 72–73
through puberty, 73
resistance to, 117–118
treatment of, 117–118
unusual forms of, 118
secretion of, 253–254
selection and use of, 28–42
sensitivity to, 88
stability of, 38
storage of, 38
strength of, 43
structure of, 251–253
substitute delivery systems of, 207–211

Injection(s), *cont.*
switch in brands of, 34
synthesis of, 255
syringes, care of, 44–45, 46
types of, 44
24-hour, 30
types of, 28, 29t, 30
characteristics of, 29t
University Group Diabetes Program study of patients receiving, 271–272
variable working hours and, 38–40
Insulin antagonists, 259
Insulin antibodies, 31
Insulin dosage, change from one to two doses daily, 37
contraindications to, 83
during "honeymoon period," 72
"fine-tuning" of, 71
following diabetic ketoacidosis, 109
for Type I adult-onset diabetics, 77, 78–79
on day of surgical procedure, 127–128
two doses daily, 35–37
variable working hours and, one dose daily, 39–40
two doses daily, 39
Insulin injection(s), of afternoon/evening dose, 36–37
of morning dose, 36
preparation for, 44–46
procedures for, 43–48
sensitivity reactions to, 38
site(s) of, choice of, 47–48
exercise and, 47, 89
in children, 47–48
rotation of, 47–48
supplementary, 37–38
technique for, 46–48
to duplicate normal physiology, 30
Insulin-dependent diabetes mellitus (IDDM). See *Type I diabetes*
Islet-cell injection, 208

Juvenile diabetes, incidence of, 68. See also *Juvenile diabetic(s); Type I diabetes*
onset of, 68–69
virus theory and, 247
Juvenile diabetics(s), brittle, 73–74
care of, 68–75
insulin requirements of, 73
newly diagnosed, 70
diabetic diary for, 71
diet of, 71
education of, 68, 71, 72
exercise for, 71
first office visit of, 72–73
follow-up office visits of, 73
"honeymoon period" of, 72
hospitalization of, 69
discharge following, 71–72
insulin requirements of, 69–70, 72–73
parents of, 71–72
urine tests for, 70
psychosocial problems of, 74–75
therapeutic program for, 68

Ketoacidosis, diabetic. See *Diabetic ketoacidosis*
Keto-Diastix, 105
Ketonemia, 153
Ketones, serum, measurement of, 105
testing for, 157, 158
Ketonuria, in diabetic, 104
in pregnancy, fetal effects of, 152, 153
management of, 157
starvation, 157
without ketonemia, 105–106
Ketosis, 157
Ketostix, 105
Kidney(s), diabetic control and, 170–171
disease of. See *Diabetic nephropathy*
impaired filtration by, 167
infections of, 134
transplantation of, diabetes following, 231
in diabetic nephropathy, 195–196
complications of, 195
Kimmelstiel-Wilson lesion, 192

Lactate-pyruvate ratio, 235–236
Lactic acidosis, dichloroacetate in, 240
differential diagnosis of, 237, 238–239t
etiology of, 236
hemodialysis in, 240
laboratory findings in, 236–237
lactate accumulation in, 235
shock in, 237
sodium bicarbonate therapy in, 237–240
symptoms of, 236
treatment of, 237–240
Lawrence type of diabetes, 233–234
Lente insulin, 28, 29t. See also *Insulin(s)*
Levulose. See *Fructose*
Lipid profile, 201
Lipids, exercise and, 87–88
measurement of, 201
Lipoatrophic diabetes, 233–234
Lipoatrophy, 118–119
Lipodystrophy, 233–234
Lipohypertrophy, 119
Limbs. See *Extremity (extremities)*

Malformations, congenital, 148, 163
Massage, value of, 142
Maturity-onset diabetes of young (MODY), 4, 250

Meal(s), carbohydrate-loaded, 10
formula for, 23
planning of, 19
Medication, discontinuance of, 12
Metabolic abnormalities, 162
Microangiopathy, 138
Microsomia, 162
Miracle fruit, 221–222
Monellin, 222
Mononeuropathy, 181
truncal, 181
Motivation, weight loss and, 123–124
Mucormycosis, rhinocerebral, 131–132
Mumps, 246

National Institutes of Health, National Diabetes Data Group of, classification of diabetes by, 2
diagnostic criteria of, 9–10
Necrobiosis lipoidica diabeticorum, 135–136
Needles, care of, 46
"Neglecters," diabetic, 152
Neonate, problems of, 162–163
Nephropathy, diabetic. See *Diabetic nephropathy*
Nerves, impaired, 138
Neuroarthropathy, 183
Neurogenic bladder. See *Bladder, neurogenic*
Neuropathic ulcers. See *Ulcers, neuropathic*
Neuropathy, diabetic. See *Diabetic neuropathy*
Nicotinic acid, 202
Non-insulin-dependent diabetes mellitus (NIDDM). See *Type II diabetes*
Nonstress test (NST), 159–160
NPH insulin, 28, 29t. See also *Insulin(s)*
Nurse(s), education for, 78
Nursing home care, 84–85

Obesity, as cause of diabetes, 121
definition of, 120
in diabetics, 120–124
consequences of, 122–123
exercise and, 91
motivation and, 123–124
pathogenesis of, 121–122
treatment of, 122–123
Type II, 80, 121, 124, 245–246
risk of, 120–121
Occupations, dangerous, 100
Occurrence of juvenile diabetes, 5
Oral contraceptives, 163
Orinase. See *Tolbutamide*
Otitis, external, 131
Overdiagnosis, conditions precipitating, 14
hazards of, 14
Oxidation, glucose metabolism and, 263

Pancreas, artificial, 7–8, 207, 211
beta cells of, 253–254
"hybrid," 211
transplantation of, 208
trauma to, 231
Pancreatectomy, 231
Pancreatitis, acute, 230
chronic, 230–231
Parents, of juvenile diabetic, education for, 71–72
guilt of, 75
Pederson's prognostically bad signs during pregnancy, 152
Penile implants, 190–191
Peritoneal dialysis, 195
Phenformin, 52, 57
Phenytoin, 182
Pheochromocytoma, 232
Phosphate depletion, 107
Photocoagulation, 173, 175, 176
Pituitary, in diabetes, 260
Pituitary ablation, in nephropathy, 194
in retinopathy, 176–177, 260–261
Platelet(s), abnormalities of, 205–206
in hyperglycemia, 169
Platelet factor(s), 205–206
Pneumonia, 132
Podiatrist(s), 142
Pork insulin, antigenicity of, 114–115
purified, 31–34
structure of, 253. See also *Insulin(s)*
Potassium, replacement of, 107
Potassium depletion, 243
Preacidosis, recognition of, 111–112
treatment of, 112–113
Precoma, 152
Prednisone, 118
Pregnancy, in diabetes, 146–164
assessment of fetal health in, 158
classification of, 146–148, 147t
complications of, 152
congenital deformities from, 148, 163
cost of, 164
diet in, 152–153
home glucose monitoring in, 156
immediate postpartum care in, 162
incidence of, 146
induction of labor or cesarean section in, 161
insulin therapy in, 154–155
ketonuria during, 152, 153
management of, 152–158
outpatient care in, 155–156
Pederson's prognostically bad signs during, 152
predelivery routine in, 160
prognosis for, 147
risk to fetus in, 147
streptococcal infection in, 133
team of specialists in, 146
timing of delivery in, 160–161

Pregnancy, *cont.*
tolbutamide during, 52
weight gain in, 153–154
screening for gestational diabetes in, 149–150
Prematurity, 162
Pressures, on foot, 143–145
Prevalence of diabetes, 4–5, 8
Progesterone, 259
Proinsulin, as indicator of insulin purity, 31, 115
composition of, 114
proteolytic conversion of, *252*, 254
structure of, *252*
Prostaglandin E, 259
Protamine zinc insulin (PZI), 28, 29t. See also *Insulin(s)*
Protein(s), glycosylation of, 167–168
insulin and, 264
pregnancy and, 153
Proteinuria, 192, 193
Proton beam therapy, 261
Psychosocial problems, of juvenile diabetics, 74–75
Pulse(s), arterial, 81
Pulse rate, 90
Pyelography, intravenous (IVP), 196
Pyelonephritis, 152

Reading list for diabetics, 277–279
Recombinant DNA insulin, 256
Recreational activities, 100
Reflex(es), of Type II diabetics, 81
squint, 95–96
Regular insulin, 28, 29t. See also *Insulin(s)*
Remission, 14
Renal failure, 192
Renal threshold, 67
Renal transplantation, diabetes following, 231
in diabetic nephropathy, 195–196
complications of, 195
Respiratory distress syndrome, 160, 161, 162
Retina, diabetic, 173. See also *Diabetic retinopathy*
Retinopathy. See *Diabetic retinopathy*
Revascularization operations, 140
Rhinocerebral mucormycosis, 131–132
Rodenticide(s), 234
Rubella, congenital, 246, 247
Rubeosis iridis, 175

Saccharin, bladder cancer and, 219, 220–221
FDA and, 219–220
sale of, 220
uses of, 218–219
Saline solution, 106
Screening test, 11
Semilente insulin, 28, 29t, 35. See also *Insulin(s)*
Serendipity berries, 222
Sexual dysfunction, female, 188
male, 188
signs of, 189–190
symptoms of, 189
Sexual therapy, 191
Shift work, insulin timing and, 38–40
Shoes, for diabetics, 141–142, 144
Skin, disorders of, 135–136
infections of, 132
of feet, burning or freezing of, 142
irritation of, foot, 141
reactions of, to insulin, 115–116
treatment of, 116
Snack(s), bedtime, 22
between-meal, 22
exercise and, 88–89
importance of, 99, 100
Sodium bicarbonate therapy, 237–240
Sodium intake, during pregnancy, 153
Somatostatin, analog, 258
functions of, 257–258
glucagon and, 251
sites of, 257
Somogyi phenomenon, 74
Sorbitol, in Schwann's cell, 179–180
oral, 224
pathway of, 168–169, 179
StatTek Twin-Beam Electronic Photometer, 214
Stillbirth, 161
Stockings, for diabetics, 141
Streptococcal infection, 133
Stress, as cause of hyperglycemia, 14
brittle diabetic(s) and, 73–74
of moderate pressure, 144
of pregnancy, 148
of surgical procedures, 125
Stress hormones, 260
diabetic ketoacidosis and, 110–111
surgery and, 125
Sucrose polyester, 202
Sugar, blood. See *Glucose, blood*
fruit. See *Fructose*
treatment of hypoglycemia with, 96
Sulfonylurea agent(s), oral, 49–58
actions of, 50t
change from insulin to, 53–54
continuing care with, 56–57
for new patient, 54
for obese diabetic, 123
second-generation, 57–58
selection of, 52–53
side effects of, 54
University Group Diabetes Program study of. See *University Group Diabetes Program (UGDP) study*
See also *Antidiabetes agent(s), oral*
Supplements, dietary, 153

Surgery, 125–130
  diabetic control during, 55–56
  elective, major, follow-up care in, 128–129
    for insulin-dependent diabetics, 127–128
    for Type II diabetics, 126–127
    preoperative preparation for, 125–126
  emergency, 129
  foot, 145
  minor, 126
  needs of diabetic(s) during, 125, 130
  scheduling of, 126
Sweeteners, non-nutritive, 217–222
  nutritive, 222–225
  substitute, 217–225
    under investigation, 222
Syringe(s), insulin, care of, 44–45, 46
    types of, 44

Tachycardia, 186
Teenagers, diabetic control in, 7, 75
Tes-Tape, 61
Test(s), in evaluation of diabetic control, 35. See also *Glucose tolerance test*
  in new juvenile patients, 69
  urine. See *Urine testing* and specific tests
Testosterone, 191
Thannhauser-Aldersberg syndrome, 201
Thigh, as insulin injection site, 47
Thyroid hormones, 259
Tinea pedis, 141
Tissues, soft, breakdown of, 144
    infections of, 132
      necrotizing, 132–133
Tobacco, 142
Toenails, care of, 141
Tolazamide, 50t
Tolbutamide, 50t, 52
  in pregnancy, 52
  University Group Diabetes Program findings on, 268
Tolinase, 50t
Travel, insulin and, 40–41
Treatment, emergency, 280–281
Triglyceride(s), determination of, 201
  elevated levels of, causes of, 201
    in hyperglycemia, 200
  exercise and, 87
  glucose metabolism and, 263
    HCF diet and, 25
    normal levels of, 201
  stores of, 86
Triopathy of complications, 165, 171
Tropical diabetes, 234
Tuberculosis, 132
Type I diabetes, adult-onset, 77. See also *Adult-onset diabetic(s), Type I*
  age distribution of, 4
  autoimmunity in, 246
  blood sugar control in, 6–7
  characteristics of, 2, 16
  dietary guidelines in, 20–22
    for new patients, 21–22
  etiology of, 245
  ideal weight and, 20
  in children. See *Juvenile diabetic(s)*
  insulin and cell receptors for, 254
  islet cell antibodies in, 246
  major elective surgical procedures in, 127–128
  urine testing in, 61
  virus theory in, 246–247
Type II diabetes, adult-onset, 83. See also *Adult-onset diabetic(s), Type II*
  blood sugar control in, 7
  characteristics of, 2–3
  diagnosis of, 15
  diet therapy for, 19
  dietary guidelines in, 22–23, 26–27
  etiology of, 245–246
  inheritance of, 249–250
  insulin receptors for, 254–255
  insulin-dependent, 127–128
  major elective surgical procedures in, 126–127
  nonobese, 3
  obesity in, 80, 121, 124, 245–246
    characteristics of, 3, 121
    consequences of, 122–123
    treatment of, 122–123
  subtypes of, 3
  suspected, 15
  urine testing in, 61

Ulcers, foot, 138
  neuropathic, differential diagnosis of, 183
    management of, 183–184
    pathogenesis of, 183
Ultralente insulin, 29t. See also *Insulin(s)*
Ultrasonography, 158
Unconsciousness, in hypoglycemia, 93, 94
Undiagnosed diabetes, 5–6
University Group Diabetes Program (UGDP) study, criticism of, 269–274
  method of, 267–268
  objectives of, 267
  position of American Diabetes Association on, 272–274
  report of, 268
    response to, 268–269
  review of, 274–275

Urinary tract infection(s), diagnosis of, 134
  treatment of, 135
    importance of, 133–134
  types of, 134
Urine, specimens of, for urine testing, 61–62. See also *Urine testing*
Urine testing, drugs and, 60t, 65
  for urinary tract infection, 134
  importance of, 59–61
    in pregnancy, 155, 157, 164
  in new juvenile diabetic(s), 70
  in Type II diabetic(s), 80
    elderly, 84
  methods of, 59–61
    compared, 60t, 64t
  prior to major surgical procedures, 128
  quantitative, 62–64
    advantages of, 63
    instructions to patient for, 63
  recording and, 64–65
    guidelines for, 65–67
  time schedule for, 61
  urine specimens for, 61–62

Vacor rodenticide, 234
Vaginal infections, 133
Valsalva maneuver, 186
Vascular disease, growth hormone and, 260–261
  peripheral, diagnosis of, 139
    management in, 139–140
    risk factors for, 139
    vessels involved in, 138–139
Virus theory, 246–247
Vitamin $B_{12}$, 182
Vitrectomy, 177
Volume depletion, 242–243

Walking, prescription for, 90
  weight loss from, 91
Water depletion, 106
Weight, gain of, during pregnancy, 154
    pattern of, 154
    recommended, 153
  ideal, 19t, 120
  reduction of, benefits of, 124
    during pregnancy, 153
    physical activity in, 91
Weight-loss program, 123–124
Working hours, insulin and, 38–40

Xylitol, 224